TISSUE HEART VALVES

By the same editor

Biological Tissue in Heart Valve Replacement
Current Techniques in Extracorporeal Circulation

TISSUE HEART VALVES

Edited by

Marian I. Ionescu, MD, FACS

Consultant Cardiothoracic Surgeon,
The General Infirmary at Leeds,

Clinical Lecturer in Cardiothoracic Surgery
at Leeds University, Leeds, England

BUTTERWORTHS
LONDON–BOSTON
Sydney–Wellington–Durban–Toronto

The Butterworth Group

United Kingdom London	Butterworth & Co (Publishers) Ltd 88 Kingsway, WC2 6AB
Australia Sydney	Butterworths Pty Ltd 586 Pacific Highway, Chatswood, NSW 2067 Also at Melbourne, Brisbane, Adelaide and Perth
Canada Toronto	Butterworth & Co (Canada) Ltd 2265 Midland Avenue, Scarborough, Ontario, M1P 4S1
New Zealand Wellington	Butterworths of New Zealand Ltd T & W Young Building, 77–85 Customhouse Quay, 1, €PO Box 472
South Africa Durban	Butterworth & Co (South Africa) (Pty) Ltd 152–154 Gale Street
USA Boston	Butterworth (Publishers) Inc 19 Cummings Park, Woburn, Massachusetts 01801

First published 1979

© Butterworth & Co (Publishers) Ltd, 1979

ISBN 0 407 00139 5

British Library Cataloguing in Publication Data

Tissue heart valves.
   1. Heart valve prosthesis
   I. Ionescu, Marian Ion
617′.412   RD598   78-40789

   ISBN 0-407-00139-5

Typeset by Reproduction Drawings Ltd, Sutton, Surrey
Printed and bound at William Clowes & Sons Limited
Beccles and London

On ne devrait s'étonner que de pouvoir encore s'étonner.
François, duc de La Rochefoucauld (1613–1680)

Foreword

It is appropriate that Marian Ion Ionescu should edit a book about biological heart valves, because his interest in these valves has stimulated a great deal of the current activity in this area. He has persuaded an outstanding group of individuals to join him in this undertaking. The book should be useful to those with either medical or surgical interests in valvular heart disease.

Birmingham, Alabama   John W. Kirklin, MD

Preface

Comme quelqu'un pourait dire de moi que j'ai seulement fait ici un
amas de fleurs étrangères, n'y ayant fourni du mien que le filet à les lier.
Michel Eyquem Montaigne (1533–1592)

Since the first valve replacements, performed more than 15 years ago, the history of heart valve surgery has been one of the most exciting, productive and challenging chapters in cardiac surgery.

Almost everything that could be imagined, invented, constructed or created has been given an experimental or clinical trial, and the number of materials, shapes and configurations used for heart valve replacement would tax the most prolific and exuberant imagination.

The experience with prosthetic and tissue valves commenced almost simultaneously with the Silastic ball valve and the aortic allograft valve. The ensuing years have been productive and an enormous amount of scientific knowledge concerning valvular and cardiac function has been accumulated during the last decade.

The three main goals set by the pioneers of heart valve substitutes namely durability, non-thrombogenicity and near normal haemodynamic performance of the artificial valves, are almost within our reach.

Through the years three basic types of prosthetic devices have been developed: the conventional ball or disc-cage valve, the cloth-covered prosthesis and the tilting or pivoting disc valves. Despite the haemodynamic shortcomings for the small sizes and the need for long-term anticoagulation, the veteran Silastic ball valve is still in clinical use. The expectation that thromboembolic complications could be minimized in the absence of anticoagulation when using cloth-covered prosthetic valves has not materialized. The need for anticoagulant treatment remains as imperative and as permanent as for any other prosthetic device.

The tilting and pivoting disc valves are at present the most accepted prostheses because of their improved haemodynamic characteristics, although they too require lifelong anticoagulation.

Despite improved materials such as pyrolitic carbon, better technology for valve fabrication, streamlined configuration and more accurate surgical techniques, the need for permanent anticoagulation of patients with prosthetic valves has not been eliminated.

The only heart valve substitutes which can be used safely without anticoagulants are the tissue valves. The initial experience with the aortic valve allografts and xenografts was sub-optimal, because of the techniques of preservation employed, and the results in the atrioventricular position have been discouraging. With the introduction of glutaraldehyde for tissue preservation, a new generation of biological valves has emerged and established itself as a standard for clinical valve replacement. The porcine aortic valve, made by three different laboratories, has been widely used, especially in the atrioventricular position. As a logical step towards simplicity of manufacture, an entirely artificially made valve was produced using xenogeneic pericardium stabilized with glutaraldehyde and moulded in a configuration more suited for improved haemodynamic performance. Finally, the glycerol treated dura mater allograft is the fourth type of tissue valve described in this volume.

With the exception of the aortic valve allograft, the other three main types of tissue valves have been in clinical use for more than seven years. All have shown an insignificant rate of thromboembolic complications even without long-term administration of prothrombin depressants, and their durability over this period of time compares very favourably with that of mechanical prostheses.

Several years ago, a period of observation of five years for heart valve substitutes '*in vivo*' would have been considered sufficient evidence of their general acceptance. At present, seven years of satisfactory clinical and haemodynamic results are certainly encouraging, but only acceptable, and a longer follow-up is always desirable.

As the tissue valves have proved to offer a better alternative for heart valve replacement, and as they are now firmly established in the armamentarium of cardiac surgeons, a detailed description of their clinical performance grouped in one volume seems appropriate. Those valves which are accepted for clinical use and which have been utilized for a period of more than seven years are presented in this book.

To establish terms for comparison, the clinical experience with a prosthetic device is described. The Björk–Shiley tilting disc valve was chosen, because it is most widely used and because in its present form, with the pyrolitic carbon disc, it has a similar period of follow-up as the tissue valves described.

Chapter 2 deals with the hydrodynamic assessment of the valves presented in this volume. Experimental and clinical data concerning the historical development of various types of tissue valves are presented in Chapter 3. The next four chapters deal with the description of, and the results obtained with the aortic valve allograft, the glutaraldehyde preserved porcine valve, the glutaraldehyde preserved pericardial xenograft and the glycerol treated dura mater allograft. Two successive chapters present data on the use of tissue valve preparations for reconstruction of ventricular pulmonary artery discontinuity. The last chapter details the intricate chemistry and biology of aldehyde treatment of biological tissue.

This book does not intend to cover the entire field of tissue heart valves, it only describes the present state of their use in cardiac surgery.

As our endeavour for perfection is never-ending, the quest for an ideal heart valve substitute will continue. Whether this ideal valve will emerge from the mechanical engineering workshop, from the biologist's laboratory or from the combined efforts of biomedical engineers remains to be seen. We hope that detailed knowledge and better understanding of the performance of tissue valves may help the next step forward towards the creation of the ideal heart valve substitute.

We take great pleasure in expressing our thanks to Professor John W. Kirklin for kindly writing the Foreword of this work. We are most grateful to all the contributors who so generously agreed to participate in this publication. To Misses Anne Tunnicliffe and Nancy Evans and Mrs Marty Pallister our deep appreciation for their competent and enthusiastic help in the preparation of the manuscript and the follow-up of our own patients.

Finally we should like to thank the publishers, Butterworth and Co. Ltd. for the many pleasant and efficient ways in which they helped with this work.

Marian I. Ionescu

Contributors

C'est une grande folie que de vouloir être sage tout seul.
François, duc de La Rochefoucauld (1613–1680)

Judith D. Angell, MS,
Director,
Cardiovascular Surgery Research,
Institute for Medical Research and Western Heart Institute,
San Jose,
California,
U.S.A.

William W. Angell, MD,
Assistant Professor of Surgery,
Stanford University,
Stanford,
California,

Chief,
Cardiovascular Surgery,
Santa Clara Valley Medical Center,

Western Heart Associates Medical Group,
San Jose,
California,
U.S.A.

Viking O. Björk, MD,
Professor of Thoracic and Cardiovascular Surgery,
Thoracic Surgical Clinic,
Karolinska Sjukhuset,
Stockholm,
Sweden.

Lawrence H. Cohn, MD,
Associate Professor of Surgery,
Harvard Medical School,

Cardiovascular Surgeon,
Peter Bent Brigham Hospital,
Boston,
Massachusetts,
U.S.A.

John J. Collins, Jr., MD,
Professor of Surgery,
Harvard Medical School,

Chief,
Cardiothoracic Surgery,
Peter Bent Brigham Hospital,
Boston,
Massachusetts,
U.S.A.

Marc R. de Leval, MD,
Consultant Cardiothoracic Surgeon,
The Hospital for Sick Children,
Great Ormond Street,
London,
England.

Axel Henze, MD,
Docent,
Thoracic Surgical Clinic,
Karolinska Sjukhuset,
Stockholm,
Sweden.

Marian I. Ionescu, MD, FACS,
Consultant Cardiothoracic Surgeon,
The General Infirmary at Leeds,

Clinical Lecturer in Cardiothoracic Surgery at Leeds University,
Leeds,
England.

Jon C. Kosek, MD,
Professor of Pathology,
Stanford University,
Stanford,
California,

Chief,
Laboratory Services,
Veterans Administration Hospital,
Palo Alto,
California,
U.S.A.

Fergus J. Macartney, MD, FRCP,
Professor of Paediatric Cardiology,
The Hospital for Sick Children,
Great Ormond Street,
London,
England.

Valentino Martelli, MD,
Senior Surgical Registrar,
National Heart Hospital,
London,
England.

Luiz B. Puig, MD,
Assistant Professor of Cardiac and Thoracic Surgery,
Hospital das Clinicas,
University of São Paulo Medical School,
São Paulo,
Brasil.

Donald N. Ross, MD, FRCS,
Director,
Department of Surgery,
Cardiothoracic Institute,

Consultant Surgeon,
National Heart Hospital,
London,
England.

Jaroslav Stark, MD,
Consultant Cardiothoracic Surgeon,
The Hospital for Sick Children,
Great Ormond Street,
London,
England.

Robert J. Szarnicki, MD,
Associate Thoracic and Cardiovascular Surgeon,
Presbyterian Hospital,
Pacific Medical Center,
San Francisco,
California,
U.S.A.

Anand P. Tandon, MD, MRCP,
Senior Cardiological and Research Registrar,
University Department of Medicine and Department of Cardiothoracic Surgery,
The General Infirmary,
Leeds,
England.

William H. Wain, PhD,
Senior Biologist,
Head, Homograft Department,
National Heart Hospital,
London,
England.

E. Aubrey Woodroof, PhD, (Woodroof Laboratories Inc.)
16646 Mt. Cachuma Circle,
Fountain Valley,
California 92708,
U.S.A.

John T. M. Wright, BSc, PhD, MIMechE, CEng,
Senior Lecturer in Bioengineering,
University of Liverpool,
Liverpool,
England.

Euryclides de Jesus Zerbini, MD,
Professor of Surgery and Director of the Instituto do Coracao,
Hospital das Clinicas,
University of São Paulo Medical School,
São Paulo,
Brasil.

Contents

1

Prosthetic Heart Valve Replacement. Nine Years' Experience with the Björk-Shiley Tilting Disc Valve

Viking O. Björk and Axel Henze

Le vrai, dans quelque sujet qu'il se trouve, ne peut être effacé par aucune comparaison d'un autre vrai, et, quelque différence qui puisse être entre deux sujets, ce qui est vrai dans l'un n'efface point ce qui est vrai dans l'autre.

François, duc de La Rochefoucauld (1613–1680)

INTRODUCTION

Nine years of surgical experience with over 1800 implants of Björk–Shiley tilting disc valve prostheses justify a detailed description of the valve design and developments, its clinical and haemodynamic performance and the late results obtained with heart valve replacement.

DESCRIPTION OF THE PROSTHESIS

The Björk–Shiley tilting disc valve prosthesis consists of a free-floating disc of Delrin or pyrolytic carbon suspended in a Stellite cage which is encircled with a Teflon sewing rim[1,2,3] (*Figure 1.1*).

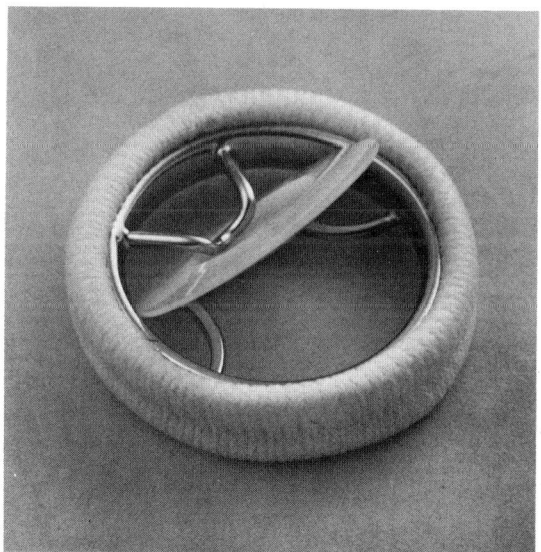

Figure 1.1 The original Björk–Shiley aortic prosthesis with the disc made of Delrin. The disc tilts open to 60°

The disc sits inside the valve ring in the closed position, leaving a minimal space between its edge and the prosthetic valve ring, thus closing with a non-overlapping mechanism. The disc opens at an angle of 60° and closes between two eccentrically situated support prongs (*Figure 1.2*). The cage of the disc valve can be rotated within its sewing rim with the aid of the valve holder, in order to ensure free movement of the disc after valve insertion.

In this particular prosthetic valve design, the circumferential seat ring for occluder contact was eliminated by means of the non-overlapping disc mechanism, whereby another 2 mm of orifice diameter were gained for a given external diameter. The Björk–Shiley prosthesis has, therefore, the highest possible orifice area-to-tissue diameter ratio. The valve is manufactured by Shiley Laboratories Inc., Irvine, California, USA.

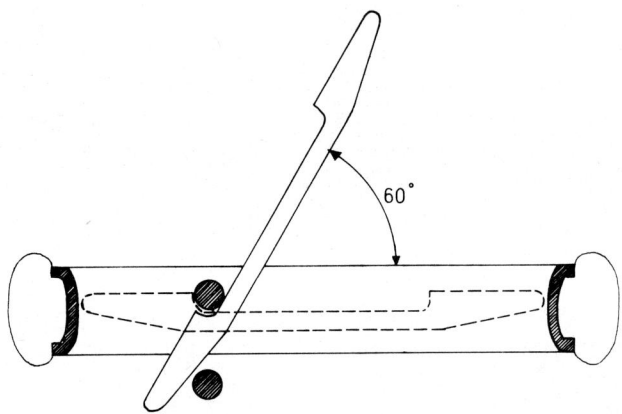

Figure 1.2 Cross-sectional view of the non-overlapping closing mechanism

Evolution and technical developments

The original Delrin disc model of the Björk–Shiley prosthesis (*Figure 1.1*) has been modified in several respects.

Disc material

In 1971, pyrolytic carbon was introduced as disc material instead of Delrin, mainly because of its longer durability[3]. A further advantage with pyrolytic carbon, in contrast to Delrin, is that it does not absorb moisture and, therefore, it remains completely unchanged in the human circulation. Accordingly, the pyrolytic carbon disc is manufactured with the least possible disc-to-orifice clearance, which, in experimental studies, has proved to minimize haemolysis and regurgitation[15].

Opening angle

The original mitral valve model had an opening angle of $50°$, which was later increased to $60°$ as in the aortic model in order to obtain optimal rheology[5].

Sewing rim

The sewing rim of the mitral valve model was designed with two flanges, which allow a wider variation of suture techniques[5] (*Figure 1.3*). Sub-annular fixation of the mitral valve prosthesis was considered essential and, therefore, the lower flange could be used for placement of the mattress sutures, which were then passed through the rim of the resected mitral valve and tied.

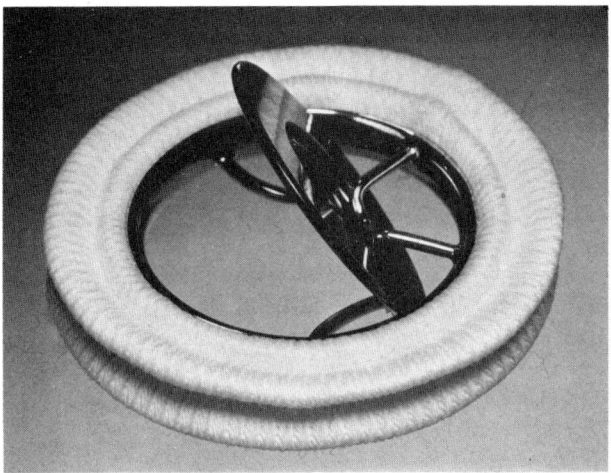

Figure 1.3 The present Björk–Shiley mitral valve prosthesis with the disc made of pyrolitic
carbon and a double-flanged sewing rim

Radio-opaque marker

The introduction of the ring-shaped radio-opaque marker within the tilting disc
occluder provides a valuable aid for instant diagnosis of prosthetic malfunction
due to thrombotic obstruction of the valve (*Figure 1.4*). The disc motion can be
easily visualized by cineradiography and fluoroscopy. These non-invasive procedures are very well tolerated, even by the critically ill patient. In the event of

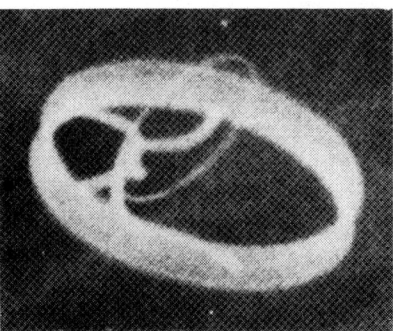

Figure 1.4 Ring-shaped radio-opaque marker incorporated into the pyrolitic carbon disc for
non-invasive control of the Björk–Shiley prosthesis function

thrombotic obstruction of the prosthesis, the motion of the tilting disc is severely
compromised. The Björk–Shiley prosthesis with the pyrolytic carbon disc and
fitted with the ring-shaped radio-opaque marker has been used in the Thoracic
Surgical Unit of the Karolinska Sjukhuset, Stockholm since March 1975[9].

Durability of the prostheses

As previously mentioned, Delrin was permanently discarded in favour of pyrolytic carbon which is a more durable material. Accelerated experimental wear tests have shown a durability corresponding to several hundred years for the pyrolytic carbon disc model of the Björk–Shiley prosthesis[2,3]. In our experience of more than 1800 implanted prosthetic valves, we have not encountered one single case of genuine mechanical valve failure. Three instances of fracture of the larger disc supporting prong or strut have been reported. These occurred in mitral prostheses of 29 and 31 mm tissue (annulus) diameter at 2, 3 and 21 months following valve insertion. This represents an incidence of three strut fractures out of 90 000 delivered valves, 16 000 of which were mitral prostheses of 29 and 31 mm tissue diameter. The probable cause of such strut fracture was a combination of factors relating to welded areas. Corrective measures have been taken to provide an even greater safety margin, in order to eliminate such accidents in the future. In one case in our series, the valve prosthesis was forcefully rotated with a clamp after it had been sutured in position, and this resulted in slight distortion of the struts. The disc loosened and the prosthesis had to be exchanged. A similar case was reported by Messmer, Rothlin and Senning[20]. The importance of careful handling of the prosthetic valve cannot be overemphasized. The prosthesis must be rotated within the sewing rim at least ten times using its original valve holder, before it is sutured in place. This loosens the metal ring from the sewing rim and facilitates rotation of the prosthesis *in situ* once it has been sutured to the heart valve annulus. Only the original valve holder should be used for this manoeuvre (*Figure 1.5*). Surgical instruments, such as forceps or clamps, may damage the metal ring and the struts in the welded area, causing strut fracture and probably initiating thrombosis.

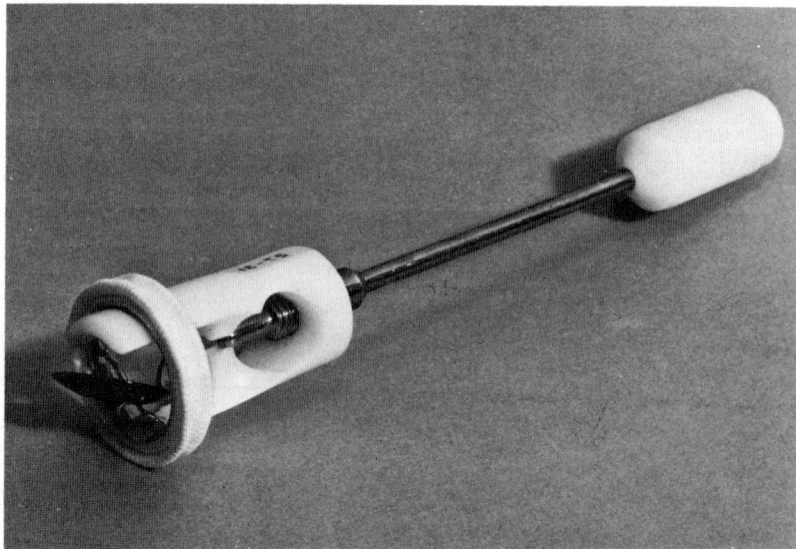

Figure 1.5 Rotation only with the original valve holder! Certain instruments, such as forceps or clamps, may cause damage leading to malfunction and thrombosis of the prosthesis

OPERATIVE PROCEDURE

In all heart valve replacement operations the heart was approached through a midline sternotomy. Total cardiopulmonary bypass with moderate generalized hypothermia to 30 °C and uninterrupted coronary circulation has been the basic principle of our perfusion technique for the isolated or combined aortic and mitral valve replacements which will be reported in this chapter. The left ventricle was always vented through the apex and ventricular fibrillation has never been induced. Selective coronary artery perfusion was employed for aortic and combined valve replacement operations (*Figure 1.6*). Long periods of aortic cross-clamping were avoided during isolated mitral valve operations. Recently, hypothermic cardioplegia has been adopted. Ringer's solution at 4 °C, containing 20 mEq/ℓ of potassium, was infused into the coronary arteries in order to obtain a myocardial temperature at, or below, 20 °C. Isolated tricuspid valve replacement was performed with euthermic perfusion. If part of a multiple valve replacement operation, the tricuspid replacement is done during the rewarming period.

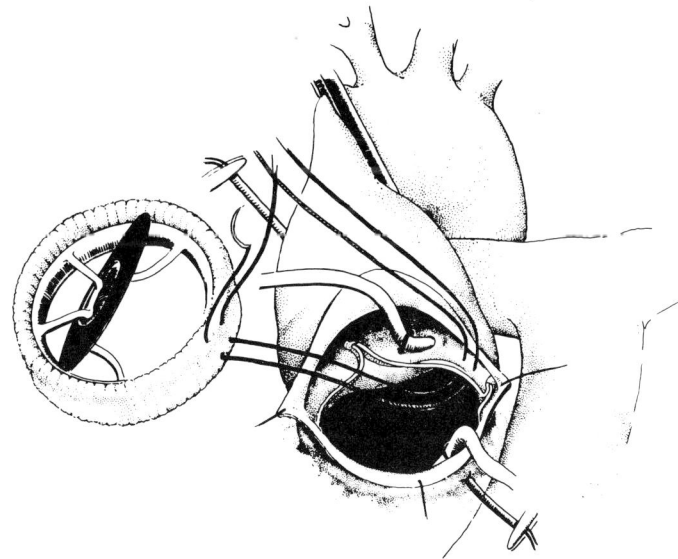

Figure 1.6 Selective coronary artery perfusion during aortic valve replacement. Isolated over-and-over sutures are used for sub-coronary positioning of the aortic prosthesis. The larger portion of the tilting disc is orientated against the commissure between the right and left coronary sinuses. (Reproduced from Åberg, B., Henze, A. and Björk, V. O.[25], by courtesy of *Scandinavian Journal of thoracic and cardiovascular Surgery*)

Sub-annular placement of the prostheses in the mitral and tricuspid positions was considered essential, as most of the strain is exerted on this junction during ventricular systole. Good fixation was obtained with 20 or more isolated mattress sutures (*Figure 1.7*). Orientation of the larger downward tilting portion of the valve disc towards the posterior mitral leaflet base was attempted in order to achieve optimal haemodynamic performance[5]. This 'posterior orientation' of the valve opening was preferred even in the tricuspid area[23].

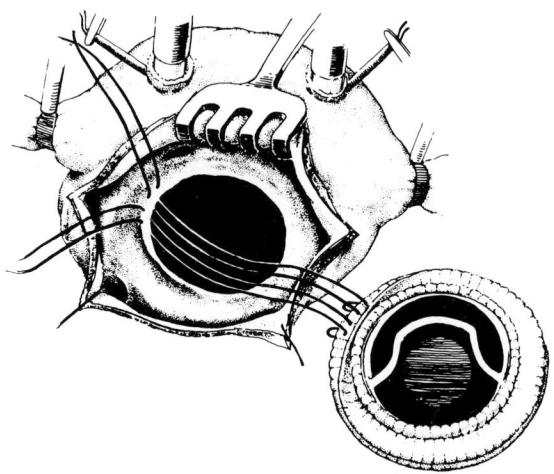

Figure 1.7 Subannular positioning of the mitral prosthesis with interrupted mattress sutures. The larger portion of the tilting disc is orientated towards the posterior wall of the left ventricle. (Reproduced from Åberg, B., Henze, A. and Björk, V. O.[25], by courtesy of *Scandinavian Journal of thoracic and cardiovascular Surgery*)

The aortic prosthesis was attached to the aortic annulus with about 30 over-and-over sutures. It was desirable to orientate the larger upward tilting portion of the disc towards the commissure between the left and right coronary sinuses, as this orientation directs the laminar blood flow to the area of the coronary ostia (*Figure 1.6*).

It must be emphasized that in patients with narrow aortic roots or valvular rings with extensive calcification or other anatomical anomalies, an absolutely free mobility of the tilting disc must have priority over the 'ideal orientations' described above. Appropriate orientation in this respect can be achieved even after the prothesis has been sutured in position, as it can be rotated within its sewing rim. As already mentioned only the original valve holder should be used for this purpose (*Figure 1.5*), because certain instruments, such as forceps or clamps, may damage the prosthesis, causing malfunction and perhaps initiating thrombosis.

HAEMOLYSIS

Almost 200 patients with mitral or aortic prostheses were investigated with respect to chronic intravascular haemolysis. Several laboratory tests were performed: haemoglobin concentration, haematocrit, blood cell counts, transaminases, serum iron and haptoglobin concentrations, serum activity of lactic dehydrogenase and total amount of haemoglobin and blood volume[8,13]. The results obtained from these investigations clearly indicated that intravascular haemolysis was of a very low degree and anaemia or iron deficiency were found only on rare occasions. On the other hand, haemolysis was a sign of periprosthetic leakage and it disappeared promptly after operative repair of the leak.

Several factors are involved in the production of haemolysis by artificial heart valves, such as turbulence, shearing stress and mechanical crushing of the red cells. There was no correlation between the size of the prosthetic valve and the degree of *in vivo* haemolysis, probably indicating that turbulence and shearing stress seldom reach critical levels around Björk–Shiley prostheses in human hearts. The fact that haemolysis increased only slightly during exercise and tachycardia lends further support to this suggestion[8]. It should also be mentioned that most patients with the 21 mm Björk–Shiley prosthesis in the aortic position (the smallest size routinely inserted) showed normal serum enzyme activities of lactic dehydrogenase. The low rate of haemolysis may also be ascribed to the non-overlapping closing mechanism of this prosthesis. Crushing of erythrocytes is minimized as the disc does not hit the valve ring during closure. This was demonstrated by means of a specially constructed test chamber (*Figure 1.8*). This apparatus permitted a normal valve function with simulated physiological left ventricular and central aortic pressures, but with a minimal volume (70 ml) of human whole blood which was exposed mainly to the movements of the occluder[18]. Non-overlapping occluders were found to cause much less haemolysis than overlapping ones and similar observations were made concerning both disc valves and ball valves[14].

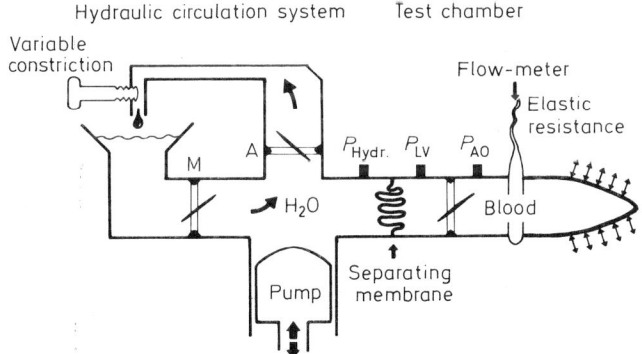

Figure 1.8 Experimental apparatus for testing the haemolysis generated by prosthetic valves with different closing mechanisms. The hydraulic circulation system is separated from the test chamber by a flaccid membrane. The test chamber was filled with 70 ml of human whole blood. With pulsatile flow through the hydraulic system, the elastic resistance of the membrane allows a certain volume displacement sufficient to open the valve during systole, while the elastic recoil permits valve closure. Pressures in the left ventricle (LV) and aorta (AO) were kept at physiological levels. (Reproduced from Henze, A. and Fortune, R. L.[18], by courtesy of *Scandinavian Journal of thoracic and cardiovascular Surgery*)

The most reliable estimate of intravascular haemolysis is the erythrocyte survival rate obtained by radioactive labelling of the red cells. This time-consuming procedure is, however, unsuitable for studies of larger series of patients. Any decrease in red cell survival will place a stress upon the bone marrow to compensate for this loss and to prevent the development of anaemia. An attempt was therefore made to calculate this bone marrow stress by converting the red cell destruction within the test chamber (per cent cells/70 ml/h) to the *in vivo* conditions, assuming a blood volume of 4800 ml, a red cell survival time of 120 days and a linear progression of haemolysis with time. The values of bone marrow stress obtained were 10 per cent of the normal bone marrow activity or red cell production rate for the non-overlapping closing mechanism, compared with 22 per cent for the overlapping one in 25 mm tissue diameter disc prostheses. Critical ranges of bone marrow stress may probably be reached if multivalvular replacements are performed with an overlapping prosthetic device. Such a critical level of stress may result in chronic haemolytic anaemia. The low rate of haemolysis calculated for the Björk–Shiley prosthesis is in accordance with our clinical findings. Haemolysis was mild and without clinical significance.

RHEOLOGY

The rheology of the prosthetic valve concerns its regurgitation and its resistance to blood flow or the trans-valvular pressure gradient.

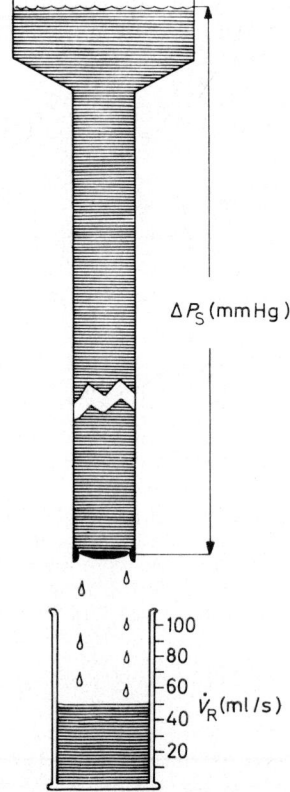

Figure 1.9 Experimental evaluation of regurgitation through the non-overlapping closing mechanism. A column of test fluid of variable height (ΔP_S, mmHg) generates regurgitation through the closed valve prosthesis ($\dot{V}_R$, ml/s). ΔP_S = driving pressure = trans-prosthetic mean systolic pressure difference in the mitral position of trans-prosthetic mean diastolic pressure difference in the aortic position. $\dot{V}_R$ = regurgitation through the non-overlapping closing mechanism with the disc seated. (Reproduced from Björk and Henze (1976) 'Flow-dynamics across the Björk–Shiley tilting disc valve in the mitral position'. *The mitral valve, a pluridisciplinary approach.* By courtesy of the Publishing Science Group, Inc.)

Regurgitation

The non-overlapping closing mechanism is, by its nature, slightly regurgitant, as some blood escapes in the retrograde direction through the circular clearance space between the disc and the valve ring, due to the driving pressure acting upon it. It might be argued that this is a disadvantage from a haemodynamic point of view, but we have learned from our experimental studies and from cardiac catheterization results that this is not the case. The regurgitation after prosthetic valve closure actually proved to be insignificant.

The relationship between the driving pressure and the regurgitation after valve closure was clarified by using a simple experimental set-up (*Figure 1.9*). The prosthesis in its closed position formed the base of a column of test fluid (human whole blood or water) of varying height. The pressure was measured directly above the valve level and the regurgitant flow was calculated by means of a graduated cylinder and a stop-watch. The driving pressure represented the trans-prosthetic mean systolic pressure difference in the mitral position and the trans-prosthetic mean diastolic pressure difference in the aortic position. Control studies were made using a pulsatile system containing human whole blood[18]. The pressure differentials were measured by planimetry of the recorded curves and the regurgitant flow was measured with an electromagnetic flow-meter. The

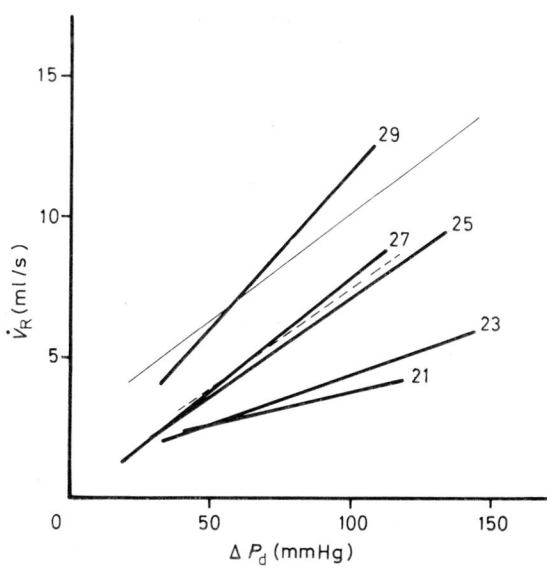

Figure 1.10 Relationship between driving pressure (ΔP_d, mmHg = trans-prosthetic mean diastolic pressure difference in the aortic position) and regurgitation after valve closure ($\dot{V}_R$ = ml/s). Thick lines represent linear regressions obtained by testing, with human whole blood, of the Björk–Shiley prosthesis with 21, 23, 25, 27 and 29 mm tissue diameter and pyrolitic carbon disc. The linear regressions are identical for corresponding sizes of the Björk–Shiley mitral prosthesis. The effect of viscosity is shown by the thin unbroken line representing the linear regression for the 25 mm prosthesis obtained by testing with water. The lower the viscosity, the higher the regurgitation for a given driving pressure. (Reproduced from Henze, A. and Fortune, R. L.[18], by courtesy of *Scandinavian Journal of thoracic and cardiovascular Surgery*)

results obtained by both these studies in a pulsatile system, as well as with the static rig, were identical.

There was a linear relationship between the driving pressure and the regurgitant flow after valve closure (*Figure 1.10*). These figures were extrapolated to the conditions obtained by cardiac catheterization in our mitral and aortic prosthetic valve patients[18]. It was found that the *in vivo* volume of regurgitant blood flow amounted to 2 per cent of the forward stroke volume for the smaller prosthetic valves and to a maximum of 5 per cent for the larger ones, both at rest and during exercise. This regurgitation is negligible from a haemodynamic point of view. On the aortogram or ventriculogram, the regurgitation appears as a slight subvalvular reflux of contrast medium (*Figure 1.11*).

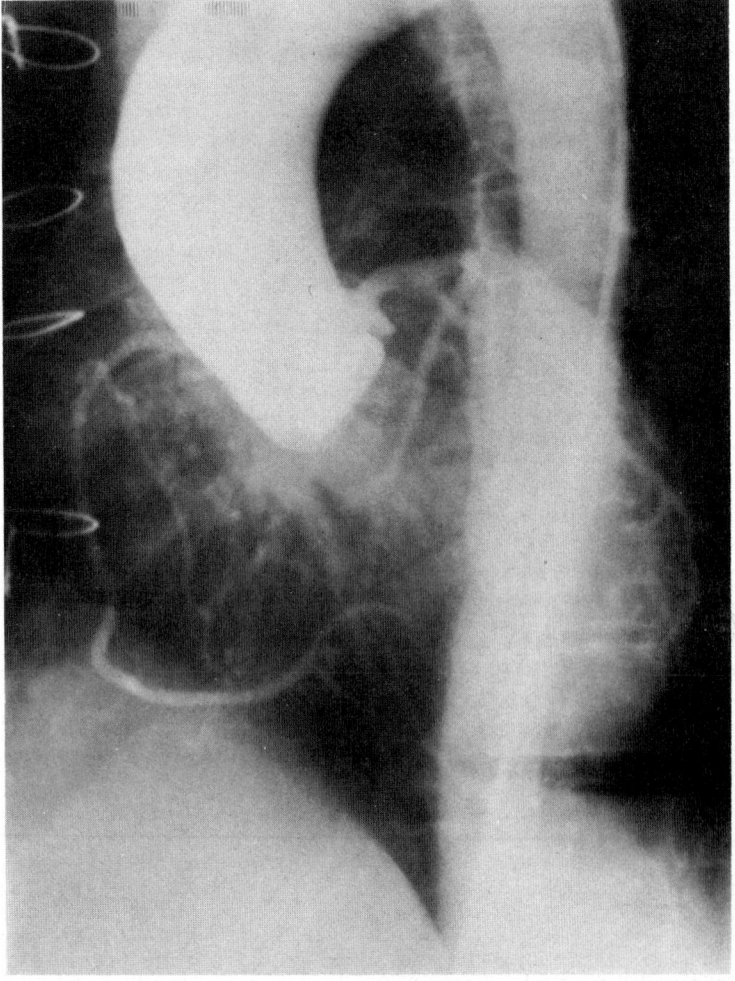

Figure 1.11 Aortic root angiogram performed seven months after aortic valve replacement with a 23 mm Björk–Shiley, Delrin disc, prosthesis for calcific aortic stenosis. There is slight subvalvular reflux of contrast medium after valve closure

Transvalvular gradient

According to the formula of Gorlin and Gorlin[16], the gradient or resistance to blood flow (in terms of a fall in driving pressure) varies directly with the flow and inversely with the fourth power of the radius of the prosthetic valve orifice. A prosthetic valve with the highest possible orifice area-to-tissue diameter ratio will therefore provide an optimal haemodynamic condition for the patient. In the construction of the Björk–Shiley prosthesis, the circumferential metal rim for occluder contact was eliminated by means of the non-overlapping tilting disc. Another 2 mm of orifice diameter were thus gained for a given external diameter.

In pulse duplicator studies, no other commercially available artificial heart valve prosthesis had such a low gradient as the Björk–Shiley prosthesis[21]. A considerable amount of work has been performed in our physiological laboratories in order to establish the *in vivo* resistance to blood flow[5,10].

A total of 90 patients were re-investigated by trans-septal left heart catheterization at rest and during exercise[10], at an average of seven months following aortic valve replacement. The mean trans-prosthetic systolic pressure difference was obtained by planimetry of simultaneously recorded left ventricular and central aortic pressure curves (*Figure 1.12*). The hydraulic valve area (A) of the prosthesis was calculated by the formula of Gorlin and Gorlin[16]:

$$A = \frac{AVF}{C\,44.5\,\sqrt{\Delta P}}$$

assuming a numerical value of 1.0 as the constant C. AVF represents the mean aortic valve flow in ml/s and ΔP the mean systolic trans-prosthetic pressure difference in mmHg. The relationship between the mean aortic valve flow and the cardiac output was obtained by the method of least squares regression between these variables.

The *in vivo* flow-driving pressure fall relationship for the aortic prosthesis was almost linear (*Figure 1.13*). The pressure difference at rest was below 10 mmHg for the 25, 27 and 29 mm valves, about 12 mmHg for the 23 mm size and 20 mmHg for the 21 mm valve. With increasing flow during exercise,

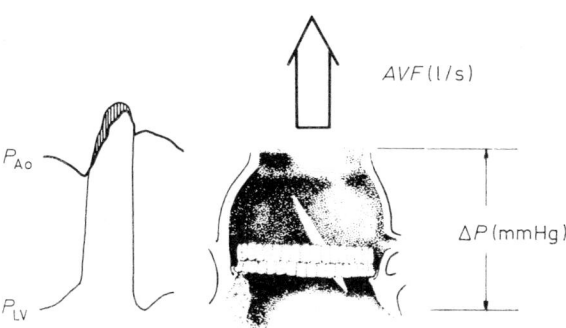

Figure 1.12 The mean systolic pressure difference (ΔP) across the Björk–Shiley prosthesis was obtained by planimetry of the demarcated area. (Reproduced from Henze, A. (1974) 'The Björk–Shiley tilting disc valve in aortic valvular disease', by courtesy of *Scandinavian Journal of thoracic and cardiovascular Surgery*)

the trans-prosthetic pressure difference increased and the slope of the line became steepest for the 21 mm valve *(Figure 1.13)*.

A total of 50 patients with mitral valve prostheses were also investigated by cardiac catheterization within one year of valve replacement[5,13]. Recordings were made at rest and during exercise and the trans-prosthetic mean diastolic pressure difference, which was obtained by planimetry of simultaneously recorded left atrial and left ventricular pressure curves, was related to the mean mitral valve flow or cardiac output in the manner described above.

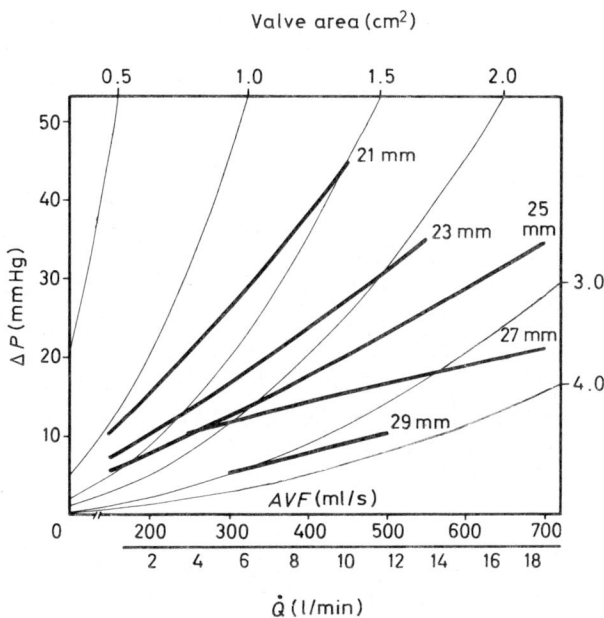

Figure 1.13 In vivo relationship between mean pressure difference (ΔP) across five sizes of the Björk–Shiley aortic prosthesis and the mean aortic valve flow (*AVF*) or cardiac output ($\dot{Q}$) shown in thick lines. The calculated prosthetic valve areas, according to Gorlin's formula are shown in thin lines. The haemodynamic investigations were performed in 90 patients with aortic valve replacement with the following sizes of Björk–Shiley prosthesis: 21 mm diameter, 12 patients; 23 mm, 26 patients; 25 mm, 33 patients; 27 mm, 12 patients; and 29 mm diameter 7 patients. (Reproduced from Björk, V. O., Henze, A. and Holmgren[10], by courtesy of *Scandinavian Journal of thoracic and cardiovascular Surgery*)

The gradient was low at rest, but rose in a linear fashion with increasing cardiac output during exercise *(Figure 1.14)*. The slope of these lines was dependent upon both the orientation of the mitral valve prosthesis and its opening angle (50° for the Delrin disc model and 60° for the pyrolytic carbon disc model). The best results were obtained with the pyrolytic carbon disc model with an opening angle of 60° and with the 'posterior orientation' of the bigger portion of the valve disc[5,13] *(Figure 1.14)*.

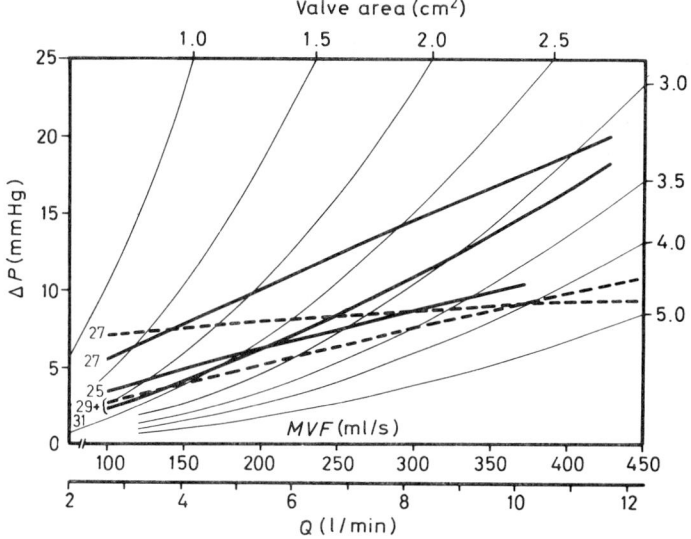

Figure 1.14 *In vivo* relationship between mean pressure difference (ΔP) across four sizes of the Björk–Shiley mitral prosthesis and mean mitral valve flow (*MVF*) or cardiac output (Q̇). Thin lines indicate the calculated prosthetic valve area according to Gorlin's formula. Thick lines represent the regression lines in 26 patients having anterior or septal orientation of the bigger portion of the Delrin disc with an opening angle of 50°. Thick broken lines represent the regression lines in 24 patients having posterior orientation of the bigger portion of the pyrolitic carbon disc with an opening angle of 60°. (Reproduced from Böök, K.[13], by courtesy of *Scandinavian Journal of thoracic and cardiovascular Surgery*)

CENTRAL HAEMODYNAMICS

Following the presentation of the rheological characteristics of the Björk–Shiley prosthesis, we now propose to describe briefly the improvements in central cardiovascular dynamics following the replacement of diseased valves with prostheses. We performed haemodynamic studies in different categories of patients, such as: patients with mitral valve disease, aortic stenosis, aortic incompetence, narrow aortic roots and in patients over 60 years of age. Detailed reports of the methodology and the results obtained have been published elsewhere[4,5,10,11,12,17]. The patients were subjected to repeat cardiac catheterization six to seven months following valve replacement, the investigations being performed at rest and during supine exercise. (The number of patients studied appears in the Figures.) The results have clearly demonstrated that, following valve replacement with the Björk–Shiley prosthesis, a considerable reduction of volume overload of the left ventricle was achieved in cases of aortic incompetence and of pressure overload in patients with aortic stenosis. A corresponding decrease in the mean left atrial pressure was obtained in cases of mitral valve disease. It is also worth mentioning that the Björk–Shiley prosthesis has given satisfactory load reduction in patients with narrow aortic roots.

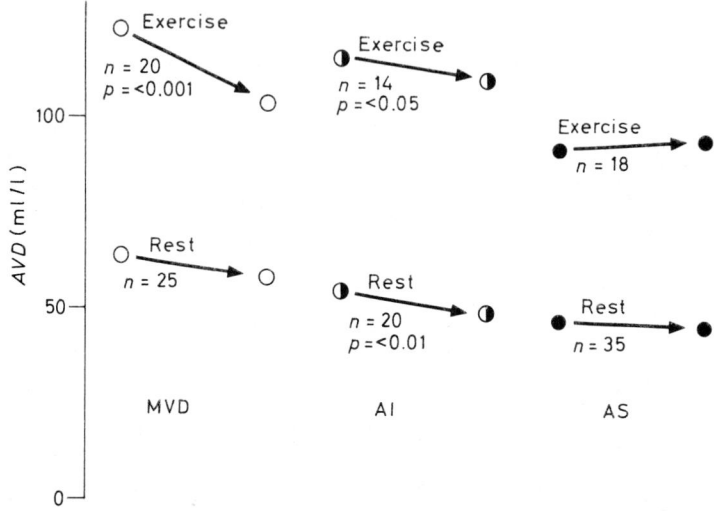

Figure 1.15 Arteriovenous oxygen difference (*AVD*, ml/ℓ) at rest and during exercise in patients with mitral valve disease (MVD), aortic incompetence (AI) and aortic stenosis (AS) before and after valve replacement with the Björk–Shiley prosthesis

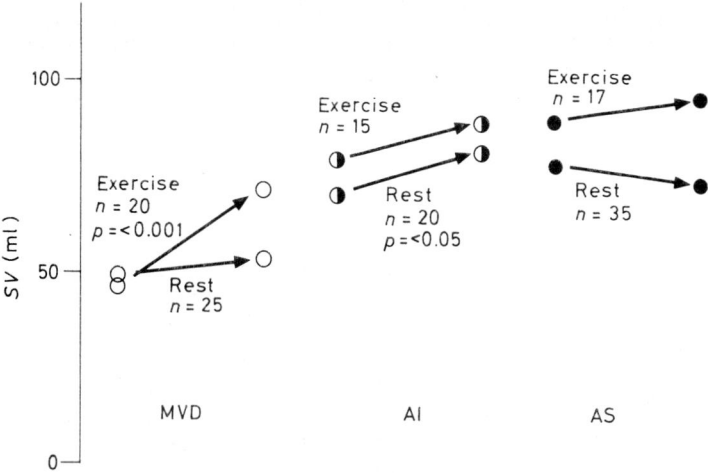

Figure 1.16 Stroke volume (*SV*, ml) at rest and during exercise in patients with mitral valve disease (MVD), aortic incompetence (AI) and aortic stenosis (AS) before and after valve replacement with the Björk–Shiley prosthesis

In order to demonstrate the post-operative haemodynamic improvement, we selected three parameters for evaluation, namely the arteriovenous oxygen difference, the stroke volume and the mean left atrial pressure.

Two groups of patients, those with mitral valve disease and those with aortic incompetence, became less hypokinetic following the operation, as the arteriovenous oxygen difference diminished. This was particularly pronounced during exercise in patients following mitral valve replacement (*Figure 1.15*).

The stroke volume increased markedly during exercise in mitral patients, while those with aortic incompetence displayed a less pronounced but obvious increase also at rest (*Figure 1.16*).

There were no statistically significant changes in either arteriovenous oxygen difference or stroke volume following valve replacement in patients with aortic stenosis. There was, however, no doubt whatsoever that the hearts of all three categories of patients were unloaded after operation as the pressure levels in the left atrium were considerably reduced (*Figure 1.17*).

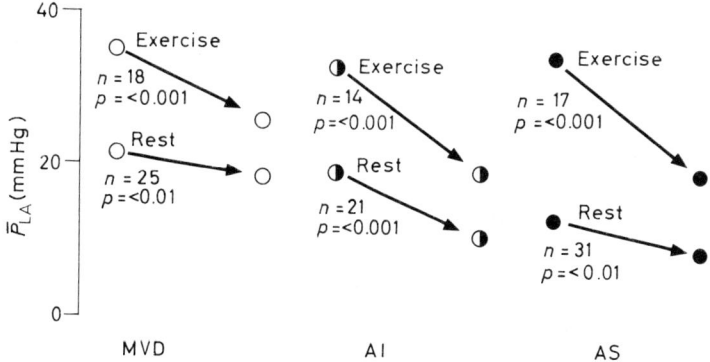

Figure 1.17 Mean left atrial pressure ($\bar{P}_{LA}$, mmHg) at rest and during exercise in patients with mitral valve disease (MVD), aortic incompetence (AI) and aortic stenosis (AS) before and after valve replacement with the Björk–Shiley prosthesis

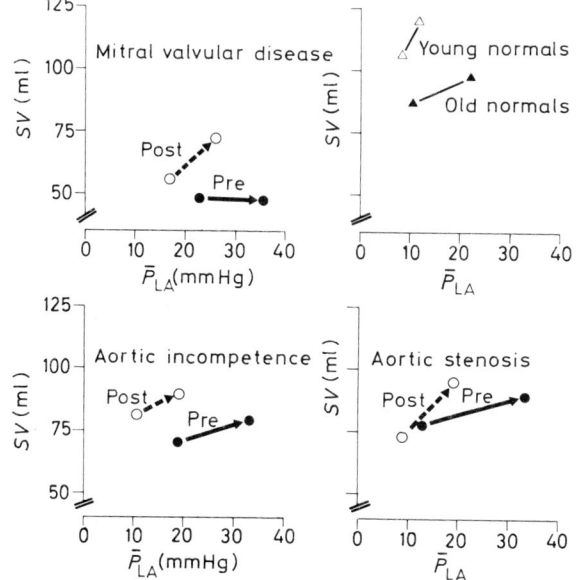

Figure 1.18 Changes in stroke volume related to changes in mean left atrial pressure ($\Delta SV/\Delta \bar{P}_{LA}$, ml/mmHg) on transition from rest to exercise in patients with mitral valve disease, aortic incompetence and aortic stenosis before and after valve replacement with the Björk–Shiley prosthesis. Figures for healthy individuals are shown for comparison

We endeavoured to outline the haemodynamic response by reproducing the change in stroke volume in relation to the change in mean left atrial pressure on transition from rest to exercise (*Figure 1.18*). This quotient, $\Delta SV/\Delta P_{LA}$, has the dimensions ml/mmHg and it was used here as an estimate of cardiac performance. Patients with heart valve disease can only increase their stroke volume very slightly during exercise, while the pressure in the left atrium rises considerably (*Figure 1.18*). The haemodynamic condition was clearly improved after valve replacement. In comparison with the performance of healthy hearts[19,24] those with different types of valve disease displayed varying degrees of improvement. In general the cardiac performance of patients with mitral valve replacement, despite post-operative improvement, remained definitely within the abnormal range of variation (*Figure 1.18*). On the other hand, patients with aortic valve disease who have undergone valve replacement, showed a higher degree of improvement. In this group of patients with aortic replacement, the haemodynamic parameters approached the values of healthy elderly persons (*Figure 1.18*).

ANTICOAGULATION AND ASSOCIATED COMPLICATIONS

The first measure to prevent thromboembolic complications was taken in the operating theatre by dipping the valve prosthesis in a heparin solution prior to its insertion. Apart from 50 000 units of heparin diluted with 60 ml of saline, this solution also contained 5 million units of penicillin. After insertion, all accessible parts of the prosthesis were again washed with the heparin solution.

Anticoagulation in the early post-operative period was considered essential and therefore intravenous heparin treatment (20 000 units/24 h/75 kg body weight) was initiated after removal of the chest drainage tubes. This was maintained until oral anticoagulation became effective.

Lifelong anticoagulant treatment in the form of dicoumarol or warfarin sodium should be attempted in all patients after valve replacement with the Björk–Shiley prosthesis. The dosage of this medication was controlled by frequent estimations of the Thrombotest index[22] (therapeutic range of 6–15 per cent in our laboratory). In a survey of the adequacy of anticoagulation it was found that on the day of admission for follow-up, 41, 76 and 80 per cent of the patients in three different series showed Thrombotest index levels indicating adequate anticoagulation[4,6,25]. At present, the majority of patients show satisfactory levels of prothrombin depression. Although thromboembolic complications still occur they are more frequent when anticoagulation is ineffective[4,6,25].

Serious bleeding complications in the form of cerebral haemorrhage occurred in 6 out of 383 anticoagulated patients, an incidence of 0.5/100 patient years, ranging from 0.4–0.8 in four different series (*Table 1.1*). The outcome was fatal in four of these six patients. From the total of six cases of cerebral haemorrhage, five were associated with anticoagulant overdosage, three were connected with systemic arterial hypertension and in three patients there was impaired hepatic function.

In an effort to eliminate the risk of bleeding complications, we decided to discontinue the anticoagulant treatment in patients with aortic valve prostheses and with either haemorrhagic episodes, unstable anticoagulation, pregnancy, or

TABLE 1.1

Incidence of cerebral haemorrhage among 383 patients having Björk–Shiley prosthetic valves and long-term anticoagulation

Valves replaced	Number of patients *	Duration of follow-up		Cerebral haemorrhage	
		Years/ patient	Patient years	Number of patients	Episodes/100 patient years
Aortic	73	5.5	402	2	0.5
Mitral	195	2.5	482	2	0.4
Mitral and aortic	68	2.4	164	1	0.6
Tricuspid (isolated or combined with other valve replacements)	47	2.7	129	1	0.8
Total	383	3.1	1177	6	0.5

* Early mortality excluded

in those requiring surgical operations. A programme with dipyridamole and acetylsalicylic acid instead of prothrombin depressant treatment was also carried out in another group of patients with aortic prostheses. As the resulting incidence of thromboembolic complications was unacceptably high (*Table 1.6 p. 22*), we discourage the interruption of anticoagulation whenever possible.

Anticoagulation should be maintained when patients with Björk–Shiley prostheses undergo surgery. A temporary reduction of the dosage in order to raise the Thrombotest index to the range of 20–30 per cent is sufficient to minimize the risk of bleeding complications. The prothrombin complex transferable by the transfusion of fresh frozen plasma assures coagulation in emergency cases.

The rare occurrence of pregnancy in patients with mechanical heart valves has become a delicate problem in view of the hazards of temporary withdrawal of anticoagulation therapy (*Table 1.6*). Our present policy is therefore a transition to heparin injected subcutaneously during the last month prior to delivery, whereafter oral anticoagulation is recommenced.

THROMBOEMBOLISM

The following report on thromboembolic complications is strictly 'prosthesis orientated', therefore only patients with valve replacement, but without other concomitant cardiac surgical procedures, were included.

Systemic embolism

This was defined by symptoms related to the sudden, total or partial, obstruction of an artery. It had a considerably variable incidence depending upon the intracardiac position of the prosthetic valve, the valve model, the underlying heart disease, cardiac rhythm and efficiency, and the maintenence of anti-coagulation.

The incidence of systemic emboli is shown in *Table 1.2*. Satisfactory results were obtained following aortic valve replacement in patients in sinus rhythm who were maintained on permanent anticoagulation. In this group there was an incidence of 0.7 emboli/100 patient years. It was noted that the incidence of embolization was highest following isolated mitral valve replacement (6.8 episodes/100 patient years), being nearly twice that following combined aortic and mitral valve replacement (3.6 episodes/100 patient years). This is probably related to the influence of the underlying heart disease.

The incidence of 6.8 episodes/100 patient years for mitral valve replacement contains data obtained both from the original Delrin disc model with an opening angle of $50°$ and from the currently available pyrolytic carbon disc model with an opening angle of $60°$. It may therefore be of interest that the pyrolytic carbon disc prosthesis $(60°)$ has clearly decreased the incidence of systemic emboli from 9.6 to 5.3 episodes/100 patient years and so far has eliminated the

TABLE 1.2
Incidence of systemic embolization among 383 patients having Björk–Shiley prosthetic valves and long-term anticoagulation

| Valves replaced | Number of patients* | Duration of follow-up | | | Systemic emboli/100 patient years | |
		Years/ patient	Patient years	Fatal	With sequelae	Without sequelae
Aortic	73 †	5.5	402	–	–	0.7
Mitral	195	2.5	482	0.8	0.8	5.2
Mitral and aortic	68	2.4	164	–	1.2	2.4
Tricuspid	9	2.6	23	–	–	–
Mitral and tricuspid	24	2.8	67	–	1.5	–
Mitral, aortic and tricuspid	14	2.8	39	–	–	–

* Early mortality excluded
† All patients in sinus rhythm

TABLE 1.3
Influence of heart rhythm on the incidence of systemic embolization in patients having Björk–Shiley prosthetic valves and long-term anticoagulation

| Valve replaced and heart rhythm | Number of patients | Duration of follow-up | | Systemic emboli (episodes/100 patient years) |
		Years/ patient	Patient years	
Aortic sinus rhythm	73	5.5	402	0.7
Aortic atrial fibrillation	10	6.1	61	6.6
Mitral	195	2.5	482	6.8

mortality due to embolization[7]. This benefit is probably related to the increased opening angle in the pyrolytic carbon disc model which causes less resistance to blood flow.

The influence of heart rhythm is demonstrated in *Table 1.3*. Patients with aortic prosthetic valves and in atrial fibrillation, as well as those with mitral prostheses, apparently show a similar rate of systemic embolization, which is nearly ten times greater than that encountered in patients with aortic prosthetic valves and in sinus rhythm.

It should be mentioned that none of the patients with tricuspid prostheses had symptoms of pulmonary embolism and screening by means of lung scintigraphy in a group of 30 patients did not show any localized perfusion defects.

Thrombotic obstruction

Thrombosis of the Björk-Shiley prosthetic valve has been the most dangerous manifestation of thromboembolism, with fatal outcome unless appropriately diagnosed and urgently treated. The incidence of prosthetic thrombosis is shown in *Table 1.4*. There was a remarkable predominance of this complication in patients with isolated mitral and particularly with tricuspid valve replacement, again indicating the influence of the underlying heart disease (*Table 1.5*). Two of the three tricuspid prosthetic thromboses were encountered in young patients

TABLE 1.4
Incidence of thrombotic obstruction in 503 Björk-Shiley prostheses implanted in 383 patients treated with long-term anticoagulation

Location of prostheses	Total number of prostheses	Duration of observation period		Prosthetic thrombosis	
		Years/ prosthesis	Prosthesis years	Number of prostheses	Episodes/100 prosthesis years
Aortic	155	3.9	605	2	0.3
Mitral	301	2.5	752	14	1.9
Tricuspid	47	2.7	129	3	2.3

TABLE 1.5
Incidence of thrombotic obstruction in 503 Björk-Shiley prostheses implanted in 383 patients treated with long-term anticoagulation; comparison between isolated and combined valve replacements

Location of prostheses	Prosthetic thrombosis (episodes/100 prosthesis years)	
	Isolated valve replacement	Combined valve replacements
Aortic	–	1.0
Mitral	2.5	0.7
Tricuspid	13.0	–

with large, dilated right atria due to Ebstein's anomaly. Thrombotic obstruction of the aortic prosthesis has not hitherto occurred in our series of patients with continuous anticoagulant treatment.

In our experience with more than 1800 implants of the Björk–Shiley prosthesis, we have encountered to date a total of 30 thrombotic obstructions. The above mentioned three tricuspid cases were re-operated upon without complications. One patient had a late recurrence which was successfully managed with thrombolytic therapy. Six out of nine patients with thrombosed aortic prostheses were referred to our clinic and re-operated upon as emergencies. All six patients survived re-operation. Only four out of 15 mitral prosthetic obstructions were recognized and operated upon, and two of them died. Both cases with mitral and aortic prosthetic thromboses were diagnosed at autopsy.

Thrombectomy was performed in the six aortic patients. It proved possible to remove the thrombotic deposits with a nerve hook and a sucker after stepwise rotation of the prosthesis within its sewing rim by using the valve holder. In contrast, a clot on the ventricular side of a mitral or tricuspid prosthesis is unlikely to be safely removed, and instrumentation may cause fragmentation and detachment of the thrombus with subsequent embolization. Thrombosed mitral prostheses should therefore be excised and replaced. A clotted tricuspid prosthesis should be first treated with thrombolytic therapy (streptokinase) through an indwelling catheter before valve replacement is attempted.

Immediate recognition of a thrombotic obstruction of the prosthetic valve is of utmost importance, as this dangerous complication can be averted by instant surgical intervention. Nevertheless, in our series, the symptoms due to a developing thrombosis were frequently mistaken for heart failure. The introduction of the ring-shaped radio-opaque marker in the tilting disc of the Björk–Shiley prosthesis has clearly increased the possibility for early diagnosis of partly or completely obstructed disc motion caused by thrombosis. Disc motion can be easily visualized by cineradiography or fluoroscopy[9] and such non-invasive procedures are well tolerated even by the critically ill patient. In the event of a thrombotic obstruction, the motion of the tilting disc is severely compromised. Early diagnosis of and emergency operation for thrombotic obstruction of the

TABLE 1.6
Influence of anticoagulant treatment on the incidence of thromboembolic complications in patients having aortic valve replacement with Björk–Shiley prostheses

Prothrombin depressant treatment	Number of patients	Duration of follow-up		Systemic emboli (episodes/100 patient years)	Prosthetic thrombosis (episodes/100 prosthesis years)
		Years/ patient	Patient years		
Long-term administration	73	5.5	402	0.7	—
None*	91	0.7	61	14.9	8.1
Discontinued	32	1.0	32	25.0	—
Re-administered	26	4.1	107	1.9	0.9

*In this group of 91 patients, 27 did not receive any anticoagulant medication while 64 patients were treated with a combination of dipyridamole and acetylsalicylic acid

prosthesis will reduce the mortality due to this dangerous complication in the future.

The importance of a careful anticoagulation programme cannot be over-emphasized and we strongly discourage interruption of anticoagulation whenever possible (*Table 1.6*). Experience has shown that thromboembolic complications still occur most frequently when anticoagulation is ineffective[4,6,25].

INFECTION

Infection, in the form of septicaemia or infective endocarditis, has been respons-ible for five deaths among 432 long-term survivors. This corresponds to 1 per cent or an incidence of 0.3 episodes/100 patient years. One further patient had recurrent septicaemia (*Staphylococcus aureus*) in association with instrumenta-tion of a lower urinary tract stricture. He was successfully managed with anti-biotic treatment. There were no re-operations because of infected prostheses. In our series prophylactic antibiotic treatment, usually with penicillin, was continued for three months post-operatively. All the above mentioned infections occurred later than one year following operation.

RE-OPERATION

Re-operations were performed because of periprosthetic leak and thrombotic obstruction of the prosthetic valve. The latter operations have already been described.

There were five perivalvular leaks in a series of 204 aortic valve replacements (2.4 per cent), four leaks in 301 mitral replacements (1.3 per cent) and none in 47 tricuspid replacements. All nine patients survived re-operation for closure of the periprosthetic leak.

MORTALITY AND SURVIVAL RATE

A total of 466 patients who underwent heart valve replacement are included in the basic data concerning mortality. Patients with concomitant cardiac surgical procedures performed at the time of valve replacement were not included in this series. All post-operative deaths which occurred during the hospitalization period were classified as early mortality. The late mortality rate was analysed in terms of incidence/100 patient years.

The early mortality rate was in the order of 5 per cent for isolated aortic and mitral valve replacement and 9 per cent for combined mitral and aortic valve replacement. The combined mitral and tricuspid valve replacement involved the highest mortality rate (27 per cent). Further details are given in *Table 1.7*.

The total mortality rate and that caused by thromboembolism are presented in *Table 1.8*. There was an incidence of 3.0 late deaths/100 patient years follow-ing isolated aortic valve replacement and 7.5/100 patient years after isolated mitral valve replacement. This comparatively high mortality in the mitral group was mainly caused by thromboembolism. Combined mitral and aortic valve replacements showed a similar trend in this respect. No fatal thromboembolic

TABLE 1.7
Early mortality in 466 patients subjected to heart valve replacement with the
Björk–Shiley prosthesis

		Early mortality	
Valves replaced	*Number of patients*	*Number*	*Per cent*
Aortic	128	6	5
Mitral	203	8	4
Mitral and aortic	75	7	9
Tricuspid	10	1	10
Mitral and tricuspid	33	9	27
Mitral, aortic and tricuspid	17	3	18
Total	466	34	7

TABLE 1.8
Late mortality in 432 hospital survivors having heart valve replacement
with Björk–Shiley prostheses

		Duration of follow-up			Late deaths/100 patient years	
Valves replaced	*Number of patients*	*Years/ patient*	*Patient years*	*Total*	*Due to thromboembolism*
Aortic	122	5.5	671	3.0	0.1
Mitral	195	2.5	482	7.5	3.1
Mitral and aortic	68	2.4	164	7.3	2.4
Tricuspid	9	2.6	23	–	–
Mitral and tricuspid	24	2.8	67	3.0	–
Mitral, aortic and tricuspid	14	2.8	39	2.6	–

complications have so far occurred following isolated or combined tricuspid
valve replacements, a fact which may be explained by very careful long-term
anticoagulation in this particular group of patients. Further information regarding survival is provided, in actuarial form, in *Figure 1.19*.

SUMMARY

This book presents the results obtained with various tissue heart valves. In order
to establish terms of comparison between the performance of tissue valves and
mechnical prostheses we have chosen to analyse the results of our own experience
with the Björk–Shiley tilting disc valve particularly with respect to those complications related to thromboembolic phenomena and to the prevention and
treatment of thromboembolism.

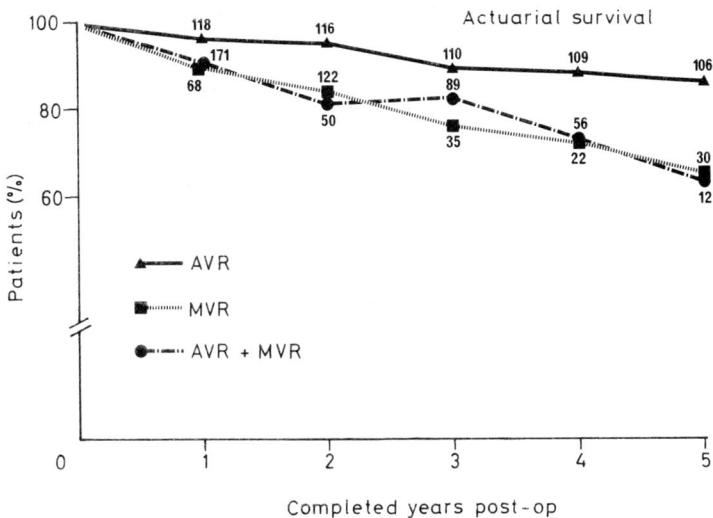

Figure 1.19 Actuarial survival rate following heart valve replacement with the Björk–Shiley prosthesis. The figures accompanying the actuarial curves denote the number of patients at risk in the three groups at the beginning of each year of observation (AVR = aortic valve replacement, MVR = mitral valve replacement)

The characteristics of the Björk–Shiley prosthesis are described and the changes made in the design of the valve are discussed. The patients' mortality, morbidity and survival rate are briefly presented. Certain complications, however, have a pronounced influence on mortality. Hence, the clinical material is summarized in such a way that late mortality, survival and complications, such as systemic embolization, re-operation, infection and haemorrhage, are reported individually (*Table 1.9*).

Thromboembolism has been and continues to remain a problem following prosthetic mitral valve replacement, while in patients with aortic valve replacement it is an extremely rare occurrence, provided that anticoagulant treatment is strictly maintained and carefully monitored. A careful and life-long anticoagulation programme is thus clearly indicated for all patients with Björk–Shiley prostheses, although our experience has shown that this therapy carried the risk of serious bleeding complications of the order of 0.5 events/100 patient years. Re-operation for periprosthetic leak in this series was performed without mortality or late complications. Infection was very unusual among the long-term survivors.

The advantages of the mechanical heart valve are obvious. The Björk–Shiley prosthesis has excellent haemodynamic properties both at rest and during exercise. Haemolysis was minimal and without clinical significance. We have not encountered any genuine mechanical failure of the prosthesis and, after almost nine years' experience with more than 1800 implants of the Björk–Shiley tilting disc valve prosthesis, we can therefore claim that it has proved its durability.

TABLE 1.9

Summary of clinical data from 432 patients having heart valve replacement with Björk–Shiley prostheses

Valves replaced	Number of patients	Age–years mean (range)	Duration of follow-up		Late deaths/ 100 patient years	Survival with complications (episodes/100 patient years)		
			Years/ patient	Patient years		Systemic emboli	Re-operation for perivalve leak or prosthetic thrombosis	Infection or haemorrhage
Aortic	122	52 (25–68)	5.5	671	3.0	0.7	0.6	–
Mitral	195	52 (7–66)	2.5	482	7.5	6.0	1.2	0.4*
Mitral and aortic	68	50 (17–67)	2.4	164	7.3	3.6	0.6	0.6†
Tricuspid (isolated or combined with other valve replacements)	47	45 (17–65)	2.7	129	2.3	0.8	2.3	–
Total	432			1446				

*Cerebral haemorrhage occurred in two patients
†Septicaemia occurred in one patient

REFERENCES

[1] Björk, V. O. 'A new tilting disc valve prosthesis', *Scandinavian Journal of thoracic and cardiovascular Surgery*, 3, 1 (1969)

[2] Björk, V. O. 'Delrin as implant material for valve occluders', *Scandinavian Journal of thoracic and cardiovascular Surgery*, 6, 103 (1972)

[3] Björk, V. O. 'The pyrolitic carbon occluder for the Björk–Shiley tilting disc valve prosthesis', *Scandinavian Journal of thoracic and cardiovascular Surgery*, 6, 109 (1972)

[4] Björk, V. O., Böök, K., Cernigliaro, C. and Holmgren, A. 'The Björk–Shiley tilting disc valve in isolated mitral lesions', *Scandinavian Journal of thoracic and cardiovascular Surgery*, 7, 131 (1973)

[5] Björk, V. O., Böök, K. and Holmgren, A. 'Significance of position and opening angle of the Björk–Shiley tilting disc valve in mitral surgery', *Scandinavian Journal of thoracic and cardiovascular Surgery*, 7, 187 (1973)

[6] Björk, V. O. and Henze, A. 'Management of thromboembolism after aortic valve replacement with the Björk–Shiley tilting disc valve', *Scandinavian Journal of thoracic and cardiovascular Surgery*, 9, 183 (1975)

[7] Björk, V. O. and Henze, A. 'Isolated mitral valve replacement with the Björk–Shiley tilting disc valve prosthesis. A six-year review and a comparison between the Delrin and the pyrolitic carbon disc models', *Scandinavian Journal of thoracic and cardiovascular Surgery*, 11, 181 (1977)

[8] Björk, V. O., Henze, A. and Carlström, A. 'Haematological evaluation of the Björk–Shiley tilting disc valve prosthesis in isolated aortic valvular disease', *Scandinavian Journal of thoracic and cardiovascular Surgery*, 8, 12 (1974)

[9] Björk, V. O., Henze, A. and Hindmarsh, T. 'Radio-opaque marker in the tilting disc of the Björk–Shiley heart valve. Evaluation of *in vivo* prosthetic valve function by cineradiography', *Journal of thoracic and cardiovascular Surgery*, 73, 563 (1977)

[10] Björk, V. O., Henze, A. and Holmgren, A. 'Central haemodynamics at rest and during exercise before and after aortic valve replacement with the Björk–Shiley tilting disc valve in patients with isolated aortic stenosis', *Scandinavian Journal of thoracic and cardiovascular Surgery*, 7, 111 (1973)

[11] Björk, V. O., Henze, A. and Holmgren, A. 'Central haemodynamics at rest and during exercise before and after operation with the Björk–Shiley tilting disc valve in patients with aortic incompetence', *Scandinavian Journal of thoracic and cardiovascular Surgery*, 7, 214 (1973)

[12] Björk, V. O., Henze, A., Holmgren, A. and Szamosi, A. 'Evaluation of the 21 mm Björk–Shiley tilting disc valve in patients with narrow aortic roots', *Scandinavian Journal of thoracic and cardiovascular Surgery*, 7, 203 (1973)

[13] Böök, K. 'Mitral valve replacement with the Björk–Shiley tilting disc valve. A clinical and haemodynamic study in patients with isolated mitral valve lesions', *Scandinavian Journal of thoracic and cardiovascular Surgery*, *(Suppl.)* 12, (1974)

[14] Fortune, R. L. and Henze, A. 'Haemolysis in ball valves with overlapping and non-overlapping closing mechanisms', *Scandinavian Journal of thoracic and cardiovascular Surgery*, 9, 1 (1975)

[15] Fortune, R. L. and Henze, A. 'Haemolysis in non-overlapping closing mechanisms of the Björk–Shiley tilting disc valve. An experimental and comparative study of Delrin and pyrolitic carbon disc prostheses', *Scandinavian Journal of thoracic and cardiovascular Surgery*, 9, 5 (1975)

[16] Gorlin, R. and Gorlin, S. G. 'Hydraulic formula for calculation of the area of the stenotic mitral valve, other cardiac valves and central circulatory shunts', *American heart Journal*, 41, 1 (1951)

[17] Henze, A. 'Aortic valve replacement in patients over the age of sixty', *Scandinavian Journal of thoracic and cardiovascular Surgery*, 8, 1 (1974)

[18] Henze, A. and Fortune, F. L. 'Regurgitation and haemolysis in artificial heart valves. An experimental study of overlapping and non-overlapping closing mechanisms and of paraprosthetic leakage', *Scandinavian Journal of thoracic and cardiovascular Surgery*, 8, 167 (1974)

[19] Holmgren, A., Jonsson, B. and Sjöstrand, T. 'Circulatory data in normal subjects at rest and during exercise in recumbent position with special reference to stroke volume at different work intensities', *Acta physiologica Scandinavica*, 49, 343 (1960)

[20] Messmer, B. J., Rothlin, M. and Senning, A. 'Early disc dislodgement. An unusual complication after insertion of a Björk–Shiley mitral valve prosthesis', *Journal of thoracic and cardiovascular Surgery*, **65**, 3 (1973)

[21] Olin, C. 'Pulsatile flow studies of prosthetic aortic valves', *Scandinavian Journal of thoracic and cardiovascular Surgery*, **5**, 1 (1973)

[22] Owren, P. A. 'The interrelationship between Normotest and Thrombotest', *Farmakoterapi*, **1**, 1 (1969)

[23] Peterffy, A., Henze, A., Jonasson, R. and Björk, V. O. 'Tricuspid valve replacement. Early and late results in 10 isolated and 51 combined cases operated upon with the Björk–Shiley tilting disc valve', *Scandinavian Journal of thoracic and cardiovascular Surgery*, **12**, 177 (1978)

[24] Strandell, T. 'Circulatory studies on healthy old men', *Acta medica Scandinavica, (Suppl.)* 414 (1964)

[25] Åberg, B., Henze, A. and Björk, V. O. 'Combined aortic and mitral valve replacement with the Björk–Shiley tilting disc valve prosthesis. Early and late results in 75 consecutive patients', *Scandinavian Journal of thoracic and cardiovascular Surgery*, **11**, 1 (1977)

2

Hydrodynamic Evaluation of Tissue Valves

John T. M. Wright

Le moment où je parle est déjà loin de moi.

Nicolas Boileau-Despreaux (1636–1711)

INTRODUCTION

The healthy mammalian aortic valve is ideally suited to meet its physiological and biological requirements. It is, therefore, not surprising that the surgeon should wish to replace a diseased heart valve with a tissue valve of similar architecture and material to that of the normal aortic valve.

In the early days of open-heart surgery this intuitive approach held out great promise, but experience showed that many of the early tissue valve replacements ultimately failed. The various reasons for failure included degradation of the leaflets (leading to cusp rigidity sometimes with calcification and stenosis), shrinkage of the cusp material (leading to insufficiency) and infection. As a result, many of these early valves had to be replaced. Fortunately tissue degeneration was usually a slow and gradual process, and in many patients re-operation could be an elective rather than an emergency procedure. A proportion of these early failures can now be attributed to the use of inappropriate tissue preservation techniques, the use of unsuitable tissues for valve construction, and probably other factors such as surgical techniques and inappropriate selection of patients. However, in recent years methods and techniques have greatly improved and as a result certain tissue valves have now become widely established as heart valve replacements of merit. This is due to the important advantages of tissue valves over mechanical prostheses. Most significant of these advantages is that generally tissue valves exhibit a low rate of thromboembolic complication; hence the patient does not require long-term anticoagulation therapy with its attendant clinical complications, financial disadvantages and patient inconvenience and anxiety. Furthermore, tissue valves are silent in operation (an advantage not fully appreciated by some), produce minimal blood trauma and have central flow paths. However, the long-term durability of the various types of tissue valves has yet to be determined. As already stated, should tissue valve failure occur this would not usually be abrupt.

Biological valves can be grouped into three categories: aortic valve allografts, aortic valve xenografts and valves constructed from non-valvular tissue.

Allograft aortic valves

Allograft aortic valves, either fresh or preserved with various techniques and chemical substances, have been extensively used by surgeons with a high individual level of success. In the great majority of clinical series these valves have been implanted as unmounted grafts in the aortic position. Few workers had used, in limited series, stent mounted aortic allografts as mitral valve replacements. These mounted valves had been preserved in various ways, none of which have given satisfactory results in the mitral position, and therefore their use was discontinued. Some authors consider that the allograft valve has the advantage of being less expensive. However, if the economics of collection, inspection, preservation, storage and wastage are taken into account, then the true cost of allografts is probably not much different from other types of valve replacements. More significant is the fact that the supply of suitable cadaver valves is such that only a few surgeons working in large population areas may be sure of a reliable supply of valves. This shortage, in turn, means that the technical standard of the valve might be less than that which would be accepted by a commercial manufacturer of xenograft bio-prostheses. Although there are no published reports of success-

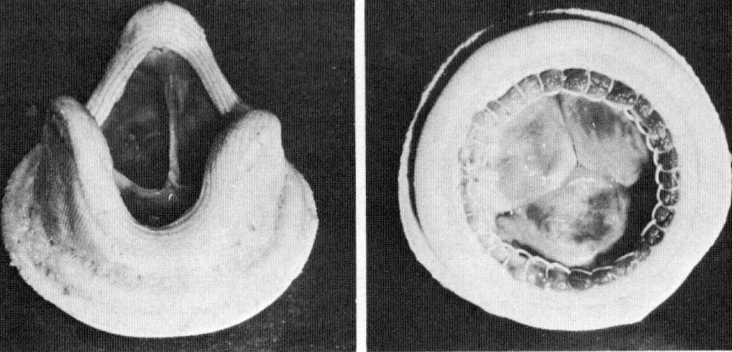

Figure 2.1 Stent mounted aortic valve allograft for mitral replacement. The valve was treated with glutaraldehyde. Implantation diameter 32 mm

ful results with either fresh or preserved stent mounted allograft aortic valves in the mitral position, two experimental allografts (*Figure 2.1*) have been tested in order to compare their hydraulic behaviour with the performance of the somewhat dissimilar, mounted aortic porcine valves.

Xenograft aortic valves

Preserved xenograft aortic valves combine the architectural advantages of the natural aortic valve, with a ready commercial availability in a wide range of sizes, and with a long shelf-life. They are mounted on a stent or frame (of plastic or metal) in order to ensure reliability of function and convenience of insertion. They are usually constructed from a single intact porcine aortic valve fixed by being subjected to a buffered glutaraldehyde solution at physiological pressure. The different manufacturers use different concentrations of glutaraldehyde and buffers (sometimes unstated for proprietary reasons). The concentration of glutaraldehyde used for fixation and storage may be different from that used for sterilization. The resulting bioprosthesis is similar in general form to the normal human aortic valve. At the time of writing, xenograft bioprostheses are produced commercially by three manufacturers. These are the Hancock valve (Hancock Laboratories Inc.), the Carpentier–Edwards valve (Edwards Laboratories Inc.) and the Angell–Shiley valve (Shiley Laboratories Inc.). In each there is no claimed difference between the individual manufacturer's aortic/pulmonic and mitral/tricuspid valve except for the sewing rim in the case of the first two makers who use different forms of suture rims for inflow and outflow valves. In the Angell–Shiley valve a universal sewing rim is used.

Unfortunately, there is a significant anatomical difference between the porcine and the human aortic valve, in the relation of the valve cusps to the septal myocardium. Because of this difference the right coronary leaflet of the porcine valve contains part of the septal shelf, which is a relatively inflexible tissue. The septal shelf is formed by the remnants of the septal myocardium, which in the pig bulges into the ventricular outflow tract. The presence of this septal shelf, which varies in size from valve to valve, reduces the active orifice

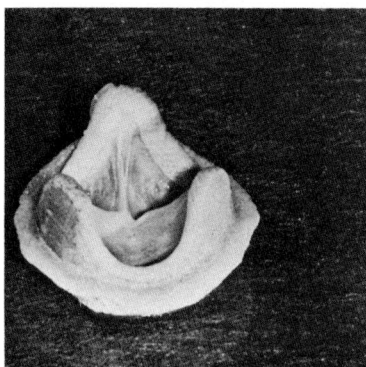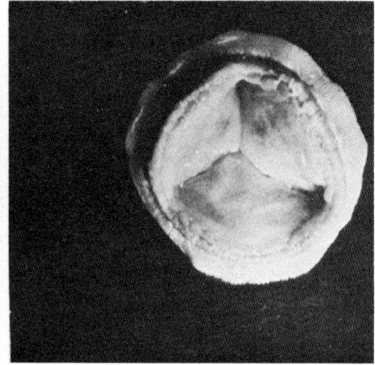

Figure 2.2 A Carpentier–Edwards stent mounted porcine bioprosthesis with aortic type sewing rim. Implantation diameter 21 mm

area of the bioprosthesis and introduces an element of variability of performance. The different manufacturers each attempt to minimize the effects of the septal shelf. In the standard Hancock valve (model 242 and 342) the protrusion of the septal shelf is slightly reduced by careful selection. In the case of the Carpentier–Edwards and Angell–Shiley valves minimization of the septal shelf is attempted by mounting the graft onto a stent with a non-circular orifice but not necessarily with hydraulic advantage. The stent of the Carpentier–Edwards valve is made of 'Elgiloy', a corrosion-resistant cobalt and nickel alloy which is claimed to have good resistance to fatigue failure. Attaching the porcine valve in such a way as to minimize the septal shelf produces an orifice which is markedly out of round (*Figure 2.2*). By contrast, in the case of the Angell–Shiley valve the sewing rim is more nearly circular, but the septal shelf is largely eliminated by attaching the right coronary leaflet to a cloth-covered protrusion moulded into the Delrin (polyacetal) flexible stent.

This has the disadvantage that, although the septal shelf is eliminated, the mounting diameter of the valve is not reduced. More important is that the non-thrombogenic material of the septal shelf has been replaced with a cloth-covered

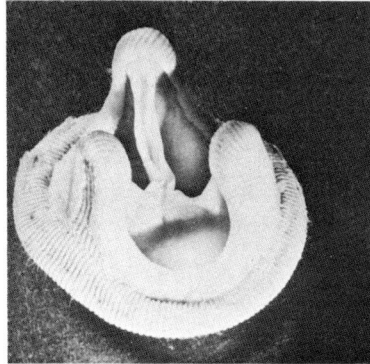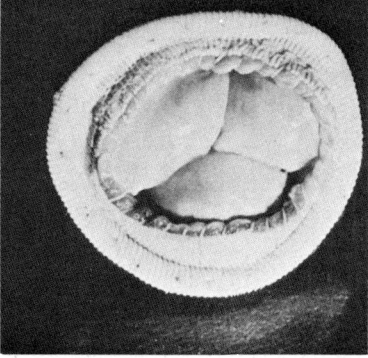

Figure 2.3 The Angell–Shiley stent mounted porcine bioprosthesis with universal sewing rim. Implantation diameter 31 mm

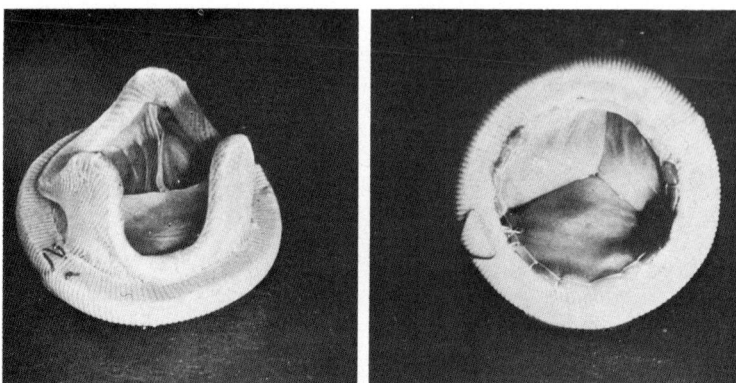

Figure 2.4 A Hancock 342 stent mounted porcine bioprosthesis with mitral type sewing rim. Implantation diameter 25 mm

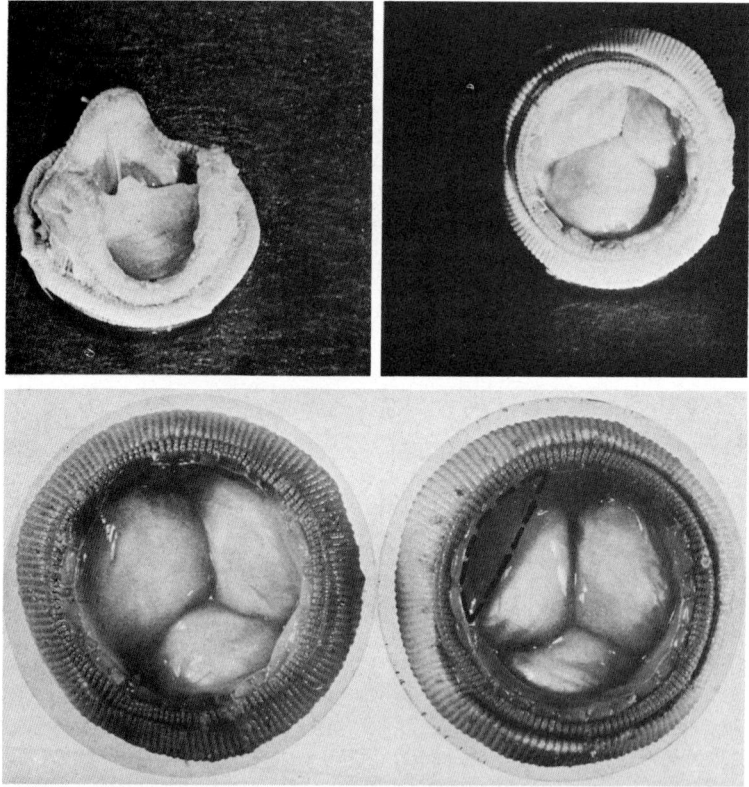

Figure 2.5 A Hancock 250 (modified orifice) stent mounted porcine bioprosthesis with aortic type sewing rim. Implantation diameter 23 mm. Top: left outflow and right inflow aspect of the valve. Bottom: a Hancock 250 modified orifice valve (left) and a Hancock 242 series valve (right). The area of the septal shelf lies approximately within the dotted line. (Lower photograph from Wright, J. T. M. 'A pulsatile flow study comparing the Hancock porcine xenograft aortic valve prosthesis models 242 and 250', *Medical Instrumentation*, **11**, 115 (1977)

plastic protrusion into the valve orifice, and this protrusion could provide a site for thrombus formation. An example of the Angell–Shiley valve is shown in *Figure 2.3*.

An alternative method of improving the active orifice area of a bioprosthesis has been made by Hancock Laboratories Inc. by the introduction of a modified orifice series of valves. In these modified valves the septal shelf has been eliminated by exercising the right coronary leaflet and replacing it with a carefully sized non-coronary leaflet from another valve. The new cusp is attached in such a way as to ensure the structural integrity of the composite bioprosthesis. The Hancock model 242/342 valve is shown in *Figure 2.4*, and the modified orifice valve in *Figure 2.5*.

Non-valvular tissue valves

The third group of tissue valves comprises those constructed from bovine pericardium, or human dura mater. These valves exhibit the non-thrombogenic properties of preserved valve tissue. However, they deviate from the geometrical form of the natural valve, and perhaps more important, from the correctly

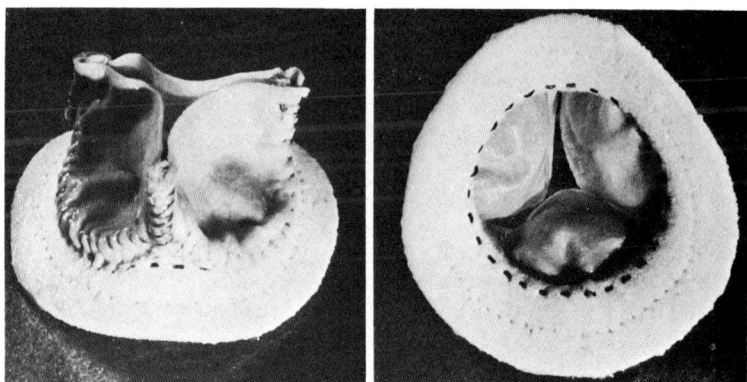

Figure 2.6 A stent mounted dura mater allograft valve for mitral replacement. Implantation diameter 31 mm (The valve was manufactured at the National Heart Hospital, London)

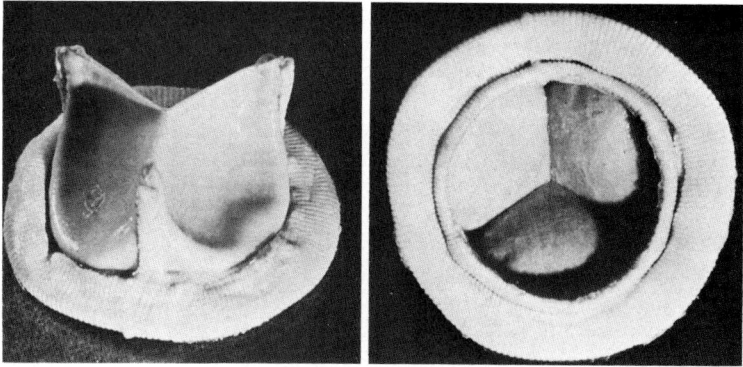

Figure 2.7 An Ionescu–Shiley stent mounted pericardial xenograft with universal sewing rim. Implantation diameter 31 mm

organized anisotropic mechanical properties of valve tissue. However, these tissue deviations may be inconsequential. The dura mater allograft valve* (*Figure 2.6*) is preserved in 98 per cent glycerol and is mounted onto a Dacron-covered metal stent. The Ionescu–Shiley pericardial xenograft (*Figure 2.7*) is mounted on a Dacron-covered titanium stent. The bovine pericardium is stabilized with buffered, purified glutaraldehyde and stored in buffered formaldehyde.

Hydrodynamic requirements of heart valve replacements

The hydrodynamic performance must be considered in selecting a substitute for heart valve replacement, but other factors, such as durability and thromboembolic incidence (which are outside the limited scope of this chapter) must also be taken into account.

Replacement of a diseased heart valve with an artificial one is usually undertaken because of a clinically significant stenosis or incompetence. One important characteristic of any substitute heart valve is, therefore, the relationship between the pressure gradient which occurs across the valve, and the rate of flow of blood through it. Ideally, the pressure gradient produced by an implanted valve would not cause clinically significant stenosis. Unfortunately, this criterion is not always achieved in aortic valve replacement, and seldom in mitral valve replacement. In the mitral region post-operative stenosis will limit the exercise potential of the patient, and a valve substitute with a low pressure gradient would, other factors being equal, give the best quality of life. A similar argument applies to patients receiving aortic valve replacement, except that gradient characteristics of the valve substitute may be more critical. For example, a patient with long-standing pure aortic insufficiency will have an enlarged heart, but the myocardial wall might be of near normal thickness. Raising the systolic ventricular pressure by implanting a valve with a significant gradient might lead to myocardial distress. This is because for the heart to contract at an increased intraventricular pressure, acting in a cavity of large cross-sectional area, the tension in the myocardial wall would have to increase. In patients with moderate or severe aortic stenosis maximum unloading of the left ventricle is required and this can only be achieved by using a valve with a minimal gradient. Thus in these two groups of patients with aortic valve disease the gradient characteristics of the implanted valve substitutes could affect life expectancy.

A second important characteristic of a valve substitute is its incompetence or insufficiency level (i.e. the total volume of blood refluxed through the valve during the closure phase and whilst shut). This level of incompetence is important because it reduces the net forward cardiac output. As a consequence the stroke volume or the pumping rate of the heart may be increased so as to compensate for this flow loss, and the extra volume pumped will cause an increase in valve gradient due to the higher flow rate through the valve. Both the extra volume pumped, and the higher resulting gradient will increase the cardiac workload.

The third characteristic of interest, which is particular to tissue valves, concerns the flexibility of the leaflets. Three factors are of significance. Firstly, at moderate cardiac output each leaflet should fully open so as to achieve the

---

* The particular dura mater allograft valve used in the study was made at the National Heart Hospital, London

maximum orifice area and hence minimum gradient. Secondly, at minimum cardiac output none of the leaflets should remain in the closed position, otherwise thrombosis might occur on the immobile leaflet. Finally, even at maximum cardiac output high speed flutter of the leaflets should not occur as this could lead to premature flexion, fatigue and failure.

It is desirable that the cardiac surgeon should be aware of the hydrodynamic characteristics of the various tissue valves which are either available commercially, or are in limited clinical use, for this information may influence the choice of valve replacement.

PULSE DUPLICATOR EVALUATION

Approximately 40 tissue valves of various types and manufacture have been tested in a pulse duplicator and the results are presented and discussed below. The valves investigated were: various porcine bioprostheses, mounted allografts and tissue valves constructed from non-valvular tissue. The porcine bioprostheses group was composed of Angell-Shiley valves (sizes 23-33 mm), Carpentier-Edwards valves (sizes 19 and 21 mm), Hancock 242 and 342 valves (sizes 19-33 mm), and Hancock 250 valves (sizes 19-25 mm). Two mounted aortic allograft valves were also studied*. One was preserved in an antibiotic solution and the other fixed in glutaraldehyde. The valves constructed from non-valvular tissue were the Ionescu-Shiley pericardial xenografts (sizes 21-31 mm) and a single dura mater valve (31 mm). All these are listed in *Table 2.1* which also shows the claimed and measured implantation (annulus) diameters of the valves.

The Angell-Shiley and Carpentier-Edwards valves had non-circular sewing rims. The circumferences of the rims adjacent to the stents were measured and the results divided by 3.14 in order to obtain the mean implantation diameters. The Ionescu-Shiley xenografts, the dura mater valve and the antibiotic preserved aortic allograft were mounted on rigid metal stents. The remaining valves used flexible plastic stents, except for the Carpentier-Edwards valves which had flexible stents made from cobalt–nickel wire.

All the valves were tested in the mitral position of the pulse duplicator. Measurements of mean diastolic pressure gradient were made at various mean diastolic flow rates over the range of 100–400 ml/s depending upon the size of the valve. The incompetence levels of the valves were also measured, at a constant rate of 100 cycles/min. Leaflet flexion was visually assessed at various pulsatile flow rates to determine the minimum flow rates that would cause the stiffest leaflet (a) just to function, and (b) to function fully. Photographs were taken of some valves at an imposed flow rate of 300 ml/s to illustrate the fully open leaflet configuration.

As a basis for comparison results of flow studies made on various mechanical mitral valve prostheses[12] with mounting diameters in the range of 29–31 mm have also been included. In addition, series of Hancock 242, Hancock 250 and Björk-Shiley tilting disc valves (size range 19–25 mm) were tested as aortic valve replacements[13], and these data enable comparisons to be made between valves tested in the mitral and in the aortic region.

Finally, certain of the tissue valves were also subjected to steady flow tests

*The two allografts were produced at Killingbeck Hospital, Leeds

TABLE 2.1
Claimed and measured implantation diameters of the tissue valves

Valve make, type and serial number	Claimed implantation diameter (mm)	Measured mean implantation diameter when used as a mitral valve (mm)	Measured mean implantation diameter when used as an aortic valve or for a subannular placement as a mitral valve (mm)
Angell–Shiley			
33ASUD5	33 ± 0.5	32.4	32.5
31ASUD4	31 ± 0.5	30.6	30.6
29ASUD14	29 ± 0.5	29.8	29.0
27ASUD22	27 ± 0.5	27.7	27.0
25ASUD20	25 ± 0.5	25.3	25.8
23ASUD4	23 ± 0.5	23.5	22.9
Carpentier–Edwards			
2625–P1601	19	—	19.3
2625–N1329	21	—	21.0
Hancock			
342AV–M7616	33	32.1	—
342AV–M8675	31	30.7	—
242A–A4980	31	31.0	—
342AV–M4528	29	28.4	—
242A–A9406	29	—	—
242A–A4922	29	28.5	—
342AV–LM4043	27	27.0	—
342AV–M7807	25	24.2	—
242A–A4668	23	—	23.0
242A–A9678	23	—	23.4
242A–A11968	21	—	21.3
242A–A10083	19	—	19.0
250A–A40913	25	—	25.0
250A–A30599	25	—	25.0
250A–A29990	23	—	23.0
250A–A39729	21	—	21.0
250A–A21153	21	—	21.0
250A–A33050	19	—	19.0
250A–A41801	19	—	19.0
Ionescu–Shiley			
31ISUD4	31	32.3	31.0
31ISU201	31	32.3	31.0
29ISUD16	29	29.8	29.0
29ISU210	29	30.4	29.0
27ISUD5	27	27.7	27.5
25ISUD3	25	25.8	24.7
23ISUD5	23	24.1	22.8
23ISU212	23	24.4	23.0
21ISU259	21	22.5	21.0
Aortic allograft			
Glutaraldehyde fixed YRTB/271	32	31.7	—
Antibiotic sterilized	26	27.9	—
Dura mater	—	31.0	—

so that a direct comparison between steady and pulsatile test methods could be made for the different valves. Flow visualization studies were made for a Hancock 342–31 valve in the mitral, and a Hancock 242–25 in the aortic position of the pulse duplicator.

Method

Tissue valves of various sizes were sutured to metal plates. The sewing rims and cloth-covered stents were then rendered impervious by sealing with self-curing silicon rubber adhesive, which had the advantage of adhering to wet cloth and would cure whilst immersed in an aqueous solution. This sealing process was important to prevent leakage occurring across the valve both for gradient and incompetence measurements. The valves thus mounted and treated were then inserted in turn into the mitral or aortic position of the pulse duplicator, which contained a flexible atrial, a ventricular, and an aortic section. The ventricular cavity was circular in cross section, of 52.5 mm diameter and contained a piston shaped like the ventricular apex. The piston was made to reciprocate sinusoidally in the cylinder a distance of 28 mm by means of a Scotch-yoke mechanism driven from a variable speed electric motor. The stroke volume of the rig was 60.4 ml. The atrial chamber was flexible and approximately spherical in shape, and the model aorta a curved tube of 28 mm bore. During mitral valve tests the outflow tract of the model left ventricle contained a pressurizing valve which caused the left ventricular pressure to rise to approximately 100 mmHg during ventricular systole. The pumping cycle period was measured by an electronic timer/counter, and the pumping speed varied to give diastolic filling or systolic ejection times over the range 516–153 ms producing mean forward flow rates over a range 100–400 ml/s.

The mean pressure gradient across the valves (the average pressure drop during the forward flow period) was measured by the method described by Wright and Brown[14]. During mitral valve tests the pressure tapping points were

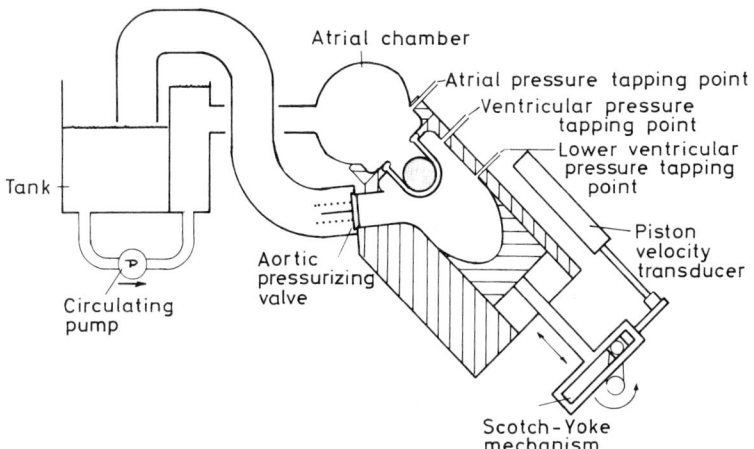

Figure 2.8 Diagrammatic layout of pulse duplicator circuit used for testing mitral valve substitutes

located in the walls of the atrial chamber and the ventricular cavity 10 mm either side of the valve under test (*Figure 2.8*). However, during aortic valve tests the pressure tapping points were located at the apex of the arch of the model aorta and in the ventricular cavity (*Figure 2.9*). These wall tapping points, with which the kinetic effects of the liquid were eliminated, approximate to those used in the clinical investigation of patients by cardiac catheterization. The test liquid used in these studies was physiological saline at 37°C. Full details of the pulse duplicator are given in Appendix 2.1.

In order to compare the effects of imposed pulsatile and steady flow on the gradients of selected tissue valves it was felt prudent to minimize the geometrical variations in the test apparatus. Therefore, the same ventricular chamber was

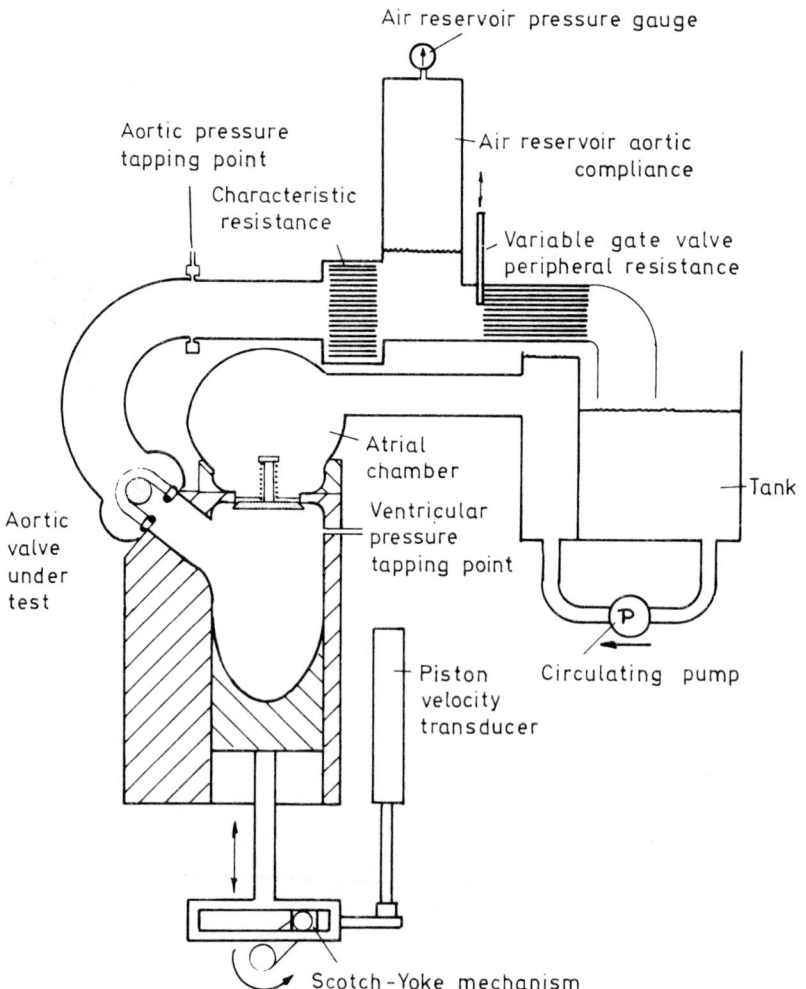

Figure 2.9 Diagrammatic layout of pulse duplicator circuit used for testing aortic valve substitutes. (Modified from Wright, J. T. M. 'A pulsatile flow study comparing the Hancock porcine xenograft aortic valve prostheses models 242 and 250', *Medical Instrumentation*, **11**, 115 (1977))

used, but the variable position piston was replaced by a fixed piston, the outflow from the ventricle being taken through a pipe fixed in its centre. The atrial chamber was replaced by a straight pipe of 57 mm bore with a flow straightener at its inlet (the characteristic resistance component of the model aortic imped-ance with its 2175 small bore tubes formed a convenient straightening section). The same differential pressure transducer as used in the pulsatile tests was employed, but with a more sensitive diaphragm fitted. The voltage output of the pressure amplifier was measured with a digital voltmeter. A Crane positive dis-placement flow meter was used to measure the steady flow rate passed through the valve under test. The hydraulic circuit diagram of the steady flow tester is shown in *Figure 2.10.*

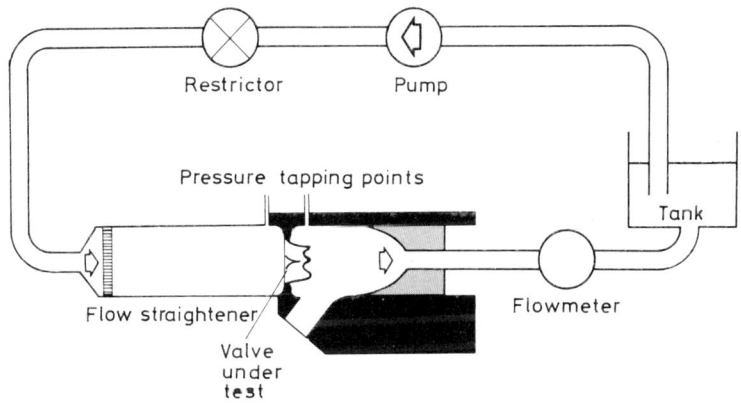

Figure 2.10 Diagrammatic layout of circuit used for steady flow testing of mitral valve replacements

The flow patterns produced in the ventricular cavity by a Hancock 342-31 mitral valve and in the aortic model by a Hancock 242-25 aortic valve were visualized by suspending a small number of white polystyrene beads (198–420 μm diameter) in a water–glycerol test liquid and shining a thin sheet of high intensity light through the central axis of the respective chamber. The resulting flow patterns were recorded by a 35 mm single lens reflex camera. The camera shutter was electrically released by a cam driven micro-switch activated off the test rig drive shaft, and the cam adjusted so that photographs were taken at chosen portions of the simulated cardiac cycle. Full details of the techniques used, together with results taken on a number of aortic and mitral valve prostheses have been previously described[15].

Results

The results of the pressure gradient measurements carried out on the 39 tissue valves are shown in *Figures 2.11* to *2.16.* In these graphs the measured mean diastolic pressure gradients have been plotted against the imposed mean diastolic flow rates. The results of the leaflet flexibility tests and incompetence measure-

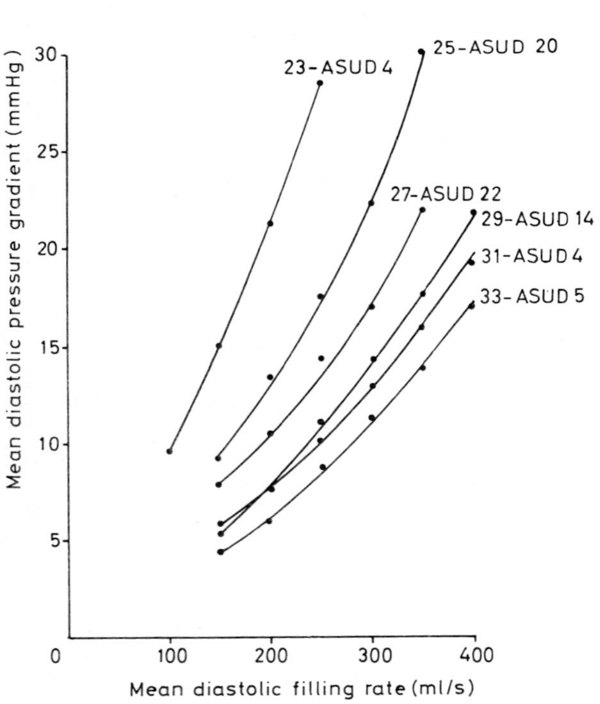

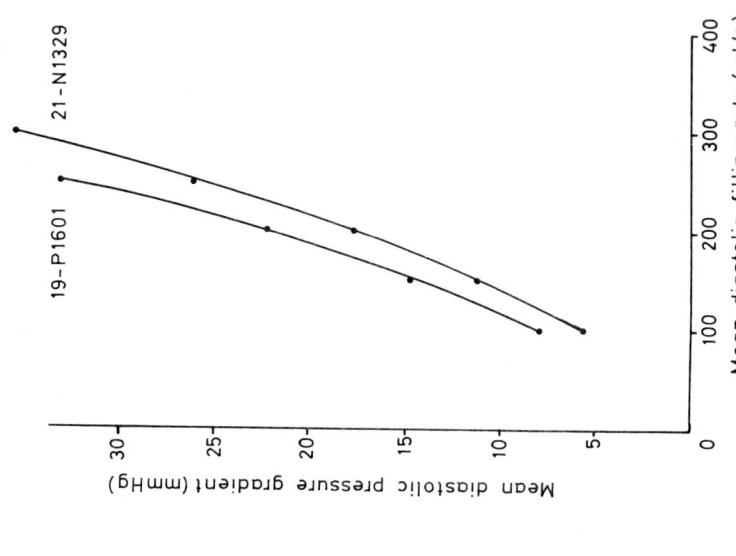

Figure 2.11 Graphic presentation of variation of mean diastolic pressure gradient with mean diastolic filling rate for the Angell-Shiley range of porcine bioprostheses (sizes 23 to 31 mm implantation diameter). Measurements were made with pulsatile flow using physiological saline at 37°C

Figure 2.12 Graphic presentation of variation of mean diastolic pressure gradient with mean diastolic filling rate for the Carpentier-Edwards 19 and 21 mm porcine bioprostheses. The measurements were made with pulsatile flow using physiological saline at 37°C

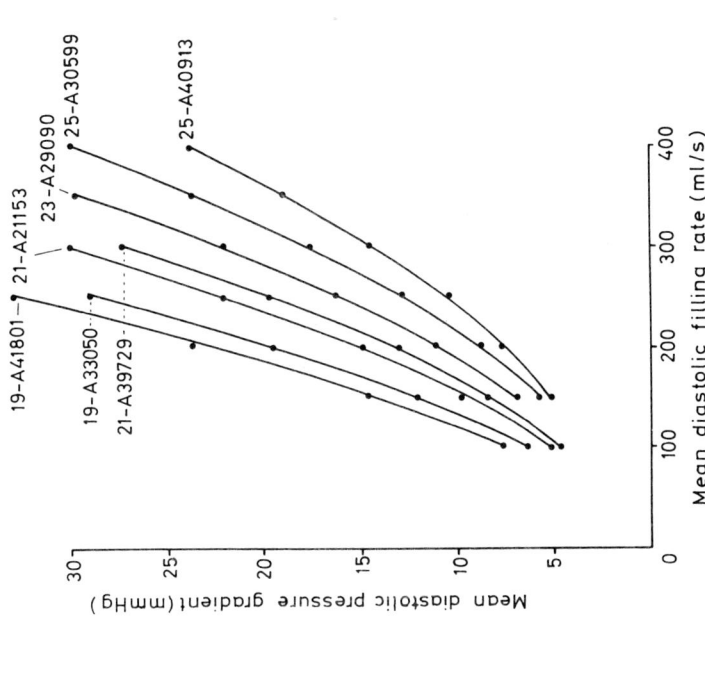

Figure 2.13 Graphic presentation of variation of mean diastolic pressure gradient with mean diastolic filling rate for the Hancock 242, 342 range of porcine bioprostheses (sizes 19 to 33 mm implantation diameter). The measurements were made with pulsatile flow using physiological saline at 37°C

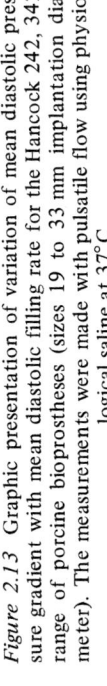
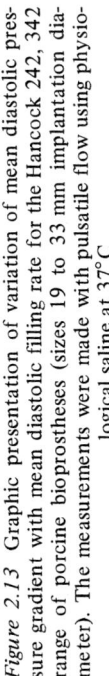

Figure 2.14 Graphic presentation of variation of mean diastolic pressure gradient with mean diastolic filling rate for Hancock 250 (modified orifice) range of porcine bioprostheses (sizes 19 to 25 mm implantation diameter). The measurements were made with pulsatile flow using physiological saline at 37°C

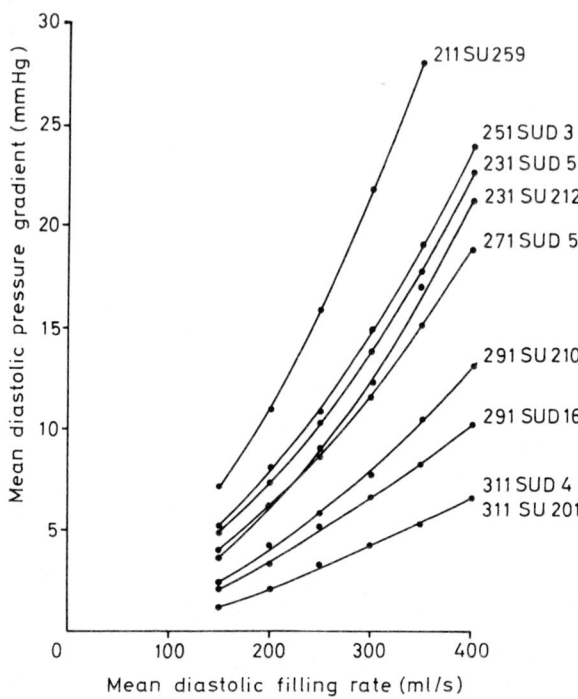

Figure 2.15 Graphic presentation of variation of mean diastolic pressure gradient with mean diastolic filling rate for the Ionescu–Shiley range of pericardial xenografts (sizes 21 to 31 mm implantation diameter). The measurements were made with pulsatile flow using physiological saline at 37 °C

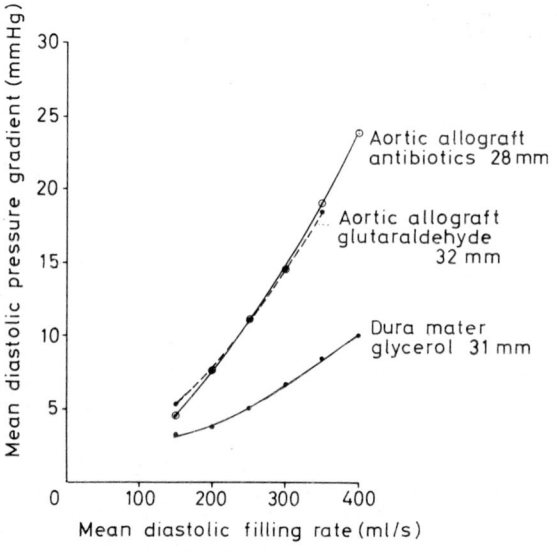

Figure 2.16 Graphic presentation of variation of mean diastolic pressure gradient with mean diastolic filling rate for the two aortic allograft valves and for the dura mater valve. The measurements were made with pulsatile flow using physiological saline at 37 °C

TABLE 2.2
Leaflet flexibility and incompetence levels of the tissue valves

| Valve make, type and serial number | Minimum peak pulsatile flow (ml/s) for 3rd leaflet to: | | Incompetence | |
	just move	fully move	Per cent of stroke volume (60 ml)	Volume reflux on closure (ml)
Angell–Shiley				
33ASUD5	101	247	5.4	3.3
31ASUD4	97	233	5.6	3.4
29ASUD14	178	210	3.4	2.0
27ASUD22	156	271	2.8	1.7
25ASUD20	156	229	3.9	2.4
23ASUD4	103	257	0.4	0.3
Mean	132 ± 35	241 ± 22		
Carpentier–Edwards				
21–2625–N1329	73	119	1.8	1.1
19–2625–P1601	35	119	3.8	2.7
Hancock				
33–342AV–M7616	77	238	2.3	1.4
31–342AV–M8675	110	165	2.9	1.8
31–242A–A4980	37	202	2.9	1.8
29–342AV–M4528	33	183	1.8	1.1
29–242A–A9406	51	196	1.9	1.2
29–242A–A4922	60	192	1.3	0.8
27–342AV–LM4043	59	192	2.1	1.3
25–342AV–M7807	73	161	2.2	1.3
23–242A–A4668	101	121	2.4	1.5
23–242A–A9678	137	156	2.1	1.3
21–242A–A11968	51	147	1.6	1.0
19–242A–A10083	31	55	1.3	0.8
Mean	68 ± 33	167 ± 46		
25–250A–A40913	60	174	2.3	1.4
25–250A–A30599	55	134	1.3	0.8
23–250A–A29990	38	156	1.7	1.0
21–250A–A39729	77	147	2.2	1.3
21–250A–A21153	42	97	1.8	1.1
19–250A–A33050	46	88	1.8	1.1
19–250A–A41801	57	159	1.2	0.7
Mean	54 ± 13	136 ± 32		
Ionescu–Shiley				
31ISUD4	24	95	10.0	6.0
31ISU201	84	293	11.0	6.7
29ISUD16	24	70	7.2	4.1
29ISU210	64	73	9.1	5.5
27ISUD5	37	92	8.6	5.2
25ISUD3	15	110	5.1	3.1
23ISUD5	44	77	6.1	3.7
23ISU212	42	110	5.1	3.1
21ISU259	48	110	3.4	2.1
Mean	40 ± 25	114 ± 69		

TABLE 2.2 (*cont.*)

Valve make, type and serial number	Minimum peak pulsatile flow (ml/s) for 3rd leaflet to:		Incompetence	
	just move	fully move	Per cent of stroke volume (60 ml)	Volume reflux on closure (ml)
Aortic allograft				
Glutaraldehyde fixed YRTB/271	33	202	3.7	2.2
Antibiotic sterilized	10	37	3.7	2.2
Dura mater	32	253*	9.9	6.0

*Second leaflet to fully open. Third leaflet did not fully open (see *Figure 2.17e*) even at a flow of 630 ml/s

ments are listed in *Table 2.2*. Firstly, the table lists the minimum peak pulsatile flow rate which would just cause the third leaflet of the valve to move, and secondly it lists that flow rate which caused the leaflet to move fully. The incompetence expressed as a percentage of the stroke volume of the ventricle (60.4 ml) is shown, as is the volume refluxed past the valve during each closure cycle. Photographs of the inlets of typical large (31 mm implantation diameter) valves and smaller (23 or 21 mm) valves are shown in *Figures 2.17 (a to f)* and *2.18 (a to e)* respectively. These photographs show valve leaflets fully open.

A comparison between the pressure gradients produced by the 31 mm implantation diameter tissue valves and typical large mechanical mitral valve prostheses are shown in *Figure 2.19*. The mechanical valves tested were the Lillehei–Kaster 25 and 22 pivoting disc valves (the numbers refer to the orifice not the implantation diameters of these valves), a Björk–Shiley 29 tilting disc valve, and a Starr–Edwards 6400-32M composite track cage ball valve. As the measurements made on the mechanical prostheses were using water–glycerol (density 1.10 g/ml and viscosity 3.0 cP) the results have been corrected to the density of blood by multiplying each pressure gradient measurement point by the factor C_{db}, where

$$C_{db} = \frac{1.05}{\text{density of the test liquid}}$$

and 1.05 is the density of blood at 37°C (for further explanation see Appendix 2.1). The volumes refluxed by the mechanical prostheses are shown in *Figure 2.20*.

The results of the tests carried out on the Hancock 242 and 250 bioprostheses and the Björk–Shiley 19-25 mm tilting disc valves in the aortic position of the pulse duplicator are shown in *Figures 2.21* and *2.22*. These pressure gradient results have also been normalized to the density of blood. The volume reflux of the Hancock aortic bioprosthesis and the Björk valve in the aortic position were measured at particular pulse rates and the results are shown in the form of a nomogram in *Figure 2.23*.

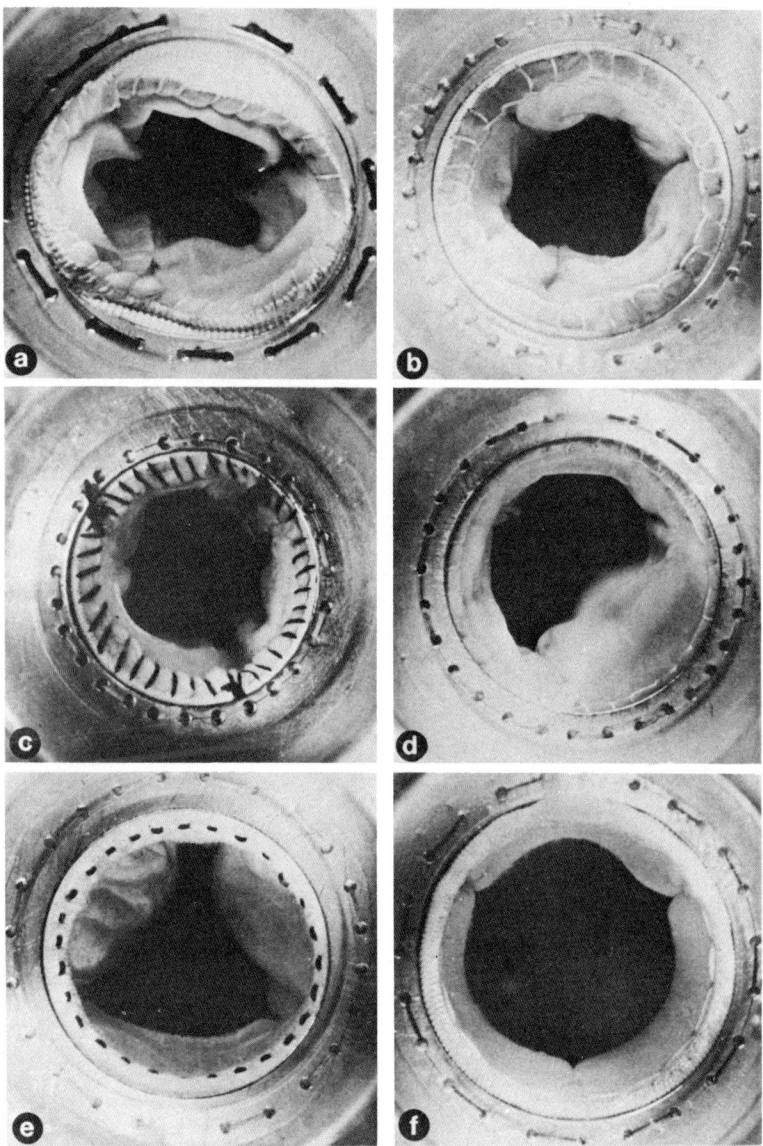

Figure 2.17 Inlet views of tissue valves at peak diastole (instantaneous flow rate, 300 ml/s: (*a*) Angell–Shiley porcine bioprosthesis 33 mm; (*b*) Aortic allograft valve (glutaraldehyde) 32 mm; (*c*) Aortic allograft valve (antibiotics) 28 mm; (*d*) Hancock 342, porcine bioprosthesis 31 mm; (*e*) dura mater valve 31 mm diameter; and (*f*) Ionescu–Shiley pericardial xenograft 31 mm

The results of some of the steady flow tests have been plotted, together with those taken under pulsatile flow conditions, and are shown in *Figure 2.24*. Finally, a single flow visualization photograph of the flow patterns produced by the Hancock 342–31 bioprosthesis in the mitral position of the pulse duplicator

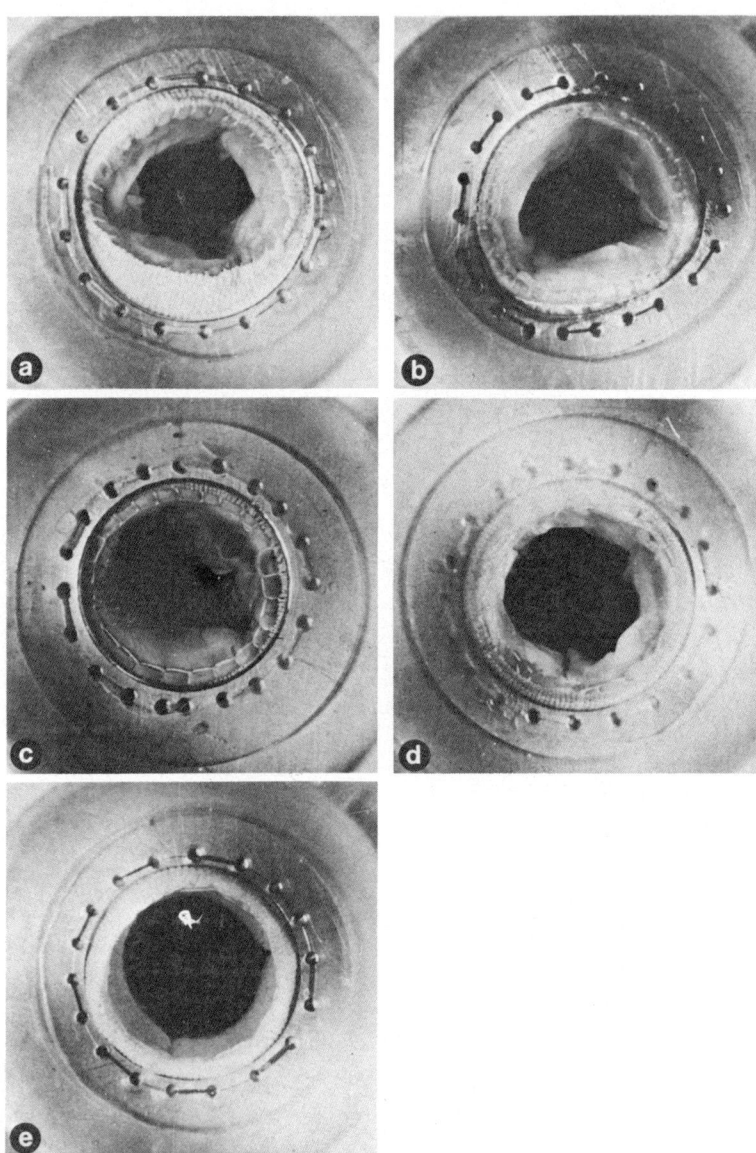

Figure 2.18 Inlet views of tissue valves at peak diastole (instantaneous flow rate 300 ml/s: (*a*) Angell–Shiley porcine bioprosthesis 23 mm; (*b*) Carpentier–Edwards porcine bioprosthesis 21 mm; (*c*) Hancock 242 porcine bioprosthesis 21 mm; (*d*) Hancock 250 porcine bioprosthesis 21 mm; and (*e*) Ionescu–Shiley pericardial xenograft 21 mm

is shown in *Figure 2.25*, and a series of flow visualization photographs taken of a Hancock 242-25 in the aortic position of the test rig in *Figure 2.26*. The numbers on the photographs show the time in milliseconds (ms) after the start of the simulated systolic period. The systolic duration in these tests was 300 ms, and a mean systolic ejection flow rate of 200 ml/s. The camera shutter speed

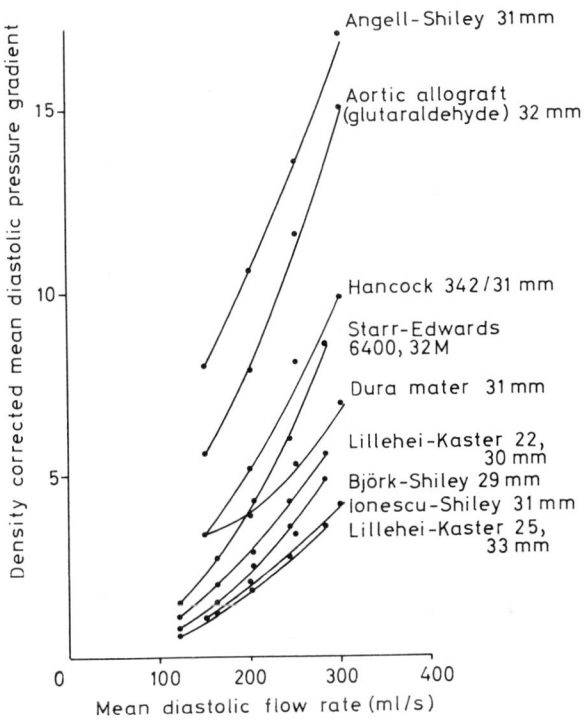

Figure 2.19 Graphic presentation of variation of density corrected mean diastolic filling rate for mechanical and tissue valve replacements. The measurements were made with pulsatile flow using water–glycerol mixture at 37°C with mechanical valves and physiological saline with tissue valves

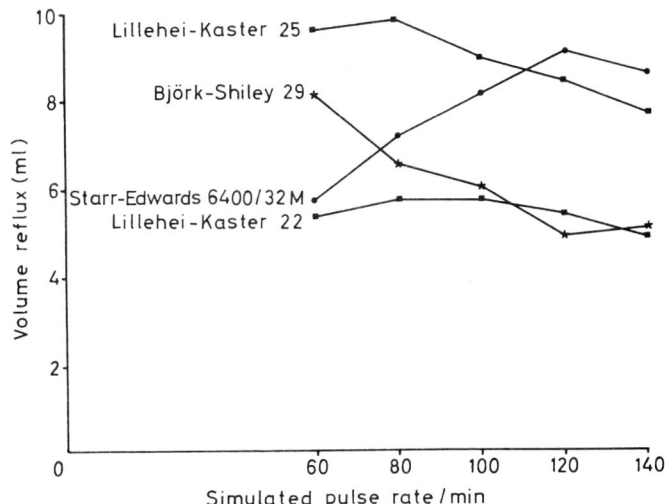

Figure 2.20 Graphic presentation of variation of volume refluxed with simulated pulse rate for various mechanical mitral valve prostheses (water–glycerol mixture 3.0 cP at 37°C). (Modified from Wright, J. T. M.[12], by courtesy of *Thorax*)

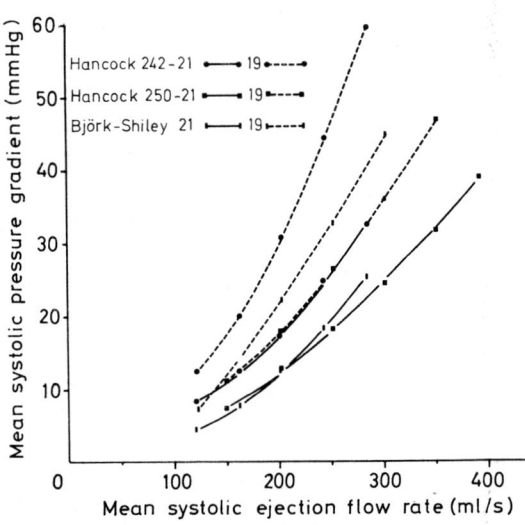

Figure 2.21 Pressure gradient characteristics of the Hancock 242 and 250 porcine bioprostheses and the Björk–Shiley tilting disc aortic valve prostheses (19 and 21 mm implantation diameter). (Modified from Wright, J. T. M.[13], by courtesy of *American Society for
Artificial Internal Organs*)

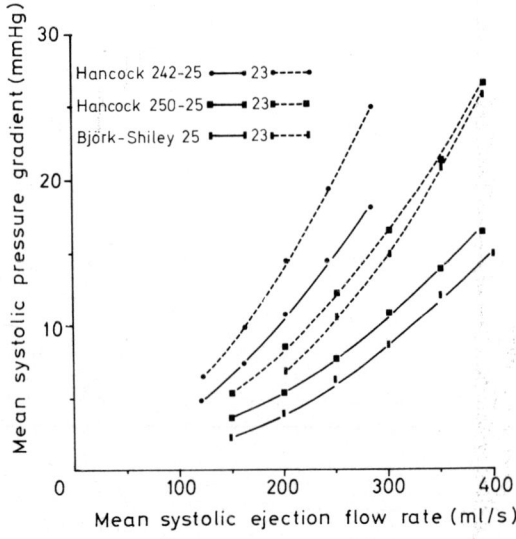

Figure 2.22 Pressure gradient characteristics of the Hancock 242 and 250 porcine bioprostheses and the Björk–Shiley tilting disc aortic valve prostheses (23 and 25 mm implantation diameter). (Modified from Wright, J. T. M.[13], by courtesy of *American Society for
Artificial Internal Organs*)

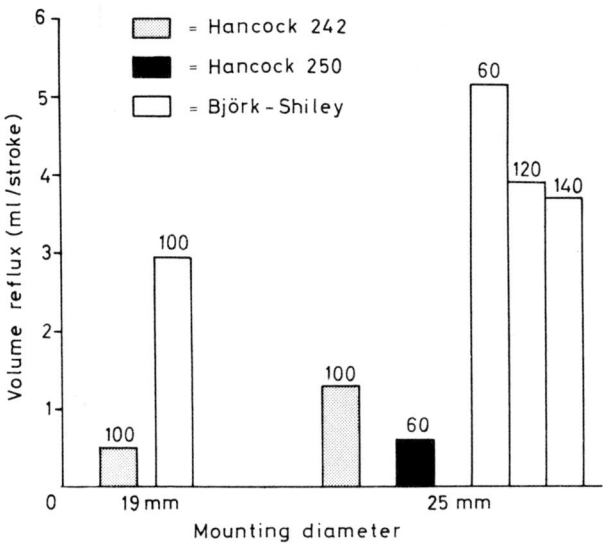

Figure 2.23 Nomogram showing the volume refluxed by various Hancock and Björk–Shiley aortic valve prostheses (the numbers above the blocks show the simulated pulse rate). (Reproduced from Wright, J. T. M.[13], by courtesy of *American Society for Artificial Internal Organs*)

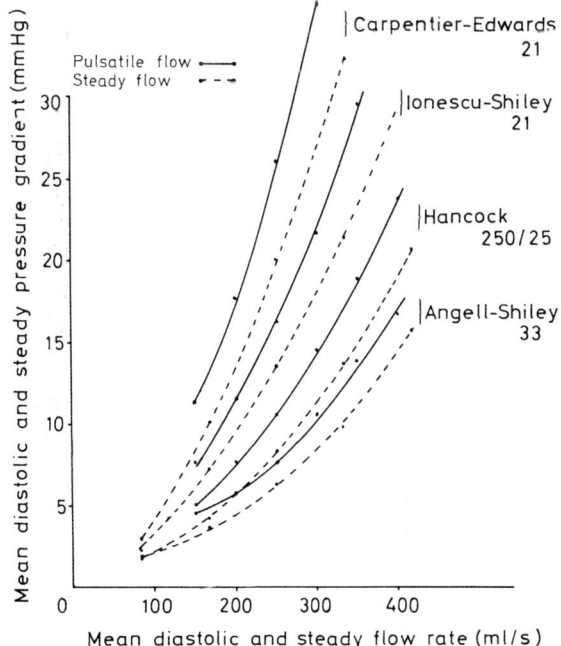

Figure 2.24 A comparison between the pressure gradients produced across four tissue valves by steady and pulsatile flow of the same mean value (physiological saline at 37 °C)

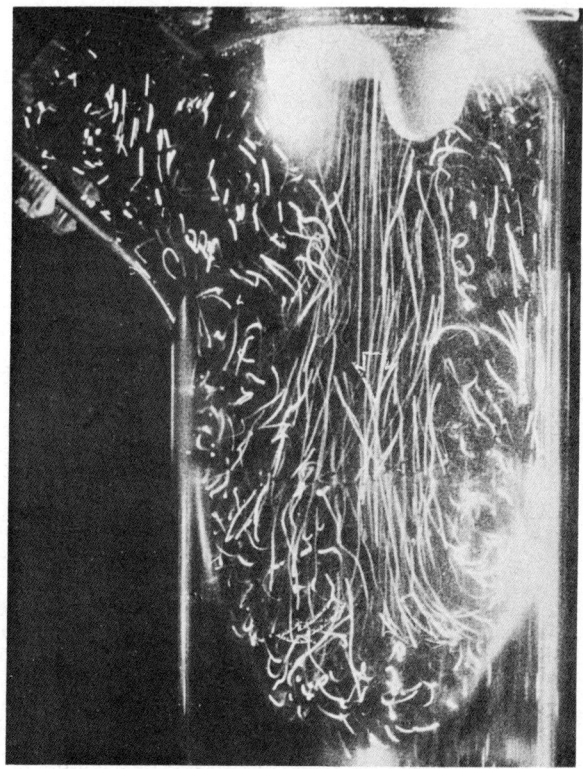

Figure 2.25 Flow patterns produced in the model ventricle by a Hancock 342 porcine bioprosthesis (31 mm implantation diameter). Arrows show direction of flow. (Reproduced from Wright, J. T. M. and Temple, L. J.[15], by courtesy of *Engineering in Medicine*)

was 1/60 s for the aortic valve study. However, *Figure 2.26* was taken with an exposure time of 1/30 s, 250 ms after the start of diastole (i.e. two thirds of the way through the diastolic period).

Discussions

The pressure gradient results of the Angell–Shiley valves are shown in *Figure 2.11*. On this and the following five graphs the variation of the mean diastolic pressure gradient has been plotted against mean pulsatile diastolic filling rate (the test liquid was physiological saline at 37 °C and the pulsatile characteristics sinusoidal). The Angell–Shiley 31 valve produced a gradient of approximately 20 mmHg at a mean diastolic filling rate of 400 ml/s. The larger 33 and smaller 29 valves had characteristics not much different, but at low flow rates the 29 valve produced a slightly lower gradient than did the 31 valve.

The pressure gradient characteristics of the Carpentier–Edwards porcine bioprostheses are shown in *Figure 2.12*. It can be seen that the 19 mm valve caused a gradient of approximately 22 mmHg at a flow rate of 200 ml/s, and the 21 mm

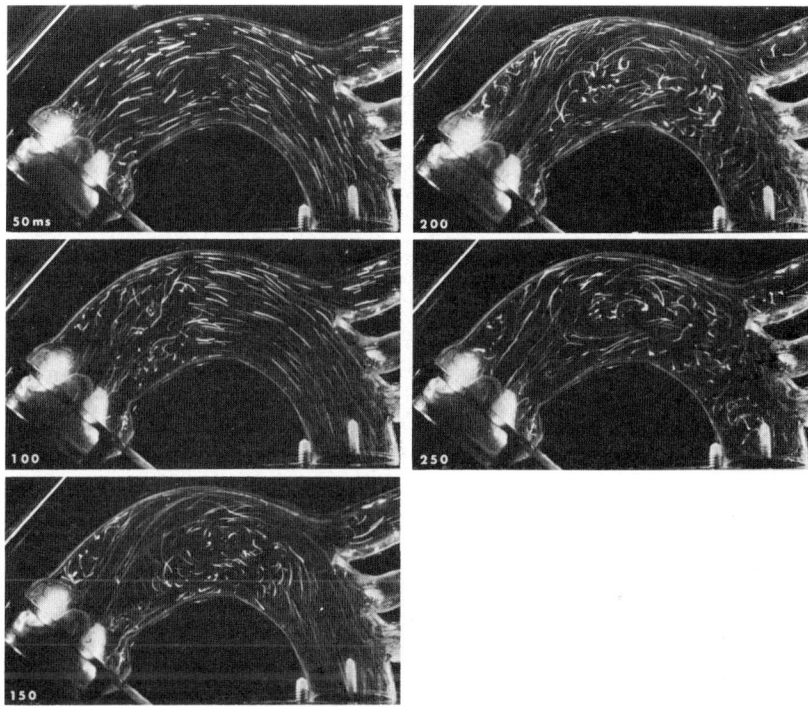

Figure 2.26 Flow patterns produced in the model aorta by a Hancock 242–25 porcine bioprosthesis (25 mm implantation diameter). The numbers in the lower left-hand corner show the time (in ms) after the beginning of systole. (Reproduced from Wright, J. T. M. and Temple, L. J.[15], by courtesy of *Engineering in Medicine*)

valve a gradient of approximately 19 mmHg at the same flow rate. *Figure 2.13* shows the gradients associated with the Hancock 242 and 342 series of porcine bioprostheses. A higher gradient was found with the 33 mm valve than with either of the 31 mm valves tested. This was not much lower than that caused by the best of the 29 mm valves. The 19 mm valve had a pressure gradient of about 32 mmHg at a flow rate of 200 ml/s, which was significantly higher than that of the Carpentier-Edwards 19 mm valve. However, the gradients produced by the larger valves (with the exception of the 33 mm size) were lower than those found with the Angell-Shiley porcine bioprostheses. The pressure gradient characteristics of the Hancock 250 modified orifice valves, sizes 19-25 mm, are shown in *Figure 2.14*. The Hancock 250 valve series produced pressure gradients similar to those observed in valves one size larger from the Hancock 242-342 range. For example valve size 23 of the 250 series had a gradient approximately the same as that of valve size 25 of the Hancock 342 series (i.e. 30 mmHg at a flow rate of 350 ml/s). One of the two 19 mm valves tested produced lower pressure gradients than did the Carpentier-Edwards 19 valve, the other caused somewhat higher gradients. The pressure gradient characteristics of the Ionescu-Shiley range of pericardial xenografts are shown in *Figure 2.15*. It can be seen that these gradients were significantly lower than those of the Hancock 242/342 or the Angell-Shiley porcine bioprostheses. The Ionescu-Shiley 21 mm valve was also markedly superior in this respect to the Carpentier-Edwards 21 valve. However, it can be seen that the Ionescu-Shiley 25 invoked a higher gradient than did either of the two Ionescu-Shiley 23 mm valves tested. One of the 23 mm valves had only a slightly higher gradient than did the 27 mm valve. The Ionescu-Shiley 21 mm valve produced a slightly lower gradient than did the Hancock 250-23 valve, but the Hancock 250-25 and the Ionescu-Shiley 25 valves had almost identical characteristics. The Ionescu-Shiley 31 valves caused a gradient of only about 7 mmHg at a flow rate of 400 ml/s, compared with a gradient of 20 mmHg found for the Angell-Shiley 31 valve and 15 mmHg for the Hancock 31 valve.

Finally, the pressure gradient characteristics of the dura mater valve, and the two stent mounted allograft valves are presented in *Figure 2.16*. The antibiotic preserved allograft valve had an implantation diameter of 27.9 mm, compared with that of 32 mm for the glutaraldehyde fixed valve, but their gradient characteristics were almost identical. Thus the antibiotic preserved valve with its more flexible leaflets had favourable gradient characteristics for its size compared with the larger glutaraldehyde fixed 32 mm allograft. The more flexible leaflets of the antibiotic preserved valve probably accounted for its reduced gradient at low flow rates compared to those valves fixed in glutaraldehyde. The dura mater valve had an associated gradient of 10 mmHg at a flow rate of 400 ml/s. Thus its pressure loss was below those found with the 31 mm porcine valves, but higher than those of the largest Ionescu-Shiley pericardial xenografts.

The insufficiency levels of the various valves listed in the last two columns of *Table 2.2* show the incompetence expressed as a percentage of the stroke volume, and the volume reflux for each closure cycle. The Angell-Shiley valves had incompetence levels of 0.4-5.6 per cent, the Carpentier-Edwards valves 1.8 and 3.8 per cent and the Hancock 242/342 valves had levels in the range of 1.3-2.9 per cent. The modified orifice range of Hancock valves (model 250) produced 1.2-2.3 per cent incompetence.

Significantly higher incompetence levels were found with the Ionescu-Shiley pericardial xenografts (3.4-11 per cent), and the dura mater valve (9.9 per cent). The two stent mounted allograft valves each produced 3.7 per cent incompetence. Clinically significant incompetence was defined by Kennedy *et al.*[8] as being more than 20 per cent of the ventricular stroke volume. All of these tissue valves were thus satisfactory in meeting this criterion.

In an attempt to clarify and compare the results obtained with the tissue valves tested in the mitral position of the pulse duplicator the mitral valve areas have been calculated according to the formula of Gorlin and Gorlin[5], and the figures are listed in *Table 2.3*.

$$MVA = \frac{Q}{44.5\sqrt{MDG}}$$

Where Q = mean diastolic ejection flow (ml/s)
   MVA = mitral valve area (cm^2)
   MDG = mean diastolic gradient

The Q quantity which has been used in the Gorlin and Gorlin formula is the reflux corrected, net (not gross) forward flow through the valve, so that the deleterious effects of valve incompetence would be taken into account. More-

TABLE 2.3
Order of hydraulic merit and calculated orifice areas of the tissue valves

Order of merit	Valve make	Model and serial number	Valve size (mm)	Calculated orifice area (cm²)
1	Ionescu–Shiley	ISUD4	31	3.0
2	Ionescu–Shiley	ISU201	31	2.98
3	Ionescu–Shiley	ISUD16	29	2.38
4	Dura mater	Glycerol	31	2.24
5	Ionescu–Shiley	ISU210	29	2.21
6	Hancock	342/M8675	31	2.10
7	Hancock	242/A4980	31	1.93
8	Hancock	342/M7616	33	1.91
9	Hancock	242/A4922	29	1.87
10	Hancock	242/A9406	29	1.86
11	Angell–Shiley	ASUD5	33	1.80
12=	Ionescu–Shiley	ISUD5	27	1.77
12=	Ionescu–Shiley	ISU212	23	1.77
14	Angell–Shiley	ASUD4	31	1.73
15	Hancock	250/A40913	25	1.69
16=	Aortic allograft	Glutaraldehyde	32	1.67
16=	Hancock	342/M4528	29	1.67
16=	Angell–Shiley	ASUD14	29	1.67
16=	Aortic allograft	Antibiotics	28	1.67
20	Ionescu–Shiley	ISUD5	23	1.63
21	Ionescu–Shiley	ISUD3	25	1.61
22	Hancock	342/LM4034	27	1.59
23	Angell–Shiley	ASUD22	27	1.56
24	Hancock	250/A30599	25	1.55
25	Ionescu–Shiley	ISU259	21	1.36
26	Hancock	250/A29990	23	1.35
27	Angell–Shiley	ASUD20	25	1.34
28	Hancock	342/M7807	25	1.33
29	Hancock	242/A9678	23	1.27
30	Hancock	250/A39729	21	1.23
31	Hancock	250/A21153	21	1.18
32	Hancock	242/A4668	23	1.13
33	Carpentier–Edwards	2625/N1329	21	1.05
34	Angell–Shiley	ASUD4	23	1.03
35	Hancock	250/A33050	19	1.00
36	Hancock	242/A11968	21	0.99
37	Hancock	250/A41801	19	0.93
38	Carpentier–Edwards	2625/P1601	19	0.91
39	Hancock	242/A10083	19	0.75

over, as the tests were all carried out using physiological saline as the test liquid (density 1.005 g/ml), and as in the clinical situation blood would be the liquid passing through the valve (density 1.05 g/ml) the quantity *MDG* in the formula was multiplied by the factor 1.05/1.005 to take account of this difference.

In *Table 2.3* the valves are listed in order of merit, a large calculated orifice area being considered advantageous. The orifice areas were calculated from the pressure gradient caused by the imposition of a mean diastolic flow rate of 300 ml/s through the valve (a lower flow rate was used in those small and stenotic valves in which the flow rate would have produced very high gradients).

The Gorlin and Gorlin formula was thus modified as follows:

$$MVA = \frac{300 \; \dfrac{(100 - \text{per cent incompetence})}{100}}{44.5 \; \sqrt{(MDG)} \; \sqrt{(1.05/1.005)}}$$

It may be seen from the table that the first five valves in the list were all constructed from non-valvular tissue, i.e. the Ionescu-Shiley 31 and 29 mm pericardial xenografts and the dura mater 31 mm valve. Had the third leaflet on the dura mater valve opened correctly it would have undoubtedly been placed higher in the order of hydraulic merit. The next five valves in the table were the larger Hancock 342-242 bioprostheses. Note that the two 31 mm valves opened to give larger valve areas than did the single 33 valve. This demonstrated the overlapping hydraulic characteristics of tissue valves in general. In other words because of the variability of the porcine aortic valve and in the methods of mounting, the clinical use of a larger valve does not necessarily mean that a lower gradient will result. However, an average large valve would be expected to produce a lower gradient than the average small valve. Possible exceptions to this were the Ionescu-Shiley 23 valves (two were tested) and the Ionescu-Shiley 25 valve, of which only one was tested. Both the 23 valves produced larger orifice areas than did the 25 valve (one had an orifice area equal to that of an Ionescu-Shiley 27 valve). In the smaller valve sizes (21 and 23 mm) the stent prongs were angled outwards some $9°$, but with the 25 mm and larger valves the stent prongs were perpendicular to the orifice. This design difference could account for the comparatively better results obtained with the smaller valve sizes.

Returning to an examination of the order of hydraulic merit table it can be seen that ranked 11th was the Angell-Shiley 33 valve with an area of 1.8 cm^2 closely followed by the Ionescu-Shiley 27 and 23 valves with areas of 1.77 cm^2. Following the Angell-Shiley 31 valve came a group of valves all with areas of 1.67 cm^2.

A nomogram depicting the calculated orifice areas of the tissue valves, which have been grouped according to their implantation diameter, is shown in *Figure 2.27*. The valves with implantation diameters of 31–33 mm were ranked as follows: two 31 mm Ionescu-Shiley pericardial xenografts, the dura mater valve, three Hancock valves, two Angell-Shiley and the glutaraldehyde fixed allograft valve. The same rank order (Ionescu-Shiley, Hancock, Angell-Shiley) was also established for the 29 and 27 mm valve sizes. However, in the 25 mm valves the rank order was Hancock 250 (modified orifice), Ionescu-Shiley, Hancock 250, Angell-Shiley, and Hancock 242 valve. In the 23 and 21 mm valve groups the Ionescu-Shiley valves led, followed by the Hancock 250 valves. Next among the 23 mm valves were the two Hancock 242 and the Angell-Shiley valve, but in the 21 mm valve group the Carpentier-Edwards was ranked fourth, followed by the Hancock 242 valve. The Hancock 250 valves led the 19 mm group, next were the Carpentier-Edwards and the Hancock 242 bioprosthesis. Thus in each group (except for the 25 and 19 mm sizes)* the Ionescu-Shiley valves produced the lowest gradients and hence the largest calculated orifice areas. Among the larger porcine bioprostheses tested the Hancock 242-342 valves produced lower gradients and larger orifice areas than did the Angell-Shiley valves. Among the

*The 19 mm Ionescu-Shiley pericardial xenograft was not available for this study

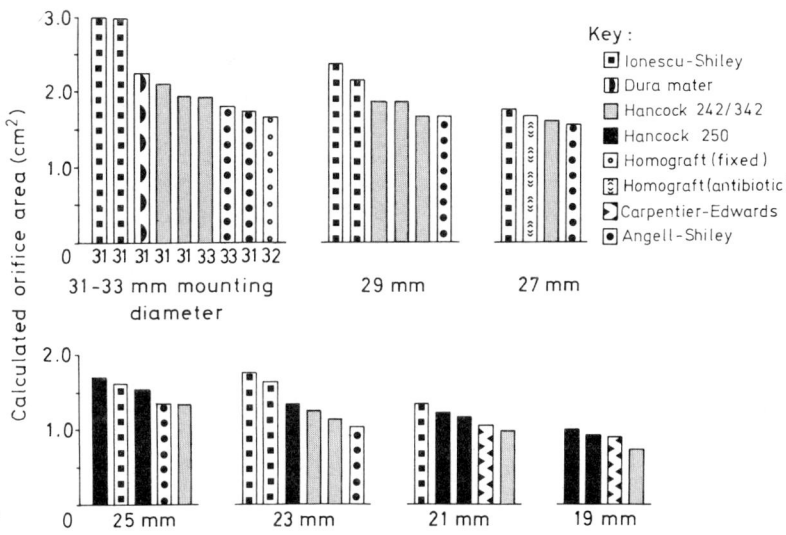

Figure 2.27 Nomogram showing calculated orifice areas (reflux and density corrected) of the tissue valves investigated. (The 19 mm Ionescu–Shiley pericardial xenograft was not available for this study)

TABLE 2.4
Variation of calculated valve areas between different valve samples

Valve make and size	Model and serial number	Calculated orifice area (cm²)	Variation of orifice area (per cent)
Ionescu–Shiley 31	ISUD4	3.0	1
	ISU201	2.98	
Hancock 31	342/M8675	2.1	8
	242/A4980	1.93	
Ionescu–Shiley 29	ISUD16	2.38	10
	ISUD210	2.15	
Hancock 29	242/A4922	1.87	0
	242/A9406	1.86	10
	342/M4528	1.67	
Hancock 25	250/A40913	1.69	8
	250/A30599	1.59	
Ionescu–Shiley 23	ISU212	1.77	8
	ISUD5	1.63	
Hancock 23	242/A9678	1.27	11
	242/A4668	1.13	
Hancock 21	250/A39729	1.23	4
	250/A21153	1.18	
Hancock 19	250/A33050	1.00	7
	250/A41801	0.93	

porcine valves below 27 mm implantation diameter the Hancock modified orifice 250 valves gave the best results. In the two smallest sizes the Carpentier-Edwards valves were ranked between the Hancock 250 and the Hancock 242-342 valves.

Unfortunately, only single samples of most of the valves were available for test. Exceptions were three sizes (31, 29 and 23 mm) of the Ionescu–Shiley and of Hancock 242-342 valves, where two samples of each size were examined (in the case of the Hancock 29 mm valve three samples were tested).

In three sizes of Hancock 250 valves (25, 21 and 19 mm) two valves of each size were also tested. The variations of the calculated orifice area between samples of the same valve size are shown in *Table 2.4*. It can be seen that the orifice areas of the three Hancock 242-342 29 mm valves varied between 0 and 10 per cent but this variation was 11 per cent between two samples of Hancock 242-23 mm valves. Variations between the Ionescu–Shiley valves were also up to 10 per cent. Measurement errors form some part of these calculated area differences, but as the repeatability of pressure measurement was typically about 5 per cent (which would produce a 2.5 per cent area change) it is clear that mostly these apparent area variations were real.

In the calculation of effective areas of the valves, using the Gorlin and Gorlin formula, two basic assumptions are made. Firstly, the formula relates the flow rate to the inverse square of the pressure gradient, and secondly a factor $(1/44.5)$ is introduced. This factor assumes that a certain coefficient of discharge is 0.88. The coefficient of discharge of an orifice is a factor which relates the flow rate through the orifice with the pressure drop across it.

The Gorlin and Gorlin formula is derived from the standard hydraulic formula for submerged small orifices

$$Q = CA \sqrt{(2gH)}$$

Where Q is the flow rate, C is the coefficient of discharge, A is the area of the orifice, g is the gravitational acceleration, and H the liquid head loss across the orifice. If the head (or pressure) loss across the orifice is measured in mmHg (redesignated *MDG*), and the area is measured in cm^2 (redesignated *MVA*) and g is 981 cm/s^2 and ρ the density of blood, then

$$Q = C \times MVA \sqrt{\left(\frac{2g \times 13.6 \times MDG}{10\rho}\right)}$$

or

$$Q = C \times MVA \times 50.41 \times \sqrt{(MDG)}$$

rearranging this we get

$$MVA = \frac{Q}{C \times 50.41 \times \sqrt{(MDG)}}$$

Hence if we assume that the coefficient of discharge is 0.88 we obtain the familiar Gorlin and Gorlin formula

$$MVA = \frac{Q}{0.88 \times 50.41 \times \sqrt{(MDG)}} = \frac{Q}{44.5 \times \sqrt{(MDG)}}$$

In practice the coefficient of discharge will vary depending on the physical shape of the orifice (valve leaflets) and to some extent on the flow rate through the valve. Thus although the formula may be useful to the cardiologist because it relates the flow rate through the valve with the pressure drop or gradient, it does not necessarily represent an accurate measurement of the area of the valve orifice. To illustrate this, the areas formed by the fully open valve leaflets (photographed in this condition with a peak flow rate of 300 ml/s—see *Figures 2.17* and *2.18*) were planimetrically measured. The calculated and measured results are listed in *Table 2.5*, together with the ratio of measured to calculated areas, and the coefficient of discharge for various valves (calculated from measurements of pressure gradient, flow rate and orifice areas). It will be noted that the calculated orifice areas of the valves do not correspond with those given in *Table 2.3*. This is because the values listed in *Table 2.5* are neither compensated for incompetence loss, nor adjusted for the density of blood. The photographic,

TABLE 2.5
Calculated and measured orifice areas of tissue valves and their coefficients of discharge

Valve make and size	Model and serial number	Calculated orifice area (cm²)	Measured orifice area (cm²)	Area ratio (measured/ calculated)	Coefficient of discharge
Ionescu–Shiley 31	ISU201	3.43	3.43	1.01	0.86
Dura mater 31	Glycerol	2.55	1.97	0.78	1.10
Hancock 242 31	A4980	2.03	1.65	0.82	1.06
Angell–Shiley 31	ASUD4	1.85	1.56	0.83	1.02
Aortic allograft	28 Antibiotics	1.77	1.63	0.87	0.93
Aortic allograft	32 Glutaraldehyde	1.77	1.38	0.78	1.10
Ionescu–Shiley 21	ISU259	1.45	1.50	1.04	0.83
Hancock 250 21	250–A39729	1.29	1.04	0.81	1.06
Carpentier– Edwards 21	2625–N1329	1.10	0.83	0.76	1.13
Angell–Shiley 23	ASUD4	1.05	0.87	0.83	1.04

planimetric and scaling techniques necessary to measure valve areas introduce errors, but these should be of an absolute rather than a relative nature. Examination of *Table 2.5* shows that the coefficients of discharge of the Ionescu–Shiley valves were slightly below that assumed by Gorlin and Gorlin, but that the discharge coefficients of the porcine bioprostheses all lay between 1.02 and 1.13. A high value for this coefficient is advantageous because a lower gradient across the valve will occur for a particular orifice area. Thus the very low gradients associated with the Ionescu–Shiley valves were due to their large orifice areas as the low discharge coefficients have adverse effects on the gradients.

The results of the leaflet flexibility test (*Table 2.2*) show that, as a group, the Angell–Shiley valves had the least mobile leaflets. The Hancock 242–342 range of valves on average fully opened at 30 per cent less flow than the Angell–Shiley xenograft, the third leaflet just moving at 48 per cent less flow. It is not clear if this was due to the differences in the methods of tissue fixation, or whether it was due to the mounting techniques. It was interesting to find that the Hancock 250 modified orifice series of valves (each constructed from two different porcine aortic valves mounted together into a stent thus eliminating the septal shelf) fully opened at a flow rate 18 per cent less than the average 242 valve. The third leaflet moved at 20 per cent less flow than the 242 valves. Thus replacement of the right coronary leaflet associated with the septal shelf produced a significantly more flexible leaflet configuration.

The valves with the greatest leaflet flexibility were the Ionescu–Shiley pericardial xenografts. These valves required, on average, only a third of the flow rate needed by the Angell–Shiley valves for the stiffest leaflet to begin to move, and less than half the flow rate for the leaflets to open fully. With only two samples of the Carpentier-Edwards valves, and only one each of the dura mater and the antibiotic and glutaraldehyde preserved allografts, comparisons cannot be made with the other valves. However, there were two exceptions to this. Firstly, the antibiotic preserved allograft had 'unfixed' leaflets that were considerably more pliable than other tissue valves tested. Secondly, the dura mater valve possessed one leaflet that would not open appreciably, probably due to a constructional defect, and a second leaflet that did not always fully open at a flow rate of 300 ml/s (*Figure 2.17e*). It can be seen from *Table 2.2* that in one of the Ionescu–Shiley 31 mm valves (serial number ISU 201) the third leaflet would only fully open at a flow rate of about 290 ml/s, nearly three times higher than for the other valves of the Ionescu–Shiley series.

These results are visual observations, and therefore subjective, and are presented as a guide to valve behaviour rather than as hard scientific data. However, they do show trends, the most significant of which is that the flexibility of valve leaflets varied with the method of manufacture, and probably fixation. However, leaflet flexibility did not seem to be related to valve size. It was expected that the smaller valves would open fully at lower flow rates than larger valves, but in none of the four main groups did this occur.

The Angell–Shiley 33 valve shown in *Figure 2.17a* had a non-circular inlet and the fully open leaflets formed a clover leaf-shaped orifice of small area when compared with the implantation area of the valve. The open leaflets were markedly corrugated as though the porcine valve was too large for the stent into which it was mounted. By contrast the two allograft valves shown in *Figures 2.17b* and *2.17c* (the glutaraldehyde and the antibiotic preserved allografts respectively) both produced almost circular leaflet openings, of smooth appearance. The effect of the septal shelf on the orifice opening of the Hancock 31 valve is clearly demonstrated in *Figure 2.17d*. Two of the valve leaflets had fully opened, but the right coronary leaflet attached to the septal shelf formed a cord across the valve inlet. The septal shelf leaflet had a blurred outline, indicating that it had moved significantly during the duration of the camera shutter opening (1/125 s). This movement or 'flutter' was confined to the leaflet associated with the septal shelf and is thought to be due to vortices shed off the protruding shelf (similar to the vortices shed off a flagpole which cause the flag to flutter in the breeze). This flutter could possibly be caused by an artifact particular to the pulse duplicator configuration. However, the effect has also been observed with some other Hancock valves and seems to be independent of angular orientation of the valve in the atrial chamber, or of the viscosity of the test liquid. For example, when testing another Hancock valve, changing the test liquid from normal saline to water–glycerol mixture of 3 cP viscosity did not noticeably reduce leaflet flutter. Some leaflet flutter was also observed when testing the Carpentier-Edwards 21 bioprosthesis. As far as is known, leaflet flutter has not been reported clinically, but if present in a patient it might be detected by a continuous wave ultrasonic doppler technique.

The dura mater valve is shown in *Figure 2.17e*. It can be seen that the lower leaflet has opened fully, but that the other two leaflets have only partially opened. The flow rate at which the photograph was taken (300 ml/s) usually just caused the right-hand leaflet to open fully. It would then appear similar to that for the lower leaflet. However, the leaflet on the left-hand side of the photograph would not open further than shown, even at a flow rate of 600 ml/s. This was probably due to inaccuracies in the valve construction. A nearly circular opening was obtained with the Ionescu-Shiley 31 valve shown in *Figure 2.17f*. It may be seen that the leaflets had opened almost symmetrically and to a greater extent than those of the other valves examined. Close examination of the photograph showed that the leaflets had rather 'furry' surfaces. These discontinuities in the surfaces could be seen to move or vibrate under the influence of flow through the valve. These 'streamers' could form emboli, but clinical experience has shown that they are sealed onto the leaflets by the deposit of fibrin within a few hours of implantation, and that the incidence of thromboembolism with the pericardial xenografts has been negligible[7].

Figure 2.18a shows the appearance of the Angell-Shiley 23 valve in its fully open position. In comparison to the Angell-Shiley 33 valve the opening is more circular, and the leaflets form a more streamlined shape. The Carpentier-Edwards 21 valve is shown in *Figure 2.18b*. It may be seen that the valve inlet is non-circular, and that the general shape of the leaflet opening follows the form of the valve inlet. Some fluttering of the valve leaflets (not easily visible in the photograph) occurred. Inlet views of the Hancock 242-21 and modified orifice 250-21 valves are shown in *Figures 2.18c* and *2.18d* respectively. In the 242 series valve the cord formed by the septal shelf is easily seen. The left-hand upper leaflet had opened fully, but the right-hand leaflet had not fully moved. By contrast in the modified orifice valve all three leaflets had fully opened to produce a nearly circular opening. Finally, the Ionescu-Shiley 21 valve shown in *Figure 2.18e* also produced a near circular form of valve opening but had the same 'furry' appearance of the Ionescu-Shiley 31 valve.

The gradients produced by the 31 and 32 mm tissue valves are compared to the gradients caused by the four mechanical valve prostheses in *Figure 2.19*. The lowest gradients were associated with the Lillehei-Kaster 25 valve (implantation diameter 33 mm) and the Ionescu-Shiley 31 mm. The dura mater valve, whose characteristic curve markedly deviated from those of other tissue valves (probably due to the leaflet opening problem) invoked a gradient higher than that of the tilting or pivoting disc valves, but lower than the Starr-Edwards ball valve prosthesis (except at flow rates of less than 200 ml/s when the ball valve produced less pressure loss). The Hancock 31, Angell-Shiley 31 and the glutaraldehyde fixed allograft all caused substantially higher gradients than the tilting and pivoting disc valves.

The incompetence characteristics of the mechanical valve prostheses are shown in *Figure 2.20*. All the prostheses produced less than 20 per cent (12 ml) reflux, and so would not be expected to cause a clinically significant level of insufficiency. The design of the Björk-Shiley valve was such that when the valve was closed a small annular leakage path existed between the disc and the orifice, thus some of the backflow did occur during the systolic part of the simulated cardiac cycle. It was for this reason that the Björk–Shiley prosthesis displayed comparatively higher levels of reflux at low pulse rates when the systolic period, and hence the leakage time, was longer. However, with sine wave flow function testing, the diastolic and systolic periods are always equal whilst in the heart, at low pulse rates the systolic period is significantly less than the diastolic period. Hence in the case of the Björk–Shiley valve the reflux level found at low pulse rates in these *in vitro* tests would be expected to be somewhat higher than that experienced *in vivo*. At high pulse rates, when systole and diastole are comparable in length, no significant error would be expected. Another difference between physiological and sine wave testing concerned the rate of change of flow during early systole. It is usually the backflow through the valve during early systole which causes closure to occur. *In vivo* an abrupt contraction of the left ventricle might produce a greater rate of change of flow than occurred with a sine wave function. However, it will be seen from *Figure 2.20* that many valves had a level or slightly falling reflux characteristic as pulse rate and hence rate of change of flow was increased. It is not therefore felt that this difference would significantly affect levels of reflux measured in these tests.

A more important variable affecting reflux values was the orientation of the ventricular chamber and the valve itself. The mechanical valve prostheses had occluders whose densities were different from that of the test liquid, particularly the tilting disc valves. Gravitational forces therefore could aid or oppose valve closure, depending on the mounted position of the valve. The angulation of the natural mitral ring varies depending on the physical characteristics of the patient and on posture. By way of compromise these tests were therefore carried out with the mitral valve angled at $45°$ to the vertical plane with the dummy aortic valve in the same horizontal plane. The tilting disc valves were then orientated as recommended by their leading proponents, i.e. the Lillehei–Kaster valve opened towards the interventricular septum, and the Björk–Shiley valve opened away from it.

Insufficiency in a prosthesis will also cause an increase in gradient, for the heart will have to increase the volume pumped to compensate for the volume refluxed past the prostheses. To allow for this effect, *Table 2.6* shows the mean

TABLE 2.6
A comparison between the density corrected pressure gradient produced by mechanical and tissue mitral valve replacements at a reflux corrected mean diastolic filling rate of 200 ml/s

Valve type	Size	Gradient (mmHg)
Lillehei–Kaster 25	33	2.4
Ionescu–Shiley	31	2.6
Björk–Shiley	29	2.9
Lillehei–Kaster 22	30	3.4
Dura mater	31	4.8
Hancock 342	31	5.4
Starr–Edwards 6400	32	5.4
Angell–Shiley	33	7.3
Aortic allograft glutaraldehyde	32	8.6
Angell–Shiley	31	8.6

diastolic pressure gradient (corrected to the density of blood) produced by the various mechanical and the 31-33 mm tissue valves at a reflux corrected diastolic filling rate of about 200 ml/s (probably equivalent to a cardiac output of about 6.5-7 ℓ/min. The Lillehei-Kaster 33 mm diameter pivoting disc valve and the Ionescu-Shiley 31 mm pericardial xenograft caused the least gradients (2.4 and 2.6 mmHg) under these circumstances. The Björk-Shiley 29 tilting disc valve and the Lillehei-Kaster 22 (30 mm implantation diameter) valve had gradients of 2.9 and 3.4 mmHg. Next came the dura mater valve (4.8 mmHg), and the Hancock 31 and Starr-Edwards 6400-32M valves, both with gradients of 5.4 mmHg. The final groups consisted of the Angell-Shiley 33 valve (7.3 mmHg) and the glutaraldehyde fixed allograft and Angell-Shiley 31 porcine valve each with gradients of 8.6 mmHg. The lowest gradient levels (around 2.5 mmHg) would probably just cause a clinically significant mitral stenosis, while the valves which produced gradients of 5-9 mmHg would be expected to cause mild to moderate degrees of mitral stenosis in patients.

The results of comparative tests between the two types of Hancock valves and the Björk-Shiley tilting disc prostheses carried out in the aortic position of the pulse duplicator showed that the pressure gradient characteristics of the Hancock 250 modified orifice valves were significantly better than those of the Hancock 242-342 series (*Figures 2.21* and *2.22*). In the smaller sizes, i.e. 19 and 21 mm, the Hancock 250 valves produced lower pressure gradients than the equivalent Björk-Shiley tilting disc prostheses. However, in the 23 and 25 mm sizes the situation was reversed. The reflux measurements (*Figure 2.23*) demonstrated that the valves tested did not produce clinically significant insufficiency, but the levels produced by the tilting disc valves were significantly higher than those of the bioprostheses. The effect of reflux in an implanted valve would probably be to cause the heart to increase its stroke volume or rate in compensation. Thus the extra volume pumped would add to the pressure gradient across the prosthesis. To allow for this effect *Figure 2.28* was drawn up. This depicts the valve replacements in order of hydraulic merit by showing the mean compensated systolic ejection flow that would cause a mean systolic pressure gradient of 20 mmHg (that being the level of pressure gradient which would just produce clinically significant aortic stenosis). This figure also shows that both the Björk-Shiley 25 and the Hancock 250-25 would allow mean systolic ejection flow rates of more than 400 ml/s (a flow rate that should allow a patient a reasonable exercise tolerance). The Björk-Shiley 23 and Hancock 250-23 would probably allow a typical patient a rather limited exercise tolerance, but at least should not produce a clinically significant aortic stenosis at rest. The smaller prostheses in these two series would probably produce aortic stenosis even at rest, and their use would normally be confined to children or to the adult patient with a small aortic root.

The small size Hancock 250-21 valve would allow 10 per cent more flow at a gradient of 20 mmHg than the Björk-Shiley 21 prosthesis, and the smallest Hancock 250-19 valve would allow 18 per cent more flow than would the Björk-Shiley 19 prosthesis. Throughout the Hancock valve range the 250 series would allow flow rates equivalent to the next larger valve in the 242 series. The smaller Angell-Shiley and the two Carpentier-Edwards porcine bioprostheses were not tested in the aortic position of the pulse duplicator, nor were the smaller Ionescu-Shiley pericardial xenografts.

Steady flow tests were carried out with the Angell-Shiley and the Ionescu-

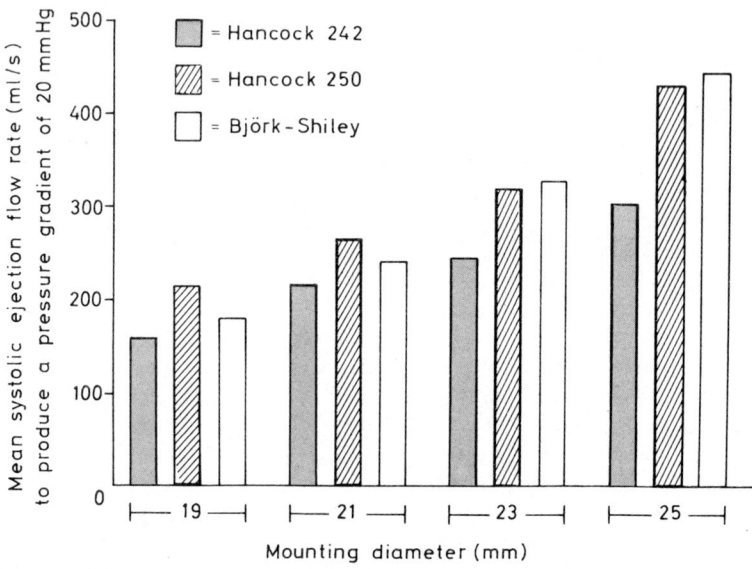

Figure 2.28 Nomogram comparing the mean systolic ejection flow rates which would just produce a clinically significant aortic stenosis by the Hancock 242 and 250 valves and the Björk-Shiley tilting disc prostheses. (Reproduced from Wright, J. T. M.[13], by courtesy of *American Society for Artificial Internal Organs*)

Shiley range of valves, and also with the two Carpentier-Edwards and a single Hancock 250-25 porcine valves. Some of the results obtained are shown in *Figure 2.24* in which the pressure gradients caused by both steady flow, and pulsatile flow of the same mean value (defined as the stroke volume divided by diastolic period) are presented. The results shown in the figure are from tests performed with the Carpentier-Edwards 21, the Ionescu-Shiley 21, the Hancock 250-25 and the Angell-Shiley 33 valves. It can be seen that in each case the gradient caused by the steady flow was less than that caused by pulsatile flow of the same value (about 15-24 per cent less).

To widen the comparison between steady and pulsatile flow tests *Table 2.7* shows the ratio of the pressure gradients caused by a steady and a mean pulsatile flow rate of 250 ml/s. The gradient values used in the calculations were taken from the experimental measured points (not from smoothed graphical lines drawn through experimental points). The average gradient difference between the two flow conditions was found to be 19 per cent for the Angell-Shiley range of valves, 30 per cent for the Carpentier-Edwards valves and 14 per cent for the Ionescu-Shiley valves. The difference associated with the Hancock 250-25 valve was 26 per cent. From these results it is clear that steady flow caused lower gradients than did pulsatile flow (a simple theoretical study indicated that 23 per cent difference should be expected—see Appendix 2.2). The gradients found with the Ionescu-Shiley pericardial xenografts, especially with the larger size valves, were so low that small experimental errors in measurement (especially caused by zero drift of the pressure transducer measuring system) would introduce large errors in the pressure drop ratios. For example measurement errors of only 0.1 mmHg on the Ionescu-Shiley 31 mm valve would vary the gradient

TABLE 2.7
Ratio of pressure gradients caused by subjecting valves to pulsatile*
and steady flow rates of 250 ml/s

Valve make and size		Model and serial number		Ratio of pulsatile/steady pressure drop at flow rates of 250 ml/s
Angell–Shiley	33	ASUD5		1.24
	31	ASUD4		1.24
	29	ASUD14		1.28
	27	ASUD22		1.29
	25	ASUD20		1.01
	23	ASUD4		1.16
			Mean	1.19 ± 0.11
Carpentier–Edwards	21	2625-N1329		1.30
	19	2625-P1601		1.33
Ionescu–Shiley	31	ISUD4		1.10
	31	ISU201		1.19
	29	ISUD16		1.10
	29	ISU210		1.07
	27	ISUD5		1.09
	25	ISUD3		1.10
	23	ISUD5		1.17
	23	ISU212		1.30
	21	ISU259		1.17
			Mean	1.14 ± 0.07
Hancock	25	250-40913		1.26
			Mean	1.19 ± 0.1

*The pulsatile flow was averaged over the diastolic filling period

ratio from 1.15 to 1.3. For this reason confidence cannot be assured in the ratios obtained with the low gradient valves. However, it did seem likely that the different ratio values found with the Hancock, Carpentier-Edwards and Angell-Shiley valves were due to the characteristics of the bioprostheses and not to the errors of the measurement system.

Flow visualization studies were only carried out with the Hancock 31 porcine valve in the mitral position of the pulse duplicator, and with a Hancock 242-25 valve in the aortic position. The results are presented to show the flow patterns associated with central orifice valves, although some differences between various types of tissue valves are to be expected. A single photograph (*Figure 2.25*) shows the flow through the Hancock 31 into the model left ventricle. The curved apex of the piston seen at the bottom of the photograph has a slightly blurred outline due to piston movement. This photograph was taken 250 ms after the onset of diastole (two-thirds of the way through diastole). It can be seen that a central jet of liquid flowed through the centre of the valve to enter the ventricular chamber until diverted by the shape of the ventricular apex. In this mechanical model the ventricular diameter was constant, but its length varied due to piston movement during the simulated cardiac cycle. In the heart the converse occurs for the ventricular length remains almost constant, but the ventricular cross-section changes during diastole and systole. For this reason one would expect the jet passing through the valve to diverge as it entered the expanding ventricle of the heart.

The flow patterns formed in the ascending aorta by the Hancock 242–25 valve are shown in *Figure 2.26*. The numbers on the five pictures show the timing of the photograph after the onset of systole (the systolic duration was 300 ms—the mean systolic flow rate being 200 ml/s). After 50 ms, fairly uniform flow velocity of about 30 cm/s existed throughout the aorta. However, 50 ms later a central jet of indeterminate velocity was passing through the valve, causing a flow disturbance to occur about 4 cm distal to the valve stent. After 150 ms a vortex had formed near to the junction of the branch representing the innominate artery. In this study 25 per cent of the flow passed through the innominate, left common carotid and left subclavian arteries. The latter two flow passages did not lie in the light beam, and so the flow was not visible in the photographs. At the commencement of these tests it was expected that the centrally opening porcine xenograft would have produced a reasonably uniform flow in the aorta. Surprisingly the flow patterns showed that a vortex was formed downstream of the bioprosthesis (*Figure 2.26*). A similar result was obtained with a Hancock 250–25 modified orifice valve, even when it was angled about $10°$ towards the inside of the curve of the aorta.

In flow visualization studies one must be aware of the shortcomings of the models, for these can markedly influence the results. The obvious limitations of the model used in this study were that the aorta was rigid, that flow was not taken from the coronary sinuses, and that the thin sheet of light was only capable of providing useful information concerning particles moving within and parallel to the light sheet. The first objection is not serious because if, for example a 10 per cent increase in the aortic systolic diameter is made, this would lead to a 20 per cent increase in cross-sectional area and hence a reduction of flow velocity of the same order. It is also unlikely that the simulation of coronary flow would have greatly changed the flow patterns during simulated ventricular systole, especially as most of the coronary flow normally occurs during diastole. Particles which travelled through the width of the sheet of light (caused by swirling components of flow) would give misleading or at least difficult to interpret tracts. However, the gravest general limitation of this method is due to the size of the particles (about 300 μm). It is clearly impossible for a bead to respond to flow fluctuations (in the form of macro or micro vortices) smaller, or even of the same size as the particles. Thus the turbulent components of the flow, which are generally vortices of small magnitude (but in which much energy is expended) remain invisible using this technique. In spite of these objections the method can give useful qualitative data provided that the shape and size of the chamber or vessel under investigation is reasonably reproduced. For example in carrying out flow visualization studies distal to heart valve prostheses straight tubes are not appropriate chambers to use.

Conclusions

The measurements performed in this study showed that in the majority of valves the implantation diameters were close or identical to those claimed by the manufacturers. The lowest pressure gradients were generally associated with the valves fabricated from non-valvular tissue. In each size (except 25 mm) the Ionescu–Shiley pericardial xenograft produced less gradient than the other bioprostheses (19 mm or smaller Ionescu–Shiley valves were not available for this study). The gradient caused by the dura mater valve, although greater than that recorded with the Ionescu–Shiley pericardial xenograft of similar sizes, was significantly lower than the gradients produced by the porcine bioprostheses. These findings indicate that the use of tissue which deviates from the anisotropic mechanical properties of normal aortic valve tissue is advantageous from the hydrodynamic point of view. Whether the *in vivo* durability and longevity of these valves will continue to equal those of the porcine valves cannot as yet be assessed. From the hydrodynamic point of view the Ionescu–Shiley pericardial xenograft and the dura mater valve look promising as cardiac valve replacements. However, the dura mater valve is treated with glycerol and the absolute effectiveness of glycerol as a sterilizing agent is questionable, while its tissue preservation qualities are not clearly defined.

Among the porcine valves the Hancock 242–342 series showed hydrodynamic advantages over the Angell–Shiley range of bioprostheses. Moreover the latter valves have the potential drawback of the cloth-covered protrusion into the valve orifice (discussed in the introduction of this chapter). Only two sizes (19 and 21 mm) of Carpentier–Edwards valves were available for investigation. Both caused slightly lower gradients than did the Hancock 242–342 valves of similar size, but both produced higher gradients than the Hancock 250 modified orifice valves. The glutaraldehyde fixed allograft produced a rather high gradient in spite of the absence of a septal shelf in the valve. The antibiotic preserved allograft, caused a relatively low gradient, probably because of its more flexible leaflets.

None of the tissue valves tested displayed clinically significant insufficiency, although the Ionescu–Shiley pericardial xenografts and the dura mater valve produced several times more volume reflux than the other bioprostheses. This was probably because their forward flow resistance (hence reverse flow resistance) was low. Thus a higher reflux flow rate was required for leaflet closure.

The leaflet flexibility tests showed that the bioprostheses with the most mobile leaflets (apart from the antibiotic preserved allograft valve) were the Ionescu–Shiley pericardial xenografts. It was not clear if this was because of different tissue mechanics, tissue fixation, or the geometric construction of the valve leaflets. The Hancock 250 range of modified orifice valves proved, on average, to have more flexible leaflets than the Hancock 242–342 valve. Thus replacement of the right coronary leaflet containing the septal shelf, with a leaflet removed from another valve, not only produced a prosthesis with a lower gradient, but one with more mobile leaflets. Whether or not this may compromise the durability of the Hancock 250 series of valves because of the new fabrication technique cannot be assessed as yet. The Angell–Shiley range of porcine bioprostheses had the least flexible leaflets of the commercially produced valves. One point of interest was that in all valve groups there was no correlation between leaflet flexibility and valve size. Thus at a given flow rate it would be just as likely for the leaflets of a large valve to function as those of a smaller one.

The tissue valves have been listed in order of hydraulic merit according to their calculated orifice areas. This was done because many cardiologists categorize their patients according to valve areas calculated using the Gorlin and Gorlin formula. Although *Table 2.3* lists calculated valve areas to three significant figures, a 1 per cent accuracy should not be assumed (the probable accuracy of calculated valve areas was 3–5 per cent). Thus small differences between calculated valve areas are not significant. There was quite good correlation between the calculated and measured orifice areas of the Ionescu–Shiley valves. However, experimentally the porcine and allograft valves produced higher coefficients of discharge than was assumed by the Gorlin and Gorlin formula. As a consequence the measured valve areas were about 19 per cent greater than the calculated valve areas, a seemingly important difference when calculated valve area is chosen as the sole criterion of excellence in patients. However, this difference will not change the rank order of the valves in *Table 2.3* (or in patients) as the Gorlin and Gorlin area really gives the square root of pressure gradient at a specified flow rate.

More than one sample of some of the Hancock and Ionescu–Shiley valves were tested. The variation in calculated orifice area between different samples of valves of similar size was up to about 10 per cent (*Table 2.4*), producing a gradient variation between samples of just over 20 per cent. Tissue valves, being individually hand-made, are bound to vary, sample to sample. The two Carpentier–Edwards porcine valves were manufactured to clinical standards and supplied from commercial stocks. Four of the Ionescu–Shiley pericardial xenografts (those without the letter 'D' in the serial number) were also made to clinical standards. The remaining valves were supplied directly from the manufacturing source, as being typical examples of valves, but not necessarily to clinical standards. For example, cosmetic or sewing rim defects were present in some of the bioprostheses, but these defects should not have affected valve performance. All the valves tested were thought to be representative of their type.

A comparison between mechanical and tissue valves with implantation diameters of 21–32 mm showed that only the Ionescu–Shiley pericardial xenograft and the dura mater valve produced gradients as low as the two tilting disc valves. The better of the two Hancock 342–31 valves caused a gradient about twice as high (at high flow rates) but similar to that produced by the Starr-Edwards 6400–32M composite track ball valve. However, the gradient caused by this Hancock 31 mm valve was 37 per cent less than that produced by the Angell-Shiley 31 bioprosthesis. Valves with the lowest gradients (the Lillehei-Kaster 25 and the Ionescu–Shiley 31) would be expected to only just cause a clinically significant mitral stenosis in patients. The 32 mm glutaraldehyde fixed allograft and the Angell-Shiley 31 valve might be expected to produce gradients equivalent to those encountered in patients with moderately severe mitral valve stenosis.

In the aortic position of the pulse duplicator only the Hancock 242–342 and the Hancock 250 series of tissue valves were tested together with the Björk-Shiley range of tilting disc valves (with pyrolytic carbon discs, but without tantalum x-ray marker rings). The Björk-Shiley range of valves varied from 19 to 25 mm implantation diameter. The two smaller sizes (19 and 21 mm) of the Hancock modified orifice 250 valve produced lower gradients than the corresponding sizes of the Björk-Shiley prosthesis. However, the gradients of these small Hancock 250 and Björk-Shiley valves were such that these valves should only be considered for use in children or small adults. Whenever possible the larger 23 mm or preferably the 25 mm sizes should be the valve replacements of choice in adult patients. In larger sizes the Björk-Shiley tilting disc valves produced slightly lower gradients than the corresponding sizes of Hancock 250 valves. These two 23 mm valves probably would not produce a clinically significant aortic stenosis in the average built adult patient at rest. The two 25 mm valves (the Hancock 250 and the Björk–Shiley prosthesis) should both allow a patient a reasonable exercise tolerance.

The results obtained when testing prostheses in the aortic position were different from those obtained in the mitral area of the pulse duplicator. Tests carried out on several Hancock valves showed that the mean systolic pressure gradient produced, at a given flow rate, in the aortic area was about 20 per cent less than the mean diastolic pressure gradient, at the same flow rate, in the mitral area. This difference in gradients is thought to be due to some pressure recovery in the ascending aorta. As liquid passes through the smallest flow area of the valve, normally the primary orifice, the velocity of the liquid is increased and so is its kinetic energy. Thus its potential energy (i.e. static pressure) must fall, on the principle of conservation of energy. Some pressure recovery will occur if, when the liquid slows downstream of the valve (because the flow area has increased) some of the kinetic energy is reconverted back to potential energy and there is an increase in static pressure distal to the valve. The amount of pressure recovery will vary with the type of prosthesis. For example when tests were carried out to determine the optimum position of the downstream pressure tapping points in the model aorta, the Hancock valves showed better pressure recoveries than did Björk–Shiley tilting disc valves[13]. For this reason caution should be used when comparing results obtained from one type of valve in the mitral position with those from another type tested in the aortic position.

Finally the 18 valves which were tested with both pulsatile and steady flow showed in every case that lower pressure gradients were obtained under steady flow conditions. On average the difference was 19 per cent, but the mean value for different valve types varied from about 10 per cent for the Ionescu–Shiley pericardial xenograft to 30 per cent for the Carpentier-Edwards valve. The average value for the whole group (19 per cent) correlated closely with the theoretical prediction of 18–23 per cent (Appendix 2.2). Results from steady flow tests can be useful but should be interpreted with caution as they differ by an unpredictable amount from the results obtained by the preferred technique of pulsatile flow testing. Moreover a simple misinterpretation in relating steady flow rate through a valve with an equivalent pulsatile flow rate can generate a 500 per cent error in the magnitude of the gradient (Appendix 2.2).

Appendix 2.1

METHOD OF TEST FOR DETERMINING THE MEAN PRESSURE DROP AND INCOMPETENCE OF PROSTHETIC HEART VALVES UNDER CONDITIONS OF PULSATILE FLOW

Introduction

The measurements of the pressure drop across a heart valve prosthesis under steady flow conditions are quite simple to perform, and represent a useful investigation during the developmental stages of a prosthesis. However, the results of steady flow tests are not always appropriate for predicting *in vivo* gradients and can sometimes be misleading. This is partly because of the discrepancy between the pulsatile flow rate and the steady flow rate which will cause the same pressure gradient across the prosthesis. Also in steady flow testing no account can be taken of the incompetence characteristics or the energy required to open the valve. Also non-linearities in valve characteristics are difficult to allow for. Pulsatile flow testing is therefore preferable when measuring valve pressure gradients, and essential when making incompetence measurements.

A method of measuring both the pressure gradient across the prosthesis and the incompetence level using a purpose-built pulsatile test rig is described below. It is recognized that the test method may not give results identical to those found in clinical use. However, the method has been designed to provide comparative results for different prostheses under conditions which approximate the clinical situation.

Basic concepts

The method of test has been based on the following concepts:

(1) The liquid used for testing should be appropriate for the prosthesis being investigated, and with certain valves, tests should be carried out at normal body temperature.
(2) The flow characteristics of the pulse duplicator should be known, should be reproducible, and should approximate to those of physiological flow.
(3) The geometry of flow passages of the pulse duplicator should approximate those of the vessels and chambers of the normal heart.
(4) The prosthesis under test should feed and should be fed from appropriate hydraulic impedances.
(5) The test rig should be capable of testing the largest and smallest mitral and aortic valve prostheses in clinical use.
(6) The orientation of the test rig should be such that similar gravitational forces influence poppet movement during test as are found in the erect patient.
(7) Suitable pressure tapping points are chosen.
(8) Mean pressure gradients are measured by a direct method.
(9) Incompetence is measured by a direct method.

Blood analogue

Although blood displays non-Newtonian characteristics in small vessels, in the major arteries and veins it can be considered a Newtonian liquid, as it behaves like a homogeneous liquid and not like a suspension of particles. The pressure loss across an open valve may be formulated as follows[9]:

$$\overline{P}_\mathrm{d} = A\dot{q} + Buq + \tfrac{1}{2}C\rho q^2$$

where $\overline{P}_\mathrm{d}$ = mean pressure gradient during forward flow phase
$\dot{q}$ = rate of change of flow rate
q = flow rate

A = liquid acceleration coefficient
(zero in a pulsatile system)
B = viscous loss coefficient
C = kinetic energy loss coefficient
u = viscosity of liquid
ρ = density of liquid

Experiments carried out in this laboratory have shown that changes in the viscosity of the test liquid have only a small effect on the pressure gradient across a prosthesis, and the major component of the pressure drop is due to kinetic energy loss, and is thus influenced by the density of the liquid. This is illustrated in *Table 2.8* which shows the viscous loss and energy loss components measured on a pivoting disc valve by carrying out pressure drop measurements over a wide range of viscosity and density variations.

TABLE 2.8
Relative viscous and kinetic energy loss of the
Lillehei–Kaster 20 mitral valve prosthesis

Mean systolic pulsatile flow rate (ml/s)	Viscous loss $B\mu q$ (μ − 3.0) (mmHg)	Kinetic loss $Cq^2\ p = 1.055$ (mmHg)
121	0.37	1.0
162	0.50	1.8
202	0.62	2.8
242	0.75	4.0
284	0.88	5.5

These tests illustrated that a 500 per cent change in viscosity altered the pressure gradient at high flow rate by only 15 per cent, while a 33 per cent change in density affected the pressure gradient by 29 per cent. Thus it is more important to match (or allow for variations in) density than viscosity. A second important consideration concerns the testing of some biological tissue valves. It has been found that the leaflets of bioprostheses preserved with glutaraldehyde or formalin appear to stiffen when exposed to a water–glycerol mixture. Thus this liquid is not an appropriate testing medium for this type of valve and physiological saline should be used in preference.

Some mechanical valve prostheses are designed so that when closed there is an annular leakage path between the occluder and the valve orifice. Thus, during the period when an appreciable back pressure exists across the valve, liquid will reflux via this path and increase the incompetence level of the valve. The rate of reflux flow through this narrow leakage path may be dependent on the viscosity of the liquid. Thus when measuring incompetence levels of this type of valve it is important to use a test liquid of appropriate viscosity (approximately 3.0 cP) and temperature (37 °C).

Because of these conflicting requirements no single test liquid can be used for all valve substitutes and compromises are necessary as follows:

(1) For pressure gradient and incompetence tests of mechanical prostheses, a water–glycerol mixture of density 1.100 g/ml at 37 °C should be used.
(2) For pressure gradient and reflux measurements of biological tissue valves, physiological saline at 37 °C (density 1.005 g/ml, viscosity approximately 0.7 cP) should be utilized.

Flow characteristics

The factors which are considered important to the flow of the blood analogue through the valve under test are: (1) the frequency of a pulsation; (2) the volume displacement per pulsation; and (3) the volume–time characteristics.

(1) The frequency of pulsation is made variable over the range 60-200 pulses/min by driving the rig with a variable speed d.c. motor. The range chosen corresponds to the probable physiological limits of a patient with heart valve replacement.
(2) The volume displacement per pulsation in the normal physiological situation varies according to the demands of the body over the range of about 60-180 ml. In order to simplify the rig construction and calibration a single stroke volume of 60 ml has been chosen. This provides a simulated cardiac output varying from 3.5 to 12 ℓ/min.
(3) Precise simulation of the filling and contraction characteristics of the heart is, unfortunately, rather difficult. The ventricle of the heart is not thought to produce a negative pressure or suction effect[6]. Thus the flow of blood into the ventricle must be a function of the pressure in the atrium and the pressure drop across the mitral valve. It follows that the filling rate of the ventricle will be dependent upon the pressure drop-flow characteristics of the mitral valve, whether it be normal, diseased or a valve substitute[4]. Thus a precise simulation is not possible. In patients with a moderate degree of aortic stenosis, the cardiac contraction characteristics deviate markedly from those of the normal subject, becoming less abrupt and more like a half cycle sine wave[1]. Finally, the ratio of diastolic to systolic period varies both with pulse rate and from individual to individual.

Some workers have attempted to simulate the heart's pumping action by enclosing a flexible ventricular chamber within an air-tight box to which alternate suction and gas pressure was applied[11,3]. Although this method gives flexibility of approach and independence between systolic and diastolic periods, it has the disadvantage that the filling and contraction characteristics of the artificial ventricle are hard to control. Moreover, because of the compressibility of the gas driving the system, the filling and contraction rates of the ventricle will vary depending on the characteristics of the valve under test, as does the normal heart. But it is also unlikely that such a system could be constructed so that the variation of filling and contraction characteristics could match those produced by the diseased heart, at least not without introducing some complexity and operator skill. The increased number of test variables would lead to some difficulty in comparing results produced by different workers.

In an attempt to overcome these difficulties, and to simplify the test apparatus as far as possible, a sine wave function has been adopted for the time-volume displacement of the rig, rather than attempting to reproduce the more complex physiological volume–time characteristics. Furthermore, it is mechanically simple to produce and reproduce a sine wave and so results of tests by different workers in different institutions will therefore be comparable.

Flow passages

Heart valves, both natural and artificial, usually generate vortices which are functions of both the valve itself and the shape of the chamber into which the liquid is flowing[2,15]. Such vortices can be important in aiding valve function. It is, therefore, necessary that the closed cavity of the left ventricle, the curve of the ascending aorta, and the aortic sinuses are reproduced in the test rig. The left ventricle fills and empties by variation of this cross-sectional diameter, its length remaining almost constant during the cardiac cycle. However, it is mechanically inconvenient to produce a test rig with this characteristic.

In order to retain both the anatomical shape of the flow passages and mechanical simplicity, the ventricular chamber of the test rig has been made in the form of a cylinder containing a piston, so shaped as to mimic the left ventricular apex. This model, the dimensions of which are shown in *Figure 2.29*, was designed from a silicone rubber injection of a cadaver left ventricle. This injection was also used to determine the size and position of the aortic outflow tract relative to that of the mitral valve. It is felt that this type of pump is a sufficiently close analogue to the left ventricle to ensure the reproduction of ventricular vortices.

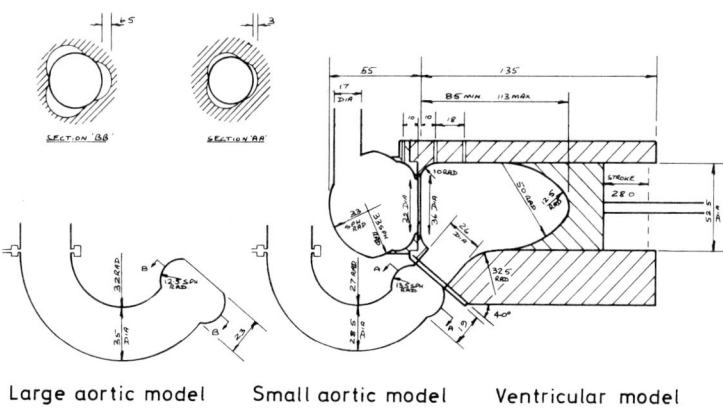

Large aortic model   Small aortic model   Ventricular model

Figure 2.29 The pulse duplicator test sections (dimensions in mm)

It is equally important that the general shape of the ascending aorta and aortic arch is reproduced. Experiments have shown that asymmetrical aortic valve substitutes such as prosthetic pivoting disc valves set up strong vortices in a model of the ascending aorta[15], and the form of these vortices depends on the angular orientation of the valve relative to the curvature of the aorta. Because these vortices are not produced in a straight pipe, and because with some types or sizes of valve the vortices may influence the pressure gradient or incompetence of the valve substitute, a straight aortic model is not appropriate. Hence the model aorta chosen for this method consists of a circular cross-section curved tube. The major branches at the apex of the aorta have not been included in the model as their absence does not substantially affect the generation of vortices in the ascending aorta.

Hydraulic impedances of the test circuit

The impedances necessary for the testing of mitral and aortic valves are different and will be considered separately.

The lungs, pulmonary veins and left atrium represent a low resistance and high compliance system and therefore no special precautions are necessary in considering the inlet connections to the mitral valve substitute except that the model atrium should be a thin-walled flexible chamber which is fed by a short pipe which represents the pulmonary veins. However, during rig systole it is important that the pressure in the left ventricle rises to physiological levels (approximately 120 mmHg) so that any retrograde flow through the valve during systole may be reproduced. At the same time, if accurate measurements of the incompetence of the mitral valve under test are to be made it is important that the aortic outflow valve should itself have not more than negligible incompetence.

To meet these two criteria a pressurizing outflow valve is inserted into the aortic valve position. This spring loaded valve and its outlet connector are shown in *Figure 2.30*. The valve is designed to open when the pressure in the ventricle reaches approximately 100 mmHg, and as its opening distance is small, the valve displaces a negligible volume of liquid. Similarly, when the rig is being used for testing an aortic valve substitute a spring loaded mitral valve is used (*Figure 2.31*), which also, because of its spring loading and low lift, displaces only a small volume of liquid. The arterial impedance is represented by a simple three-element model[10] consisting of a characteristic impedance, a compliance and a peripheral impedance. The characteristic impedance is composed of 2175 parallel stainless steel tubes, each measuring 0.725 mm bore by 28 mm long. The compliance is represented by a reservoir with a free air space of 900 ml. This arrangement is shown in *Figure 2.32*, together with the peripheral resistance,

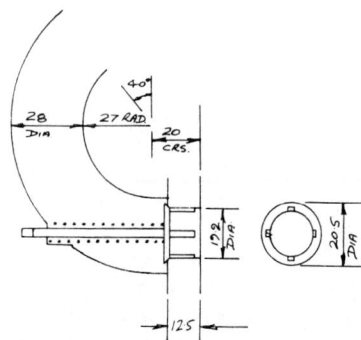

Figure 2.30 Spring loaded outlet valve (dimensions in mm). Spring to be such that the valve starts to open with an axial load of 200 g, and is fully open with an applied load of 350 g

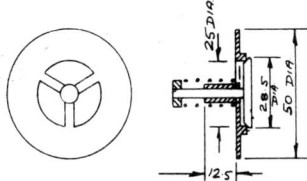

Figure 2.31 Spring loaded inlet valve (dimensions in mm). Spring to be such that the valve starts to open with an axial load of 70 g, and is fully open with an applied load of 120 g

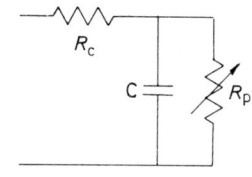

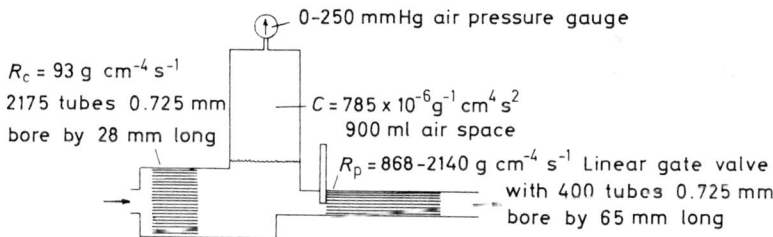

R_c = 93 g cm^{-4} s^{-1}
2175 tubes 0.725 mm
bore by 28 mm long

0-250 mmHg air pressure gauge

C = 785 x 10^{-6} g^{-1} cm^4 s^2
900 ml air space

R_p = 868-2140 g cm^{-4} s^{-1} Linear gate valve
with 400 tubes 0.725 mm
bore by 65 mm long

Figure 2.32 Arterial impedance components

which is represented by a partially closed laminar flow gate valve constructed from 400 parallel stainless steel tubes, each measuring 0.725 mm bore by 65 mm long and packed into a 25 mm bore pipe of the same length. A sliding gate controls the value of the resistance. The calculations of the physical dimensions of the components making up the arterial impedance have been based on the assumption that the test liquid will have a viscosity of 3 cP (an appropriate liquid for the incompetence testing of mechanical valve prostheses). When a physiological saline solution is used for testing biological tissue valves, the arterial impedance will theoretically introduce some errors, but because of the low values of incompetence of biological valves these errors will not normally be significant. In pressure gradient measurements the accuracy of measurement is not influenced by the linearity of the arterial impedance.

Size range of valve substitutes

A wide range of sizes of aortic valves are available. To accommodate these, two sizes of model aortae are necessary. The smaller model is suitable for testing aortic valve substitutes with an implantation (tissue/annulus) diameter of 24 mm or less, whilst the larger model is suitable for valves with implantation diameter in the range of 24-31 mm. The analogue of the smaller model was designed from a silicone rubber injection of a cadaver aorta, and the larger model was scaled up from the smaller one. The dimensions of the model aortae are shown in *Figure 2.29.*

Orientation of the test rig

In many current valve substitutes the density of the occluder is markedly different from that of blood, and therefore gravitation effects can influence poppet movement, especially at low pulse rates when hydraulic forces are minimal. The main axis of the heart in an erect subject varies from individual to individual depending on physical characteristics. For example, in ectomorphic subjects the main axis of the heart is nearly vertical, but in endomorphs the axis is nearly horizontal. As a compromise it was decided that mitral valve substitutes would be tested with the ventricular cavity inclined at an angle of 45° and with the axis of the aortic valve in the same horizontal plane. However, when aortic valves are to be tested the ventricle is positioned vertically.

Location of pressure tapping points

The pressure tapping points used in this test method on mitral valves are in the walls of the atrial chamber and in the ventricle. The points are situated 10 mm either side of the valve mounting plate. However, valve flow visualization studies[15] have shown that with disc valves the liquid stream is diverted by the disc to impinge onto the ventricular wall in this region. Thus, when testing disc valves the pressure tapping point is subjected to kinetic energy from the liquid and a false, low value of gradient is obtained. In such cases the ventricular pressure tapping point should be moved sufficiently far downstream (usually 28 mm will suffice) so that this effect is nullified. For aortic valve pressure gradient measurements the ventricular wall is chosen as one pressure tapping point, and a ring tapping point situated at a place equivalent to the apex of the aortic arch is used for the other tapping. These two points are used for the following reasons. In the heart the left ventricular wall contraction is opposed by the internal pressure in the ventricular cavity, and the major baroreceptors are placed at the apex of the aortic arch. Also this latter point is sufficiently far downstream so that the major part of any pressure recovery distal to the valve will have occurred. The positions of pressure tapping points are shown in *Figures 2.8* and *2.9.* The ring tapping point was made up from four holes equally spaced around the circumference of the model aorta. The holes feed into a manifold to which the pressure transducer is connected.

Direct method of measuring valve gradient

Unfortunately, the forward pressure drop produced by the valve under testing may be very small compared to the pressure across the valve when it is closed. Thus the measuring system has to cope with a large dynamic range and, with some valve substitutes, fast transients. In selecting a suitable transducer these requirements must be considered.

In pulsatile testing the duration of the forward flow phase depends both on the pulse rate of the rig, and the closure delay time of other valves incorporated in the pulse duplicator circuit. It is therefore necessary to have a method of selecting (gating) just that proportion of the pressure gradient waveform which is to be processed, and determining the mean value of the pressure waveform[14].

The pressure drop across the valve under test is continually monitored and fed to the processing unit, shown diagrammatically in *Figure 2.33*. The signal from the differential pressure transducer–amplifier is fed into the input amplifier and gated in such a way that only the portion of the differential pressure signal produced by forward flow through the valve is passed through the gate. The gate is actuated by a variable position micro-switch driven by a cam (cam 1) on the drive shaft of the test rig. A d.c. reference voltage, but of opposite polarity is also simultaneously gated. The sum of these two signals is integrated by feeding each, via its resistor R to a common capacitor C. The reference voltage is varied to reproduce zero net charge on capacitor C. The mean value of the forward flow pressure signal will then be equal to the value of the reference voltage, and since both signals are gated for identical periods, the relationship is valid at all speeds of operation. A non-linear amplifier driving a centre zero meter is used to indicate zero voltage across the capacitor C. This gives high sensitivity about the null point, but low sensitivity at extreme ends of the meter scale.

The gated pressure signal is displayed on a variable persistence oscilloscope via a switched low pass filter (which allows high frequency noise and transients to be removed from the displayed signal). The gate opening time and duration is set by adjusting the angular and radial position of the micro-switch on cam 1. During mitral valve tests this micro-switch is adjusted so that the gate opens at that instant when the ventricular pressure (which has been approximately minus 120 mmHg relative to the atrial pressure during systole) first becomes equal to the atrial pressure, and the gate closes when the flow through the mitral valve

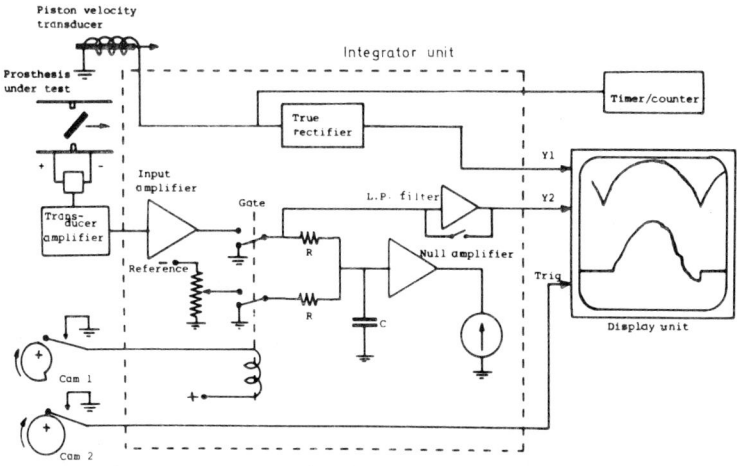

Figure 2.33 Block diagram of the monitoring system. (Reproduced from Wright, J. T. M. and Brown, M. C.[14], by courtesy of *Medical Instrumentation*)

falls to zero at end diastole. This latter point is determined by observing the voltage generated by a transducer used to measure piston velocity. The output of this velocity transducer is passed through a true rectifier to provide a signal on which the zero velocity points can be readily identified. The velocity signal is also fed to a counter-timer for measurement of cycle time and hence rig speed. A second rig driven micro-switch is used to synchronize the oscilloscope.

Circuit details

The circuit diagram is shown in *Figure 2.34*. The input amplifier has gain and zero offset controls. A zero button can be used to check input offset from the pressure amplifier. The reference voltage is derived from a high linearity, multi-turn potentiometer fitted with a digital indicator. The voltage supply to the potentiometer is stabilized by a zener diode. The gate switching is performed by a two-way two-pole reed relay or a high speed mercury wetted relay. A test button allows the gate to be closed with the rig stationary. The two 47 KΩ resistors feeding the integrator capacitors are matched, and two values of integrator time constant may be selected by a 'normal–fast' switch. The 'fast' position is used during calibration and when making initial adjustments of the reference potentiometer. The 'normal' position is used for final measurements. An internal null button discharges the integrator capacitors during setting up and measurements.

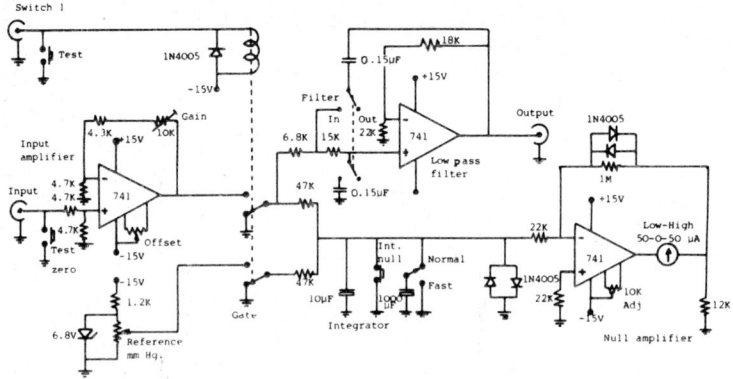

Figure 2.34   Circuit diagram of the integrator. (Reproduced from Wright, J. T. M. and Brown, M. C.[14], by courtesy of *Medical Instrumentation*)

Calibration

The processor is calibrated as follows. With the internal null button pressed, the centre zero meter is brought to null by the offset adjustment of the non-linear amplifier. The reference potentiometer is set to zero and the gate closed. Zero pressure difference is then applied to the transducer and the input offset control varied to give a null reading on the meter. A known pressure difference is then applied to the transducer (20 mmHg), the reference potentiometer set to indicate this value, and the gain of the input amplifier varied to give null deflection on the meter. This completes the calibration.

The differential pressure transducer

A differential pressure transducer should be used for measurement of valve gradient in preference to two individual pressure transducers, because non-linearity in individual transducers, zero drift and unmatched transient response will all lead to increased measurement errors. The transient pressures developed during the opening of some prostheses require that the pressure transducer can cope with frequencies many times the pulse frequency. It is also important that the transducer be capable of sustaining the relatively high pressure drop across the valve when it is in its closed phase, and the transducer should have minimal hysteresis. With some transducers some form of damping is necessary to prevent step changes in pressure exciting the transducer to ring at its resonant frequency. Electrical damping by a low pass filter in the transducer amplifier output may be used, but this introduces phase shift in the output, thus leading to errors when setting gating time. An alternative method which introduces less phase shift is to apply hydraulic damping to the pressure transducer connecting tubes. The frequency response of the differential pressure transducer and its associated pipes and taps should be such that a flat response to at least 15 Hz is obtained. This is the minimum requirement. A response of 100 Hz is preferable to capture any opening transients which may be present in some valve substitutes.

Usually the use of short, stiff and relatively thick-walled plastic pipes are preferable for making pressure connections between the test rig and the transducers. Standard medical pressure monitoring uses three-way Luer taper taps from a convenient part of the connection system.

The transducer used in the studies carried out in this laboratory is a Validyne DP9 fitted with a 10 or 20 psi diaphragm. In spite of the stiffness of the diaphragms, this transducer is capable of making pressure measurements of less than 0.1 mmHg.

With most transducers, it is important that gas bubbles should be eliminated from the transducer and its connecting tubing and this may be accomplished by flushing the system with ethyl alcohol and filling it with de-aerated water, produced by evacuating water down to its water vapour pressure and holding at this pressure for about ten minutes. A filter pump connected to a cold water tap will conveniently provide this vacuum. An additional advantage of using de-aerated water is that any small bubbles remaining in the transducer system will tend to be re-absorbed. When the rig is being used to test aortic valves the transducer is connected to pressure tapping points on either side of that valve (in the ventricular wall and at the aortic ring tapping point). When mitral valves are being investigated the tapping points in the ventricular and atrial walls are used.

Direct measurement of valve incompetence

The incompetence of the valve is measured by weighing the quantity of liquid ejected from the ventricle for 100 strokes of the piston with the previously determined quantity displaced by the piston. The difference between these two values is due to retrograde flow through the prosthesis. Clearly some retrograde flow is always needed to close a valve.

Description of the test rig

The hydraulic components of the test rig consist of a tank, an atrial feed reservoir, a flexible atrial chamber, a ventricular piston pump and an aortic outflow section. A thermostatically controlled heater maintains the test liquid in the tank at $37\,^\circ C \pm 1\,^\circ C$. A circulating pump is used to pump liquid from the bath into the atrial feed reservoir, and the level is maintained by a simple overflow (the excess runs back into the tank). Liquid is fed by a short 17 mm bore tube to the flexible atrium from the atrial reservoir. The flexible atrial chamber is manufactured by multiple dip coating a former in a polyurethane solution (15 per cent polyurethane in dimethyl formamide). The ventricular chamber manufactured from clear methyl methacrylate, contains a cylinder 52.5 mm diameter which incorporates a piston shaped like the left ventricular apex. When the piston recedes in the cylinder, liquid is drawn through the inlet valve and hence into the ventricle. When the piston advances in the cylinder, the liquid displaced is ejected from the ventricle through the outlet valve and hence returns to the tank via the outlet pipe. The stroke displacement of the piston is approximately 60 ml, the actual displacement being measured under static conditions. The dimensions of the ventricular section and piston are shown in *Figure 2.29*.

   The piston is driven by a Scotch yoke mechanical sine wave generator with a stroke displacement of 28 mm. Alternatively, because a long connecting rod (approximately 140 mm) may be used, a negligible deviation from a sine wave will occur if a simple crank mechanism is used. The mechanical sine wave generator is driven by a variable speed d.c. shunt motor controlled by a thyristor motor speed controller. When the rig is being used to test aortic valves the inlet spring loaded valve is used and the circuit is as shown in *Figure 2.9*. The gate valve is adjusted so that the mean aortic pressure is approximately 100 mmHg. This may conveniently be monitored by using an air pressure gauge to measure the air pressure in the air reservoir. A change of rig speed will necessitate further adjustment of the gate valve. When mitral valves are being tested, the spring loaded outlet valve is used and the circuit is connected as shown in *Figure 2.8*.

Preparing the valve substitute for test

Before the valves can be tested they have to be suitably mounted in the rig. The aortic valves are each attached to a flat stainless steel plate 0.75 mm thick (except when the larger aortic model is being used when the mounting plate is of 4 mm thick plastic), the valve being recessed into the plate. The plate is pierced with a round hole, larger than the valve orifice, but small enough so that the orifice body could rest against the plate. The hole is surrounded by a ring of 1 mm diameter holes about 3 mm apart, through which the valve is sutured. Leakage around the sewing ring is prevented by sealing it with a self-curing silicone rubber compound. The aortic valve plates are located between the ventricular outflow tract and the model aortic section. Mitral valves are similarly mounted on circular plates and located between the atrial and ventricular sections of the pulse duplicator. The valves, mounted in this manner, can quickly and easily be interchanged. External leakage is prevented by thin rubber gaskets either side of the valve plates.

Preparing the pulse duplicator

The rig is prepared for testing by mounting the valve under investigation and the appropriate spring loaded valve in the pulse duplicator. The rig is filled with the appropriate test liquid and the circulating pump started. The temperature is adjusted to 37 °C (and when water-glycerol mixture is being used, the density of the test liquid checked). Air is bled from the ventricular and atrial cavities and the drive motor started. The rig is run for several minutes, to give time for conditions to stabilize, and then stopped. The tests carried out are described below.

Measurement of mean gradient

Before running the test rig it is necessary to ensure that the pressure transducer gives zero output at zero flow even though the tapping points might not be in the same horizontal plane. When setting the transducer amplifier zero control it is important to see that no static pressure difference exists across the valve, either by observing that the valve is open, or by making a temporary hydraulic connection between one side of the valve and the other. The test rig is run at the desired speed and the gated pressure gradient signal is monitored on the oscilloscope. Also monitored is the rectified signal from the velocity transducer. The angular position of the micro-switch is adjusted so that the gate opens at zero

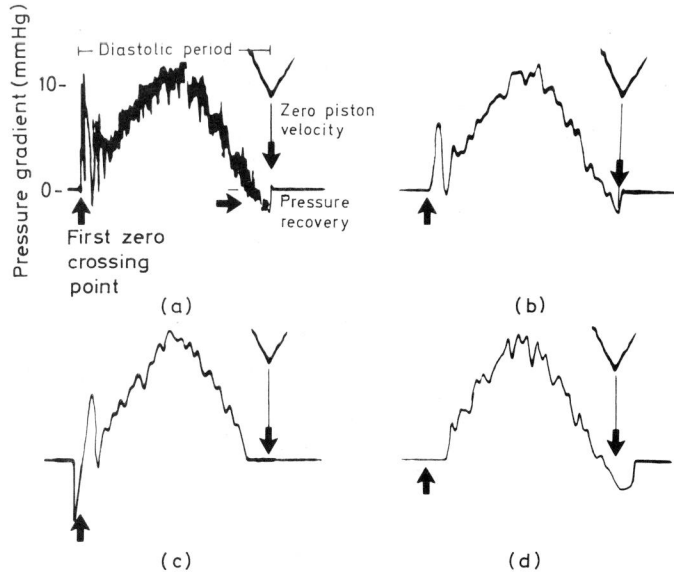

Figure 2.35 Correct and incorrect settings of the electronic gate. (*a*) Correctly gated unfiltered signal; (*b*) correctly gated filtered signal; (*c*) incorrectly gated filtered signal—gate closes and opens too early; (*d*) incorrectly gated filtered signal—gate closes and opens too late. (Reproduced from Wright, J. T. M. and Brown, M. C.[14], by courtesy of *Medical Instrumentation*)

flow (as determined from the velocity signal). The radial position of micro-switch 1 is then adjusted so that the gate closes to coincide with the first zero crossing point of the pressure signal. Correct and incorrect settings are illustrated in *Figure 2.35*. Depending on the amount of high frequency noise that may be present the low pass filter is usually switched in. However, because of phase shift introduced by the low pass filter, the gate opening and closing points are always checked with an unfiltered signal. With the integrator time constant set to 'fast' the approximately correct reference pressure is identified when the null meter oscillates roughly about the centre. On switching to 'normal' time constant the meter creeps slowly up or down, indicating the adjustment required to correct the error. The null button brings the meter quickly back to the centre. Adjustment of the reference potentiometer is made until the meter remains in the central region (a 0.1 mmHg band) for 30 cycles. The mean pressure drop can now be read from the reference potentiometer.

Measurement of valve incompetence

The outlet pipe from the appropriate aortic section directs the ejected liquid back into the tank, but when required the liquid can be collected in a separate container to be weighed.

Calibration of dynamic displacement

The dynamic displacement of the rig may be checked by fitting both spring loaded inlet and outlet valves, running the rig at the desired speed, and weighing the liquid collected by 100 pumping cycles. Typically the dynamic displacement is approximately 1 per cent less than the static displacement, and is not influenced by the speed of the test rig. The dynamic displacement is used when calculating the percentage incompetence of valve prostheses.

Valve incompetence measurements

The rig is started and the required speed set. The aortic return tube is transferred from the bath so that the ejected liquid is collected in a weighing tank. The systolic ejections are counted and when the required number of 100 is reached the outlet tube is quickly returned to the bath. The tank is then weighed both with and without the collected liquid. The incompetence level of the valve (expressed as a percentage of the stroke volume of the rig) is calculated as follows:

$$\text{Percentage incompetence } (I) = \frac{Y - W}{Y} \times 100$$

where:

W = weight of liquid collected (kg)/100 strokes of piston with valve under test.
Y = weight of liquid collected (kg)/100 strokes of piston with both spring loaded valves.

The incompetence of the valve, expressed as volume loss/stroke is calculated from:

$$\text{Incompetence (ml/stroke)} = \frac{W \times I}{10\rho}$$

where:

I = percentage incompetence calculated above
ρ = density of test liquid (g/ml)

Presentation of results

Mean pressure gradient

To present results so that different valves tested with various test liquids may be directly compared it is necessary to correct the measured mean systolic or diastolic gradient for variations in the density of the test liquid from that of blood as follows:

$$\overline{P}_{dc} = \frac{1.055}{\rho} \times \overline{P}_d$$

where:

$\overline{P}_{dc}$ = density corrected mean pressure gradient (mmHg)

$\overline{P}_d$ = measured mean pressure gradient (mmHg)
ρ = density of test liquid at test temperature (g/ml)
1.055 = density of blood at $37\,^{\circ}$C

Appendix 2.2

A THEORETICAL COMPARISON OF THE EFFECTS OF PULSATILE AND STEADY FLOW ON THE PRESSURE GRADIENT PRODUCED ACROSS A HEART VALVE PROSTHESIS

The general expression for the pressure gradient across an open prosthetic heart valve subject to flow was given by Sauvage et al.[9] as follows:

$$\overline{P}_d = A\dot{q} + B\rho q + C\mu q^2 \qquad (1)$$

where $\overline{P}_d$ = mean pressure gradient during forward flow phase
$\dot{q}$ = rate of change of flow rate
q = flow rate
A = liquid acceleration coefficient
B = viscous loss coefficient
C = kinetic or turbulent loss coefficient
μ = viscosity of liquid
ρ = density of liquid

In the pulse duplicator the volume-time displacement characteristics and hence flow fluctuations were of half wave rectified sinusoidal form.
i.e.

$$q(t) = \hat{q} \sin \omega t \qquad \text{from } (t = 0 \text{ to } t = \pi/\omega)$$

and

$$q(t) = 0 \qquad \text{from } (t = \pi/\omega \text{ to } t = 2\pi/\omega)$$

where $q(t)$ means flow as a function of time, and $\hat{q}$ = peak pulsatile flow rate. Now assuming that the pressure gradient needed to open the prosthesis fully is negligible then substituting in equation (1).

$$\overline{P}_d = A\omega\hat{q} \cos \omega t + B\mu\hat{q} \sin \omega t + C\hat{\rho}q^2 \sin^2 \omega t$$

$$\overline{P}_d = \frac{\omega}{\pi} \int_0^{\pi/\omega} (A\omega\hat{q} \cos \omega t + B\mu\hat{q} \sin \omega t + C\rho\hat{q}^2 \sin^2 \omega t) \, dt$$

$$\overline{P}_d = \frac{\omega}{\pi} \int_0^{\pi/\omega} [A\omega\hat{q} \cos \omega t + B\mu\hat{q} \sin \omega t + \tfrac{1}{2} C\rho\hat{q}^2 (1 - \cos 2\omega t)] \, dt$$

$$\overline{P}_d = \frac{\omega}{\pi} \left[A\hat{q} \sin \omega t - \frac{B\mu\hat{q}}{\omega} \cos \omega t + \frac{C\rho\hat{q}^2}{2} \left(t - \frac{\sin \omega t}{\omega} \right) \right]_0^{\pi/\omega}$$

$$\overline{P}_d = \frac{\omega}{\pi} \left(0 - \frac{B\mu\hat{q}}{\omega} (-1 - 1) + \frac{C\rho\hat{q}^2}{2} \frac{\pi}{\omega} \right)$$

$$\overline{P}_d = \frac{2 B\mu\hat{q}}{\pi} + \frac{C\rho\hat{q}^2}{2} \tag{2}$$

To relate steady flow q_s with a pulsatile flow $\hat{q} \sin \omega t$ of same mean value

$$q_s = \frac{\omega}{\pi} \int_0^{\pi/\omega} q \, dt \tag{3}$$

$$q_s = \frac{\omega}{\pi} \int_0^{\pi/\omega} \hat{q} \sin \omega t \, dt$$

$$q_s = \frac{\omega\hat{q}}{\pi} \left[- \frac{\cos \omega t}{\omega} \right]_0^{\pi/\omega}$$

$$q_s = \frac{2\hat{q}}{\pi}$$

Hence

$$\hat{q} = \frac{\pi q_s}{2} \tag{4}$$

Substituting equation (4) in equation (2)

$$\bar{P}_d = B\mu q_s + \frac{C\rho\pi^2}{8} q_s^2$$

$$\bar{P}_d = B\mu q_s + 1.23 C\rho q_s^2 \tag{5}$$

Now the pressure gradient caused by a steady flow will be

$$P_{ds} = A\dot{q} + B\mu q + C\rho q^2$$

where P_{ds} = pressure gradient across the fully open valve due to steady flow q_s
but since $\dot{q} = 0$
then

$$P_{ds} = B\mu q_s + C\rho q_s^2 \tag{6}$$

Experiments carried out in this laboratory on prosthetic mechanical and tissue valves have shown that the term $B\mu q$ is small compared to $C\rho q^2$ at high flow rates.

If $B\mu q$ is neglected and equation (5) is divided by equation (6)

$$\bar{P}_d = 1.23 P_{ds}$$

However, if it is assumed that $B\mu q_s$ is approximately 15 per cent of $C\rho q_s^2$ then

$$\bar{P}_d = 1.18 P_{ds}$$

In summary from these equations one would expect:

(1) The term $A\dot{q}$ to have no effect on the mean pressure gradient under steady flow, or a complete half cycle of pulsatile flow.
(2) The mean pressure gradient to be directly related to the mean flow rate. A given change in flow rate could be by a change in stroke volume or in simulated pulse rate. The effect on the gradient will be the same in either case.
(3) That the mean pressure gradient produced by a pulsatile flow to be 18-23 per cent greater than that caused by a steady flow of the same *mean* value (taken over the half cycle). For example assume that a pulsatile test rig has a stroke volume of 60 ml and the rig is run at a simulated pulse rate of 100/min. The total simulated cardiac cycle time is 0.6 s, and the forward flow time is 0.3 s. The mean pulsatile flow rate will therefore be

$$\frac{60}{0.3} = 200 \text{ ml/s } (12\ell/\text{min}) \text{ } NOT \text{ } 60 \times 100 = 6 \text{ } \ell/\text{min}$$

If a steady flow of half the correct value was used equation (3) would become

$$q_s = \frac{\omega}{2\pi} \int_0^{2\pi/\omega} q \, dt$$

Hence equation (4) will become

$$\hat{q} = \pi q_s$$

and equation (5) will become

$$\bar{P}_d = 2B\mu q_s + 4.93 C\rho q_s^2$$

Thus the pressure drop due to pulsatile flow would be about five times the gradient produced by the steady flow of the same value averaged (incorrectly) over the whole simulated cardiac cycle. In examining steady flow pressure gradient curves the range of flow rate of interest should be about 8-18 ℓ/min for mitral valves and about 10-25 ℓ/min for aortic valves.

Acknowledgements

The generosity of the manufacturers and hospitals in providing the bioprostheses for evaluation is gratefully acknowledged. Without their cooperation this work could not have been carried out.

SUMMARY

In vitro pulsatile flow studies have been carried out on approximately 40 tissue valves of various makes, types and sizes. Included in the study were commercially available Angell-Shiley, Carpentier-Edwards and Hancock porcine xenograft bioprostheses and Ionescu-Shiley pericardial valves. Also examined were an experimental dura mater valve from the National Heart Hospital, London and two mounted homograft valves from Killingbeck Hospital, Leeds. All the valves were investigated in the mitral position of the pulse duplicator, and some of the smaller Hancock 242 and 250 type valves in the aortic position. In the mitral valve tests measurements were made of pressure gradient, incompetence level and leaflet mobility. From the results effective valve areas were calculated using the formula of Gorlin and Gorlin, and the valves ranked in order of hydraulic merit. Selected valves were photographed at peak diastolic flow and the orifice areas measured planimetrically. Comparisons were then made between the calculated and measured areas so that the discharge coefficients of the valves could be obtained.

The hydraulic characteristics of the bioprosthetic mitral valves in the size range 31-32 mounting diameter were compared with those of mechanical prostheses in the size range 29-33 mm mounting diameter. In the aortic region the Hancock 242 and 250 xenograft valves were compared with Björk-Shiley tilting disc valves in the size range 19-25 mm diameter. In addition, some flow visualization studies carried out on a 31 mm Hancock mitral valve and on a 25 mm aortic valve are reported. Finally, some of the tissue valves were tested in the mitral position using steady flow and the results compared to those obtained using pulsatile flow on the same valves.

The results of all these investigations are described in detail and discussed in the context of *in vitro* performance of the valves.

REFERENCES

[1] Bache, R. J., Wang, Y. and Jorgensen, C. R. 'Haemodynamic effects of exercise in isolated valvular aortic stenosis', *Circulation*, **44**, 1003 (1971)

[2] Bellhouse, B. J. and Talbot, L. 'The fluid mechanics of the aortic valve', *Journal of Fluid Mechanics*, **35**, 721 (1969)

[3] Cornhill, J. F. 'An aortic left ventricular pulse duplicator used in testing prosthetic aortic heart valves', *Journal of thoracic and cardiovascular Surgery,* **73**, 550 (1977)

[4] Folts, J. D., Young, W. P. and Rowe, G. G. 'Phasic flow through normal and prosthetic mitral valves in unanaesthetized dogs', *Journal of thoracic and cardiovascular Surgery,* **61**, 235 (1971)

[5] Gorlin, R. and Gorlin, S. G. 'Hydraulic formula for the calculation of the area of stenotic mitral valve, other cardiac valves and central circulatory shunts', *American heart Journal,* **41**, 1 (1951)

[6] Henderson, Y. 'The volume curve of the ventricles of the mammalian heart, and the significance of this curve in respect to the mechanics of the heart beat and the filling of the ventricles', *American Journal of Physiology,* **16**, 325 (1906)

[7] Ionescu, M. I. Personal communication (1977)

[8] Kennedy, J. W., Yarnall, S. R., Murray, J. A. and Figley, M. M. 'Quantitative angiocardiography IV. Relationship of left atrial and ventricular pressure and volume in mitral valve disease', *Circulation,* **41**, 817 (1970)

[9] Sauvage, L. R., Viggers, R. F., Robel, S. B., Wood, S. J., Berger, K. and Wesolowski, S. A. 'Prosthetic heart valve replacements', *Annals of the New York Academy of Sciences,* **146**, 289 (1968)

[10] Westerhof, N., Elzinga, G. and Sipkenma, P. 'An artificial arterial system for pumping hearts', *Journal of applied Physiology,* **31**, 776 (1971)

[11] Wieting, D. W. 'Dynamic flow characteristics of heart valves', *Ph.D Thesis, University of Texas at Austin* (1969)

[12] Wright, J. T. M. 'An *in vitro* assessment of the hydraulic characteristics of the Mark II Abrams–Lucas mitral valve prosthesis', *Thorax,* **32**, 296 (1977)

[13] Wright, J. T. M. 'An *in vitro* comparison between the hydrodynamic characteristics of the Hancock 250 (modified orifice) xenografts and the Björk–Shiley aortic valve prostheses', *Transactions, American Society for Artificial Internal Organs,* **23**, 89 (1977)

[14] Wright, J. T. M. and Brown, M. C. 'A method for measuring the mean pressure gradient across prosthetic heart valves under *in vitro* pulsatile flow conditions', *Medical Instrumentation,* **11**, 110 (1977)

[15] Wright, J. T. M. and Temple, L. J. 'A flow visualization study of prosthetic aortic and mitral valves in a model of the aorta and left heart', *Engineering in Medicine,* **6**, 31 (1977)

3

Clinical and Experimental Comparisons Establishing the Glutaraldehyde Treated Xenograft as the Standard for Tissue Heart Valve Replacement

William W. Angell
Judith D. Angell
and Jon C. Kosek

Le temps met tout en lumière.

Thalès de Milet (640–547 av. J.C.)

INTRODUCTION

The ideal cardiac valve substitute remains the goal for those seeking to improve the clinical results of valve replacement surgery. The generally accepted characteristics of the ideal heart valve substitute are: proven structural durability over a period of 10 to 20 years, central flow orifice without transvalvular gradient, absence of host reactivity deleterious to valve function, non-thrombogenicity without the use of anticoagulants, resistance to infective endocarditis and ready availability and ease of surgical implantation.

While we have continued over the last 11 years to evaluate clinically and experimentally the available valve replacement devices, we have retained the prejudice that the tissue valve has a greater potential for achieving these objectives than does the mechanical prosthetic valve. Glutaraldehyde fixation of tissue has solved most of the problems associated with the use of these valves. Sterility is guaranteed and the capability of prolonged storage ensures ready availability. Most significant, however, is the fact that the glutaraldehyde treated valve has been proved durable in all intracardiac positions for eight years[3,25,27,58]. Although the clinical series followed for this interval is small, few patients are reported to have suffered valve failure due to tissue deterioration. This is in direct contrast to previously reported tissue valve experiences where the primary mode of failure after five years was the structural deterioration of the valve tissue. This chapter describes the clinical and experimental evolution of the glutaraldehyde-treated tissue valve. A comparison with other valve substitutes indicates that the glutaraldehyde xenograft fulfills many of the criteria for an ideal valve substitute and is rapidly becoming the new standard for heart valve replacement.

BACKGROUND

Interest in the clinical use of tissue valves was kindled by Lam, Aram and Munnell who, in 1952, successfully implanted fresh aortic allografts in the descending thoracic aorta of dogs[34]. This technique was modified and applied clinically by Murray, Heimbecker and Bigelow[43] and several of these patients are known— some 20 years post-implantation—to have functional valve leaflets[29]. A method for sub-coronary implantation of the fresh aortic allograft was experimentally developed by Duran and Gunning[26], and in 1962, the first successful clinical orthotopic implantation of an allograft valve in the aortic position was accomplished by Ross[48]. In this same year, Brian Barratt-Boyes[14] employed the fresh homograft using the present two suture-line implantation method in a series of 16 patients. A number of patients from these early groups have valves functioning for over 15 years without evidence of tissue failure[16,49]. Subsequent to these initial reports, allograft aortic valve implantation was enthusiastically undertaken by several other groups[19,30,38].

Our own interest in the use of the fresh aortic allograft as a replacement for damaged cardiac valves began 12 years ago at Stanford University Medical Center, following an analysis of a clinical series of 1000 patients who had undergone mitral valve replacement with the Starr–Edwards prosthesis. The hospital mortality rate in this group of patients was 15 per cent while 20 per cent of patients experienced thromboembolic or haemorrhagic complications during the first 24 post-operative months. The four-year survival rate of less than 65 per cent in this series was due to complications associated with chronic anticoagulation as well as mechanical dysfunction of the prostheses and valve infection. These suboptimal results increased our dissatisfaction with the performance of prosthetic devices and prompted a trial of the tissue valve[12].

THE AORTIC ALLOGRAFT VALVE

Early in 1966, a series of animal experiments were designed to compare the various methods of preparation and storage employed by those centres using aortic allograft valves. The five types of canine aortic valves used in this experiment included fresh, sterile procured valves, beta propriolactone sterilized valves and valves that had been stored either by refrigeration, deep freezing or freeze-drying.

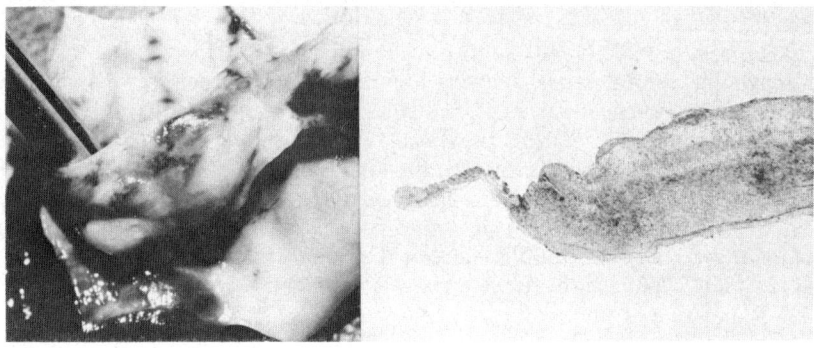

Figure 3.1 Fresh canine aortic valve allograft. Macroscopic aspect of cusp thickening and shortening, rendering the valve incompetent (left). Microscopic section of a similar canine aortic allograft cusp showing persistent donor cellularity and fibroblastic proliferation (right). Haematoxylin and eosin stain × 30, reduced by $\frac{1}{3}$ in printing. (Reproduced from Angell, W. W., Pillsbury, R. C. and Shumway, N. E.[10], by courtesy of *Archives of Surgery*)

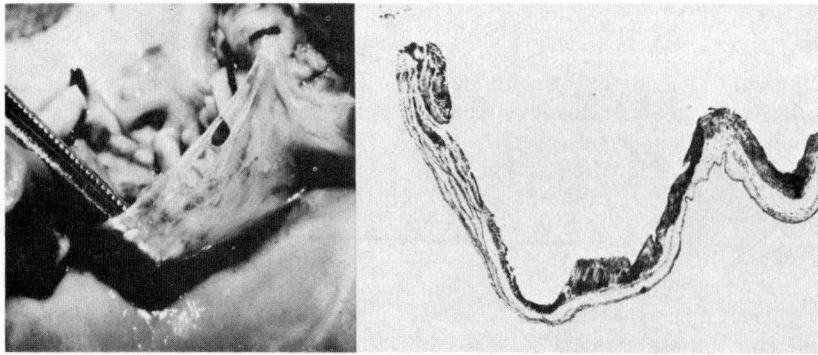

Figure 3.2 Stored in canine aortic allograft. Macroscopic appearance of thinned, perforated cusp (left). Microscopy showed lack of cellularity and absence of fibroblastic reaction or invasion of the cusps. The tissue integrity is disrupted (right). Haematoxylin and eosin stain × 30, reduced by $\frac{1}{3}$ in printing. (Reproduced as *Figure 3.1*)

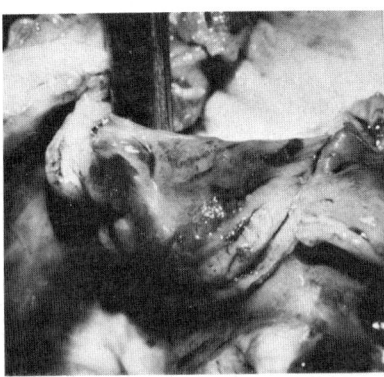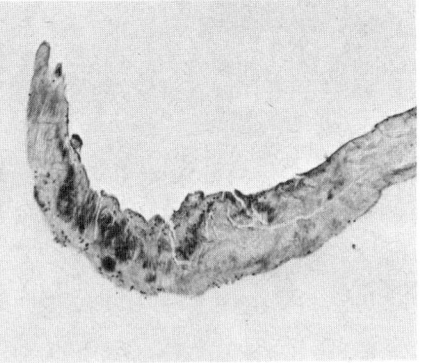

Figure 3.3 Frozen canine aortic allograft. The thickening of the valve cusp is evident. The histology is similar to the one observed in frozen valves except for the thickening of the cusp. Haematoxylin and eosin stain × 30, reduced by $\frac{1}{3}$ in printing.
(Reproduced as *Figure 3.1*)

The valves were implanted in the sub-coronary position of 56 dogs and the results concerning both valve function and gross and microscopic appearance of the valves were analysed and compared[10]. Histological examination of the fresh aortic valve allograft revealed persistent donor cellularity and a progressive fibroblastic proliferation resulting in cusp thickening and shortening with a troublesome incidence of valve insufficiency (*Figure 3.1*). Tissue integrity, however, was good, and although some acellular areas of collagen were present, perforations through these were not found. Conversely, the stored, frozen, freeze-dried and beta-propiolactone sterilized valve cusps were shown to have been rendered completely acellular by these methods. Histologically, no fibroblastic reaction or invasion of the cusps was observed, and this loss of tissue integrity combined with disruption of the collagen matrix led to cusp perforation and dehiscence with resultant functional inadequacy (*Figures 3.2, 3.3* and *3.4*).

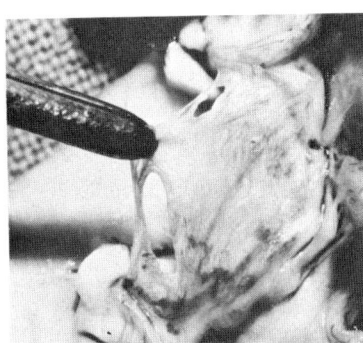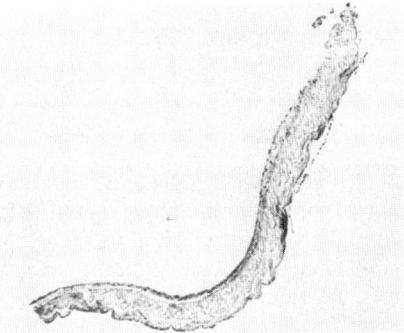

Figure 3.4 Canine aortic allograft sterilized with beta-propiolactone or freeze dried. The macroscopic (left) and microscopic (right) appearances are very similar to those of frozen valves (*Figure 3.2*). Haematoxylin and eosin stain × 30, reduced by $\frac{1}{3}$ in printing.
(Reproduced as *Figure 3.1*)

The fresh aortic allograft valve

Based on the experimental results mentioned above, a series of 40 patients received, early in 1967, fresh, aortic allograft valves procured under sterile conditions. The valves were implanted as free grafts in the sub-coronary position[51]. During a follow-up interval of 11 months there were five hospital deaths and one late death, none due to allograft dysfunction. All 34 surviving patients were either asymptomatic or greatly improved. Seven patients developed early diastolic murmurs from one week to four months post-operatively, but none had signs of significant aortic incompetence. The results of this clinical series and of continued experimental follow-up prompted the construction of premounted fresh allograft valves on a stent to enable the insertion of allografts in other intracardiac positions (*Figure 3.5*). A series of 13 canine implants in the mitral position were done with no mortality and good haemodynamic function, and thus, in March 1967, this frame mounted preparation was employed clinically[12].

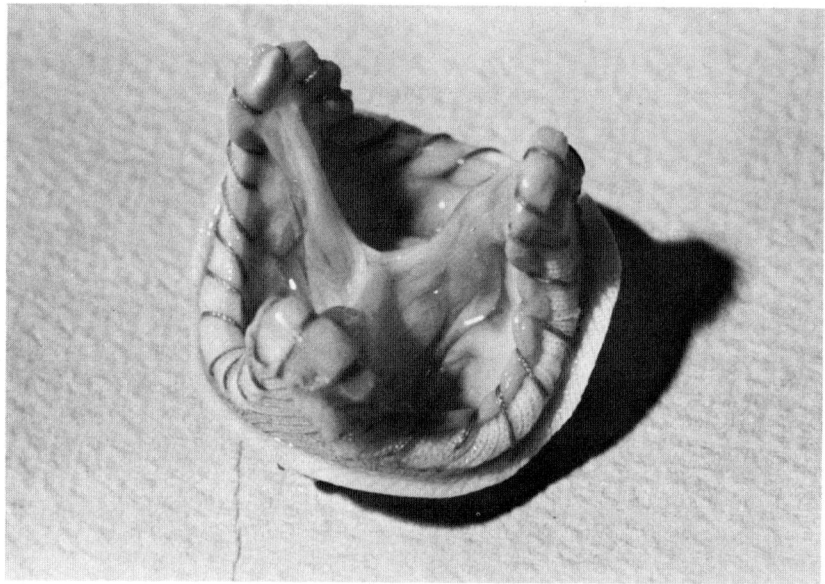

Figure 3.5 Outflow aspect of a fresh aortic allograft mounted onto a cloth-covered symmetrical metal support. (Reproduced from Angell, W. W., Angell, J. D. and Sywak, A.[3], by courtesy of *Surgery*)

During the following year, 31 patients received fresh aortic allograft valves mounted on a cloth-covered symmetrical metal support. The valves were implanted in the mitral position. The early results were good and the patients experienced considerable post-operative haemodynamic improvement with no significant transvalvular gradients. The incidence of mitral incompetence was low and not considered haemodynamically significant or symptomatic in any patient. Of greatest importance was the fact that for the first time mitral valve replacement was performed without the need for chronic anticoagulation and without an incidence of valve-related thromboembolism[8,28]. The natural consequence of this experience was the use of mounted allograft valves for multiple valve replacement, and the results with a series of six patients who underwent combined mitral, aortic and tricuspid replacement between June 1967 and March 1968 were excellent with no deaths and with marked improvement in all patients[9,52]. The fresh aortic allograft, having enjoyed a gratifying one-year experience, was felt to offer significant advantages over the existing prosthetic devices. Widespread use of tissue valves thus became feasible and prompted efforts to solve the problems of guaranteed sterility, prolonged storage and ready availability.

The antibiotic sterilized aortic allograft valve

The choice of technique for sterilization and storage of fresh tissue valves is largely dependent upon whether or not the preservation of tissue viability and thus the maintenance of normal cell morphology is considered essential to the long-term function of the graft. While not generally accepted by other authors, our clinical and experimental histological studies indicated that fresh grafts retain viable fibrocytes following implantation and that these cells, albeit abnormal, are capable of proliferation and elaboration of ground substance and collagen which are essential to the maintenance of valve integrity and function (*Figure 3.6*). Viable cells have never been present in those areas of the valve where stretching, thinning and attenuation of the leaflets occurred. Furthermore valves prepared by severe techniques such as exposure to ethylene oxide or beta-propiolactone sterilization, irradiation, freezing and freeze-drying were found to develop clinically significant regurgitation at a rate of 10 per cent/year or more with the acellular valve leaflets becoming focally thinned, fenestrated or ruptured.

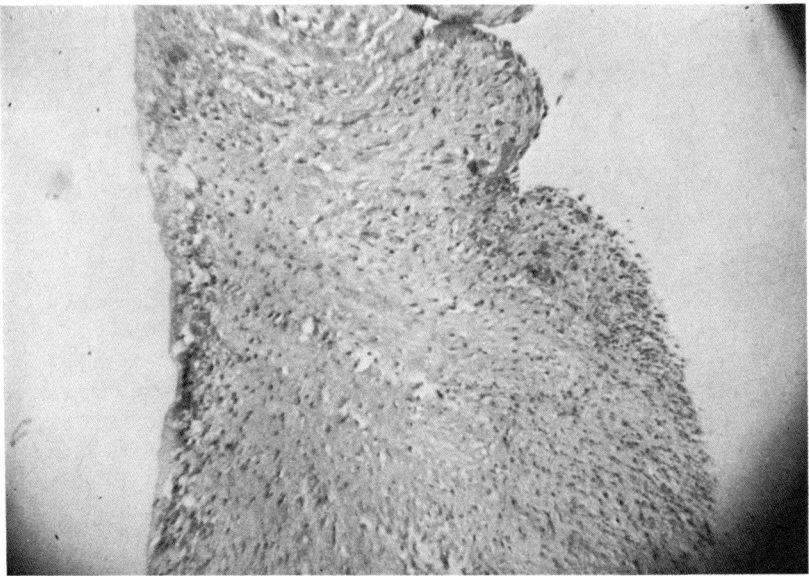

Figure 3.6 Microscopic appearance of a cusp from a fresh aortic allograft valve. The cusp contains viable fibrocytes. Haematoxylin and eosin stain × 50, reduced by $\frac{1}{3}$ in printing

   The failure of valves treated by these traumatic techniques was accompanied by a growing realization of the inadequacy of the method used for 'fresh' valve preparation. Between January 1967 and March 1970, over 500 fresh aortic allograft valves were removed from human donors under sterile conditions and stored in solutions containing penicillin (100 units/ml), streptomycin (100 μg/ml) and amphotericin (0.25 μg/ml) at 4 °C for two to five days prior to use. In all, 237 of these allograft valves were implanted clinically. At three years of follow-up this series revealed an incidence of tissue failure of 12.2 per cent and an incidence of valve related mortality of 1.3 per cent. The incidence of infective endocarditis was 4.2 per cent with an associated mortality of 3.8 per cent[4]. Thus, methods of sterilization and storage were sought which would maintain valve viability and, at the same time, solve the following significant problems:

(1) the inability to ensure sterility of the valves as evidenced by a persistent incidence of infective endocarditis;
(2) the small, but troublesome incidence of tissue failure attributed either to preparation techniques, *in vivo* haemodynamic trauma and/or a chronic rejection phenomenon;
(3) the significant loss of valves due to 'storage death' which thus precluded the establishment of a 'valve bank' and ready availability;
(4) the logistically difficult and laborious technique of sterile valve procurement.

   In late 1969, a technique of surface sterilization of valves using formalin vapour was tried. It was felt that this method would be effective against surface contamination occurring during procurement and, at the same time, kill only the superficial endothelial cell layer of the valve which was known to be destroyed, in any case, by the current methods of handling and storage. An experimental series of 35 canine aortic allograft valves sterilized in this manner, were successfully implanted in the mitral position. However, clinical results revealed this method to be difficult, not absolutely reliable and to cause extensive cell death with concomitant tissue deterioration and valve failure. Of the 19 valves implanted clinically, four failed in less than two years, two became infected and five patients died[11].

   In comtemplating other reliable methods of sterilization, the use of *in vitro* antibiotics seemed the most logical remaining course. Antibiotic sterilization was being simultaneously employed by Barratt-Boyes'[15], Mohri's[42] and Bolooki's[21] groups. The concentrations of the antibiotics used were high and while efficacious for sterility, these methods consistently yielded non-viable valves. Our first successful method of antibiotic sterilization evolved by early 1970 and consisted of non-sterile procurement and euthermic (37 °C) incubation of the valves in tissue culture solutions containing physiological doses of selected antibiotics. A wide range of antibiotics was examined, and on the basis of their effectiveness against the types of contaminant micro-organisms most commonly encountered, lincomycin* and gentamicin* were chosen. Their therapeutic index was found to lie between 10 and 150 μg/ml, and the optimal concentration for maintenance of good cell viability was determined by tissue culture to be

*Lincomycin,. Upjohn Co., Kalamazoo, Michigan
*Gentamicin,Schering Corp., Kenilworth, New Jersey

50 μg/ml. This technique was used with 134 allograft valves, and the results revealed an unacceptable level of contamination due to the persistence of significant numbers of resistant bacteria. The antibiotic solution was, therefore, modified to include kanamycin*, colistimethate* and amphotericin B*, and the final formula of the solution is described in *Table 3.1*. Of the 170 human aortic valves subjected to this method, 143 (84.5 per cent) were effectively sterilized.

TABLE 3.1
Allograft antibiotic sterilization solution†

Colistimethate	25 μg/ml
Gentamicin	25 μg/ml
Kanamycin	75 μg/ml
Lincomycin	250 μg/ml

†Contained in TC-199 HEPES buffer with
glutamine and fetal calf serum

Thirteen of the 27 contaminated valves were found to be resistant to all anti-biotics. The persistence of an acceptable degree of viability was documented by *in vitro* tissue culture and histological evaluation of 26 similarly treated canine aortic valve implants examined at the time of sacrifice of the animals (*Figure 3.7*). The experimental success of this technique led to its clinical application in March 1970. Between March 1970 and October 1971, 181 patients received aortic allograft valves sterilized by this method. Although consistent positive tissue cultures from implanted valves were difficult to obtain, the clinical results with this valve were good[6,13].

Subsequent analysis of the five years' experience (1967 to 1972) with 368 patients receiving the 'viable' aortic allograft valve and a comparison of these patients with a retrospectively matched series of 369 patients receiving Starr–Edwards prostheses showed the allograft valve to have a slight advantage in terms of actuarial survival (*Figure 3.8*). While only 1.5 per cent of the deaths in this allograft series were directly related to tissue failure, the incidence of murmurs and re-operation due to tissue failure was significant[5,11], making it far from the ideal valve replacement.

Protocols were thus established for the re-evaluation of the selection of anti-biotics. Their bactericidal rates against representative bacteria were determined relative to antibiotic concentration and combination and to temperature and duration of exposure, and these were then evaluated on the basis of their effect on fibroblast viability. Four representative bacteria were chosen on account of the frequency of their appearance in the more than 800 valves that had been procured over the previous five years. These included *Escherichia coli, Klebsiella pneumoniae, Streptococcus viridans*, and *Enterococcus*. Consideration was given to more than 15 commonly used antibiotic agents. Their spectrum of activity and mechanism of action were examined and those agents that did not require cell wall formation or organism growth to effect a rapid and irreversible bacteri-cidal effect were given prime consideration. The following antibiotics were chosen for this study; colistimethate, gentamicin, kanamycin and lincomycin. Cell densities of 5×10^4 and 5×10^6 organisms/ml were tested against the

*Kanamycin, Bristol Myers Co., Syracuse, New York
 Colistimethate, Warner Chilcott, Morris Plains, New Jersey
 Amphotericin B, Squibb Laboratories, Princeton, New Jersey

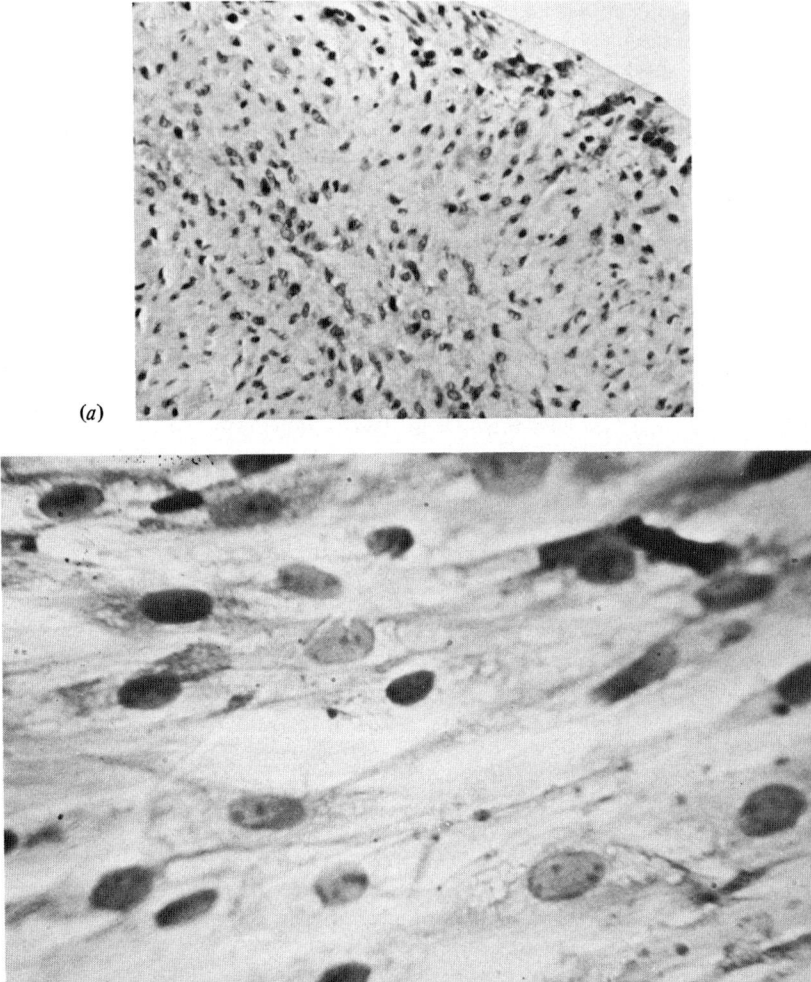

Figure 3.7 Microscopy of antibiotic sterilized canine aortic allograft valve. The histology of a cusp removed from the animal one month following implantation shows persistence of an acceptable degree of viability (*a*). Haematoxylin and eosin stain × 100, reduced by $\frac{1}{3}$ in printing. Tissue culture of a similarly treated canine aortic valve cusp shows tissue viability on microscopical examination (*b*). Methylene Blue × 150, reduced by $\frac{1}{3}$ in printing

single antibiotics, as well as a combination of antibiotics in concentrations ranging from 25 to 200 µg/ml. The results of this study revealed the chosen antibiotics and concentration range to be effective in eradicating the respective bacteria and this was found to be most rapidly accomplished after incubation at 37 °C for 24 h. Antibiotic tissue toxicity was examined using 11 human aortic valves providing 82 tissue specimens. Viability was assessed by comparing pre- and post-treatment tissue culture following exposure to antibiotic concentrations ranging serially from 50 to 1500 µg/ml. The maximum antibiotic concentrations

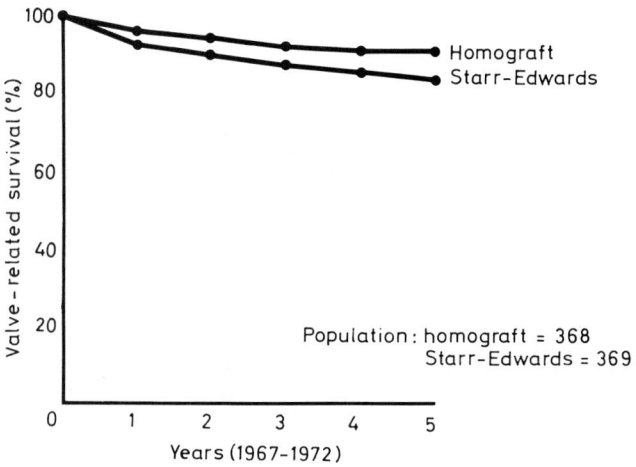

Figure 3.8 Actuarial survival rate curves for two retrospectively matched series of patients with 'viable' aortic allografts (368) and Starr–Edwards prostheses (369), both followed-up for a period of five years. (Reproduced as *Figure 3.5*)

In vitro–in vivo triple cusp preparation

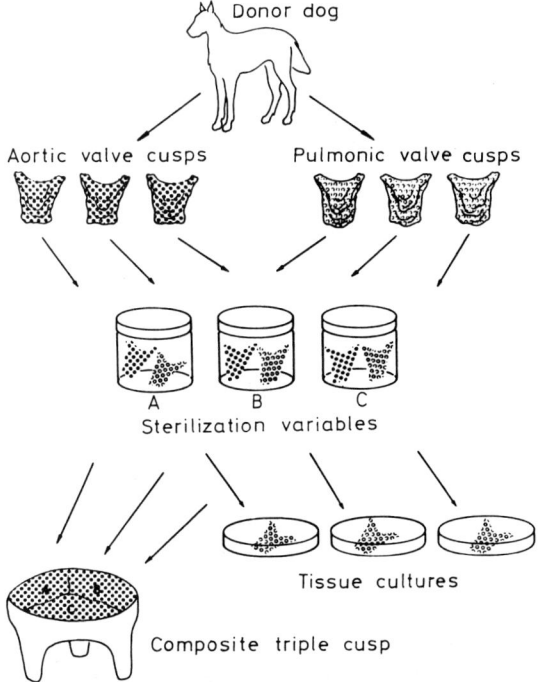

Figure 3.9 Composite triple cusp valve. Experimental chimera for evaluating the effect of different antibiotic sterilization techniques on allograft valve viability

tolerated without loss of fibroblasts was thus determined. The *in vivo* effect of the antibiotic concentration, incubation temperature and duration of exposure on valve viability was examined using the triple cusp valve preparation (*Figure 3.9*). Canine aortic valves were procured under sterile conditions and carefully divided along the commissures into their three component cusps. Each cusp was then sterilized in a different manner with respect to one of the variables of antibiotic concentration, incubation temperature and of duration of incubation. Following sterilization, the three cusps were then reconstructed into a composite valve by mounting them together onto a support frame. These composite valves were implanted in the mitral position of 35 dogs and observed for periods of time from one to three months. Viability following implantation was evaluated by tissue culture and histological sections of each aortic valve cusp. The results indicated that of the four antibiotics tested, colistimethate was the most toxic. The remaining three antibiotics all exhibited similar cytocidal effects. The sterilization solution described in *Table 3.1* is the result of correlating these data[7]. Of the 129 human aortic valves successfully sterilized using this technique, all were seen to experience a reduction in viability by less than 15 per cent as compared to pre-sterilization controls. It was believed that the implantation of valves containing a higher percentage of viable fibroblasts would aid in reducing the incidence of valve tissue failure.

Sterility testing

Examination of the five-year clinical series had also revealed a distressingly persistent occurrence of infection secondary to valve contamination. Four cases of infection (3 per cent) due to implantation of valves contaminated after sterilization, were reported. Furthermore, it was found that, in the presence of antibiotics, some organisms would remain viable but dormant on the valve and persist undetected because the technique of bacteriological and mycological control of the valves used in this series involved culturing only the valve-containing solution. The various methods of bacteriological control were examined and the final technique was reorganized after the standard method of Millipore filtration, as described by the US Pharmacopeia and required by the US Food and Drug Administration, for the commercial preparation of sterile solutions. As amended, this method includes filtration of all valve preparation solutions including a piece of minced pulmonic valve tissue which has accompanied the valve through all preparation steps. More than 364 valves have been submitted to this procedure and in no instance has a contaminant been found in the valve or valve solution when culture of the filter was negative. Even more important is the fact that none of the patients receiving valves tested with these techniques has suffered from infection.

Long-term storage of the aortic allograft valve

The problem of developing a method of long-term storage that would increase the viable lifetime of the valve beyond two to five days and thereby allow for the establishment of a valve bank capable of maintaining an adequate clinical supply has been less easily met. Early efforts to attain this objective were sought in the area of organ culture or hypothermic (4 °C to 10 °C) storage with augmentation of the storage solution (TC 199 Hanks base salts)* by the addition of fetal calf serum* and glutamine*. The results of these efforts served to prolong the storage interval of fresh tissue to the extent that viable cells were demonstrated four to seven weeks following procurement. In spite of this enhancement, however, viability was found to decrease steadily over this interval with a reduction of 23 per cent after one week of storage at 10 °C and with only 25 to 33 per cent of cells remaining viable at the end of seven weeks. Insofar as bacteriological control techniques required three weeks for determination of valve sterility, the time available for use of the valve (one to four weeks) was not sufficient to establish functional reserves.

The success of cryopreservation techniques is well documented in the transplantation literature. Functionally competent cells such as sperm[45], white blood cells[1], red blood cells[36] and bone marrow cells[35] have been preserved at −196 °C for extended periods of time without loss of vital function[31,32,33,34]. More complex systems such as skin and cornea were also found to withstand freeze storage without substantial loss of viability and successful transplantation[22,31]. A series of studies were thus designed to examine all aspects of a freezing technique including the freezing media, the type, concentration, equilibration and re-equilibration of cryophilactic agents and the freezing and thawing velocity.

The protection afforded by penetrating, hydrophilic, non-electrolytes such as glycerol, glucose and dimethylsulphoxide (DMSO) is well documented[39]. It is important that the cryoprotectant freely penetrates the cell and is not toxic in the concentrations necessary for cellular protection. In so doing, these agents guard against the formation of ice crystals and changes in intracellular volume concentrations, both of which have deleterious intra- and extracellular implications. Because of its positive influence on similar cell types, dimethylsulphoxide was chosen and its effective concentration was determined to be 7.5 per cent. Equilibration to this concentration and re-equilibration to isotonicity was established at 15 min for each process. The optimal freezing rate was determined to be 1 °C/min with thawing accomplished as rapidly as possible. Augmentation of the freezing solution (TC 199 Hanks base salts, glutamine and fetal calf serum) with Hepes buffer* served to maintain the pH of the freezing solution at 7.4 and to eliminate the previously observed increasing acidity of this solution following freezing. Although these techniques were determined to have the least deleterious effect on allograft viability, tissue culture of frozen valves has continued to reveal a 40–60 per cent reduction in the number of viable fibroblasts following freezing. Thirty-three patients have received valves prepared by this method and the results at three years' follow-up were comparable to those obtained with the fresh allograft valve. The final series of allograft valves implanted at our centre were these antibiotic sterilized and frozen valves.

Allograft rejection

Another aspect in the development of a technique for establishing the human aortic valve allograft has been the question of the presence of an immunologically induced process of tissue deterioration. Several studies have been undertaken to

*Grand Island Biological Co., Oakland, California

detect the presence of allograft valve rejection. Mohri *et al.*[41] examined the allograft antigenicity in both sensitized and non-sensitized dogs and found no differences in the two groups. Baue, Donawick and Blakemore[17] observed accelerated rejection in cusps placed in subcutaneous pockets of sensitized and non-sensitized animals, but found no differences when the grafts were implanted in the pulmonary valve area. Lower, Stofer and Shumway[37] compared ortho-topic pulmonic valve autografts with allografts and found the autografts to be thickened but otherwise normal. A significantly higher rate of valve survival was found by Kwong, Paton and Hill[33] in animals which were treated with Imuran.

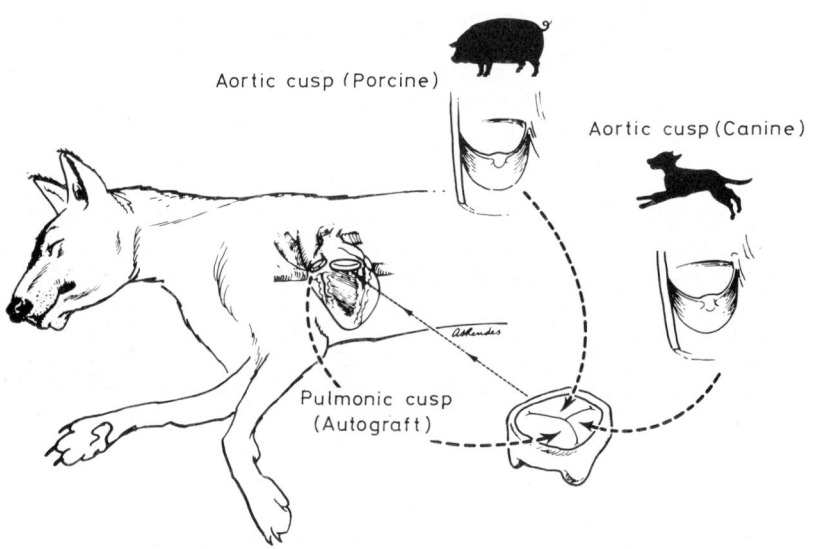

Figure 3.10 Composite triple cusp valve. Experimental chimera for evaluating the role of mechanical trauma and rejection reaction on the viability of the allograft aortic valve. (Reproduced from Buch, W. S. *et al.*[24], by courtesy of *Journal of thoracic and cardiovascular Surgery*)

Ongoing morphological studies of fresh allografts from our series have reveal-ed significant structural alterations, some of which, according to Kosek *et al.*[32], are suggestive of a host rejection reaction. However, the effects of preparation techniques, surgical trauma, stent mounting and changed haemodynamic stress, particularly for valves inserted into the mitral position, could not be disregarded when interpreting the observed response. In an effort to clarify this issue, we developed, in early 1970, an experimental chimera. It consisted of a stented composite triple cusp valve formed with one cusp each from a canine aortic allograft, a porcine aortic xenograft and a pulmonic autograft (*Figures 3.10* and *3.11*). Each cusp was treated in an identical manner with regard to preparation, handling and haemodynamic environment, and thus represented a different antigenic challenge to the host. These composite valves were implanted in the mitral position of 20 dogs which were sacrificed at intervals ranging from five days to one year post-operatively. The allograft cusps exhibited general fibro-plasia with thickening and neocollagen formation, simultaneous with endothelial

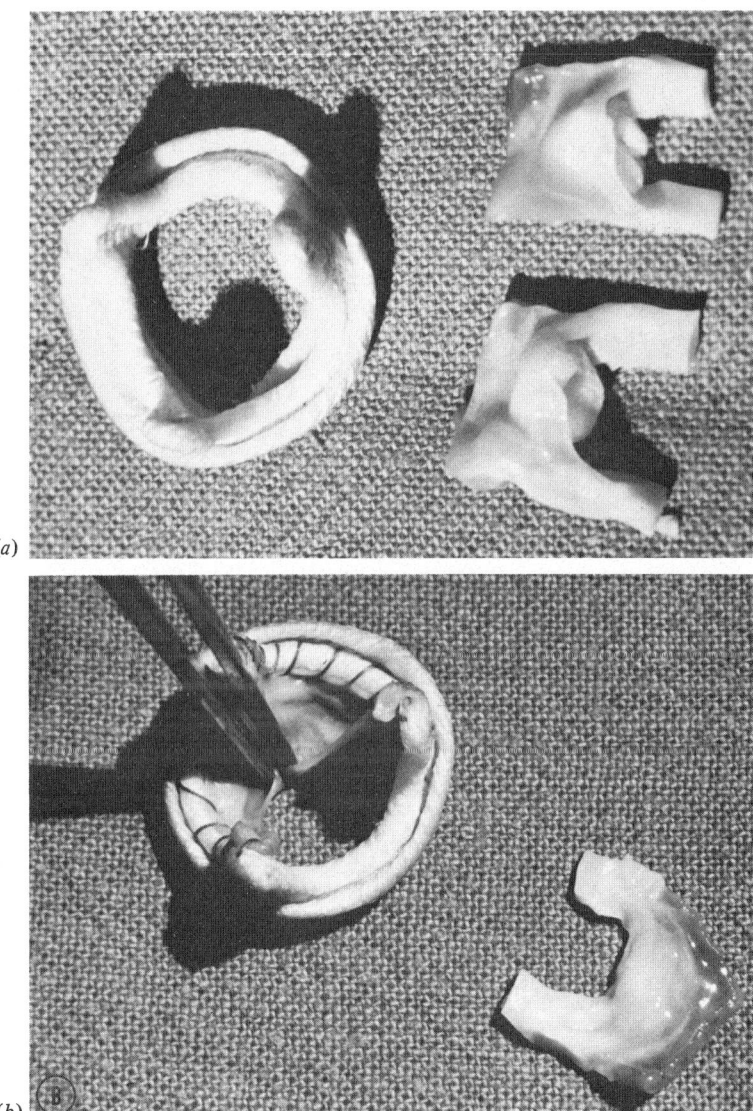

Figure 3.11 Construction of the composite triple cusp valve. The cloth-covered metal support frame is shown together with a canine aortic allograft cusp and a porcine aortic xenograft cusp prior to mounting (*a*). The two cusps have been attached to the support frame and held together with a forceps. An autogeneic pulmonary valve cusp was prepared to complete the experimental chimera (*b*). (Reproduced as *Figure 3.10*)

destruction, acellularity, fibroblastic dysfunction and occasional necrosis. This initial exuberant fibroplasia was also observed in both the autograft and xenograft cusps, but to a lesser extent in the former and a greater one in the latter. Since the distortion of connective tissue is known to stimulate collagen synthesis, this reaction was attributed to the abnormal haemodynamic forces encountered in the mitral position. However, unlike the autograft, which represents a non-immunologic control, both the allograft and the xenograft cusps exhibited degenerative changes suggesting rejection. These alterations were much less severe in the allograft. Endothelial destruction was observed in both grafts, but contrary to the xenograft, the allograft showed only superficial accellularity, fibroblastic destruction and rare host round cell infiltration (*Figure 3.12*).

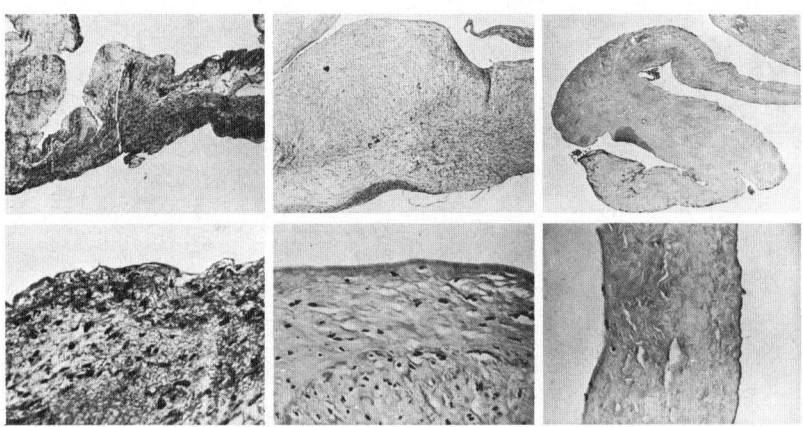

Figure 3.12 Histology of leaflets from a composite valve examined one year following insertion in the canine mitral position. From left: the autograft cusp shows hyperplasia with a normal endothelium; the allograft cusp shows hyperplasia with fibroblastic dysplasia and distorted collagen fibres and; the xenograft cusp shows complete acellularity (top row magnification × 63, reduced by $\frac{1}{3}$ in printing; bottom row magnification × 1000, reduced by $\frac{1}{3}$ in printing). (Reproduced as *Figure 3.10*)

These changes were in every way similar to those occurring in the allografts implanted in humans. The fact that these changes may represent low-grade rejection is exemplified by their close similarity to valves of rejected whole heart allografts[24]. Experiments designed to seek a method of minimizing the extent of this immunological response were centred around short- and long-term post-operative immunosuppressive therapy using Solu-Medrol* and Imuran*. While difficulty was experienced in obtaining a significant number of surviving animals due to a high rate of death from infection, histological examination of specimens revealed no significant difference in the extent of host round cell infiltration and fibroblastic destruction between treated and untreated animals. This fact coupled with the well-known potential clinical complications of immunosuppressive treatment caused us to reject this technique as a possible solution to allograft antigenicity. Because of the disastrous whole organ effect of ABO incompatibility, we did however attempt to match valve recipient patients with respect to this parameter during the later phases of the allograft implantation programme.

To determine the magnitude and to quantitate the precise extent to which preparation and storage techniques, stent mounting, altered haemodynamic stress and host immunological response may contribute to tissue deterioration

*Solu-Medrol, Upjohn Co., Kalamazoo, Michigan
Imuran, Burroughs Wellcome Co., Research Triangle Park, North Carolina

and thus affect the long-term function of the fresh aortic allograft valve, was difficult to assess and even more difficult to control. The prudent avoidance of major ABO group incompatibilities between donor and host and the continual development of more refined and less traumatic methods of tissue preparation was considered to have perhaps only prolonged the inevitable failure of many of these fresh tissue valves. These factors in combination with the ever-present logistical difficulties of procuring human tissue and storing an adequate supply of valves in the viable state led us, as well as other investigators earlier on, to seek alternative valve sources.

THE FORMALDEHYDE PRESERVED XENOGRAFT

The xenograft valve offered an attractive alternative to the allograft because of the ease of procuring an adequate number of valves of required sizes and good quality. In addition, the already applied clinical technique of treating these valves with a potent chemical agent which served to both sterilize and render the valve non-viable while preserving the natural cell architecture of the tissue promised to solve other problems associated with the fresh allograft. The original clinical experiences with this valve belong to Binet *et al.*[20] who used mercurial salts to sterilize the xenograft and to O'Brien and Clarebrough[44] who employed a 4 per cent buffered formaldehyde solution. Our experience was begun in 1968 with the experimental implantation of some 115 whole and composite triple cusp porcine aortic valve xenografts treated with 4 per cent buffered formaldehyde following the method of O'Brien and Clarebrough[44]. Although initial results with 32 valves implanted clinically were excellent, formalin fixation by

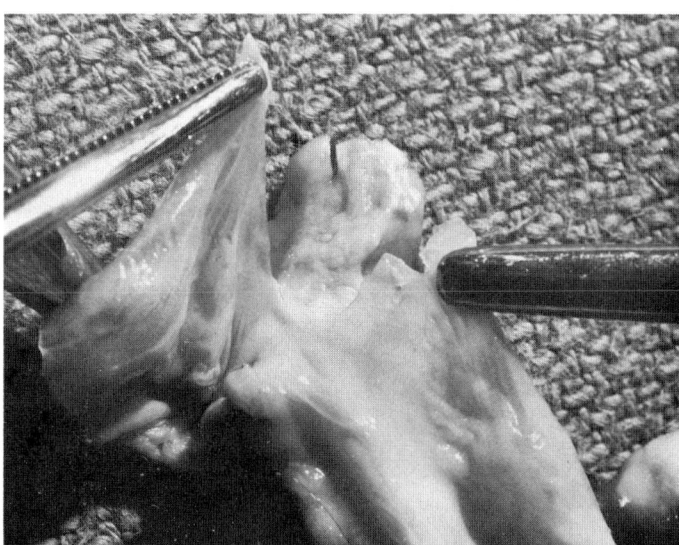

Figure 3.13 Macroscopic appearance of a xenograft aortic valve treated with formaldehyde. The deterioration of tissue is shown with thinning and tearing of the cusps near to a commissure. (Reproduced from Buch, W. S. *et al.*[23], by courtesy of *Journal of thoracic and cardiovascular Surgery*)

cross-linking of valve collagen was found to be reversed *in vivo* and to result in valve deterioration and incompetence with stretching, thinning and tearing of the leaflets (*Figure 3.13*). The mechanism of failure resulting from this reversible binding of formalin with valve protein was felt to be a combination of mechanical disruption of the deteriorated collagen and immunological rejection due to the presence of unbound, antigenically active proteins. Microscopically, the specimens examined were totally acellular. Macrophage activity was profound,

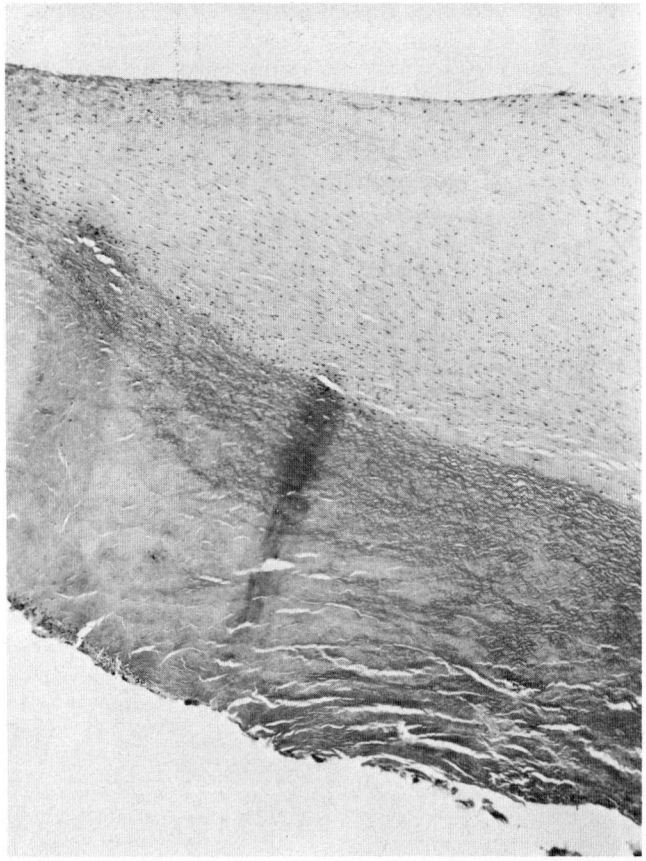

Figure 3.14 Microscopy of a cusp from a formaldehyde treated xenograft aortic valve. The host sheath along the base of the leaflet is seen. Haematoxylin and eosin stain × 50. (Reproduced from Angell, W. W., Buch, W. S. and Iben, A. B. 'Formalin preservation of porcine heterografts'. In *Biological Tissue in Heart Valve Replacement*. Ed. by M. I. Ionescu, D. N. Ross and G. H. Wooler, pp. 543–552. London; Butterworths (1972)

and collagen was seen to be disordered, fibrillar and vacuolated. Although a superficial sheath of host tissue was present at the base of most leaflets, it never extended over more than 1/3 of the cusp and did not appear to be repopulating the native collagen (*Figure 3.14*). This diffuse deterioration was found to occur in 60 per cent of the valves at two years' follow-up[23] and, by six years, all 32 valves implanted had failed.

THE GLUTARALDEHYDE PRESERVED XENOGRAFT

Simultaneous with the experimental and clinical application of the formaldehyde treated xenograft, the tanning properties of glutaraldehyde were also
examined. Thirty-four porcine aortic xenograft valves were treated with buffered
glutaraldehyde solutions of varying concentrations from 0.5–10 per cent and
were implanted in the mitral position of dogs. Histological examination of these
xenografts revealed them to be qualitatively quite similar to the formalin treated
valves. There was infiltration of macrophages onto the cusp surfaces of all
specimens although more superficial and quantitatively less prominent than in
the formalin treated tissue. These similarities and the observed late failure of
many of the formalin valves led to the cautious clinical application, during 1970,
of six porcine xenografts, sterilized and preserved with 0.5 per cent buffered
glutaraldehyde. Careful follow-up of these six patients over the next two and a
half years revealed excellent function with no evidence of valve failure and, in
1972, the use of this valve preparation was enthusiastically increased. At the
same time, studies were begun in order both to define the complex and poorly
described chemistry of glutaraldehyde and its reactions with tissue proteins and
to improve the haemodynamics of, and reduce the physical stress on, the stent
mounted valve.

The anatomic stent

The functional significance of recreating or maintaining the natural anatomic
configuration of the valve tissue became evident early in the experience with
tissue valves. The double, as opposed to the single, suture line technique for
insertion of 'free' valves in the aortic root of experimental animals improved the
overall results. Those valves anatomically resuspended as 'free grafts' produced
markedly improved haemodynamic results, as well as a greater longevity of
function when compared with valves mounted in a rigid symmetrical stent
which produced sub-optimal central coaptation, poor lateral leaflet alignment
and general annular distortion. The effect of deforming the aortic allograft
resulted in a significant incidence of leaflet prolapse, central regurgitation and
cusp disruption along with dehiscence of the valve from the support ring at the
inflow and outflow attachments due to the presence of abnormal physical stress
at these points (*Figure 3.15*).
  Precise anatomic reconfiguration can be accomplished either by employing a
'free graft' in the aortic position inserted with a specialized technique which is
difficult, lengthy and thus compromising in the hands of the inexperienced, or
by mounting the valve onto an asymmetrical stent produced from moulds of the
naturally occurring aortic root. The latter was sought as a solution. Some 640
porcine aortic valves were measured and an attempt was made to analyse mathe-
matically these data in order to devise a series of stents calculated to fit the
greatest number of valves occurring in each of the 15 clinically used diameters.
However, configurations were found to be too variable for mathematical averag-
ing even when 38 different variables were measured. Castings were thus made of
the most frequently occurring and anatomically acceptable valves in each size
which had a regular annulus and symmetrical cusps. This has resulted in a number
of anatomically varied stents for each of the 15 annulus sizes, and made available

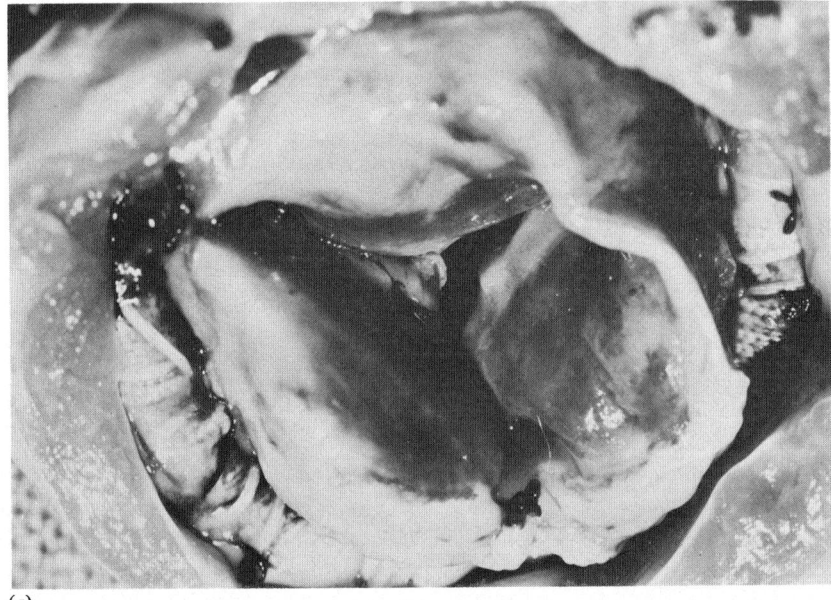

(*a*)

Disparity between valve and ring

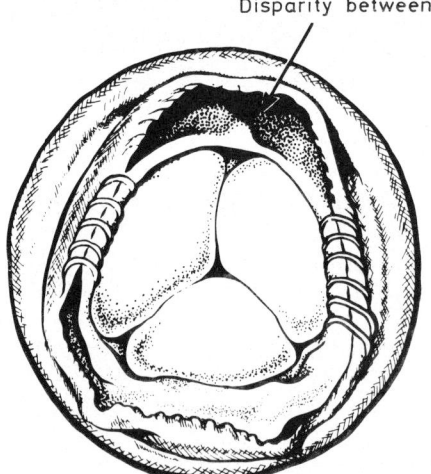

(*b*)

Figure 3.15 (*a*) Aortic allograft valve examined at seven months following implantation. The valve became detached from the support frame along the inflow orifice. (*b*) Drawing demonstrating the cause and mechanism of dehiscence. (Reproduced as *Figure 3.5*)

more than 70 stents to provide natural support of the porcine aortic root (*Figure 3.16*). The use of the anatomic design and the fabrication of these stents from Delrin plastic* made it possible to maintain proper cusp alignment during mounting and thus aid in preserving the natural opening and closing character- istics of the valve leaflets. When compared in an accelerated pulse duplicator

*Dupont, T. M., Wilmington, Delaware

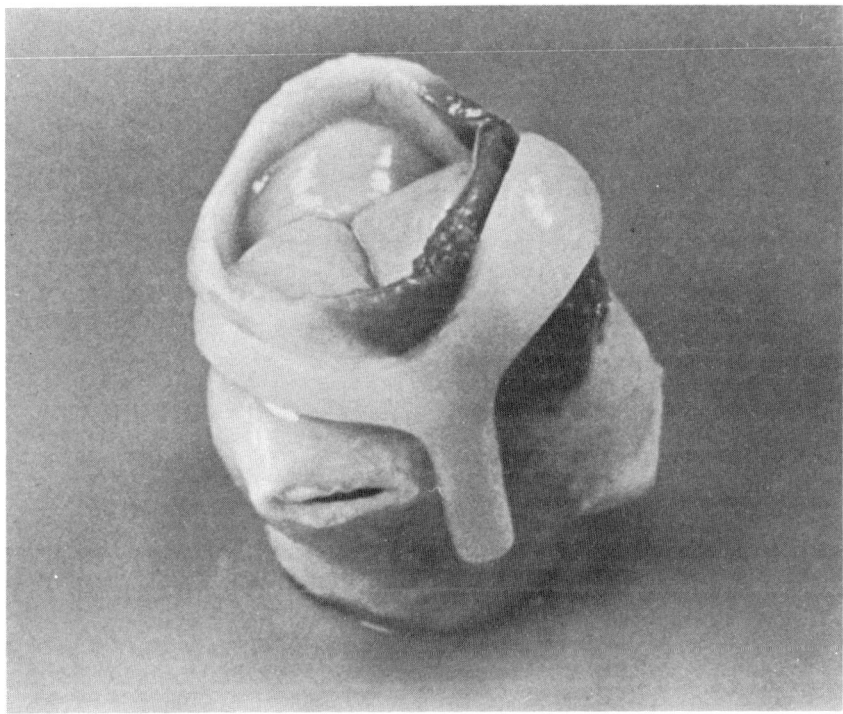

Figure 3.16   The Angell-Shiley flexible anatomic support frame positioned over a porcine aortic valve. (Reproduced as *Figure 3.5*)

with valves mounted on rigid symmetrical metal support frames, the anatomically supported xenograft was found to be effective in reducing abnormal stress on the tissue thereby preventing dehiscence of the valve from the stent as well as cusp distortion or perforation.

Glutaraldehyde chemistry

While the successful use of glutaraldehyde over the past eight years to sterilize and stabilize heart valve connective tissue has been widely recognized, the chemistry of its solutions, its stabilizing reactions with connective tissue proteins and its effect on the antigenicity of transplanted connective tissue have been poorly described.

Although the glutaraldehyde monomer (*Figure 3.17*) is a simple dialdehyde, its tendency to polymerize in solution makes the understanding of its interactions with tissue proteins complex. Polymerization of monomeric glutaraldehyde is known to occur through different reactions. One of them is by cyclic hydration to form hemiacetal monomeric glutaraldehyde. These cyclic hemiacetals then react by the formation of additional hemiacetal bonds to form polymeric glutar-aldehyde (*Figure 3.18a*). Beyond four monomer units, these polymer chains become insoluble in aqueous solution and reversal is accomplished only by heating or increasing the acidity. A second one is by interactions of monomeric

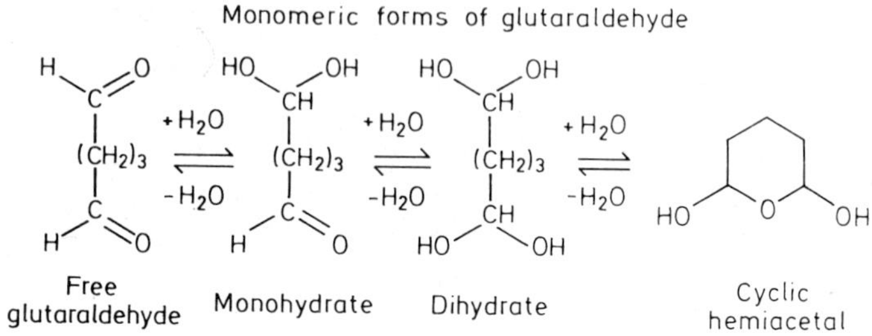

Monomeric forms of glutaraldehyde

Free glutaraldehyde   Monohydrate   Dihydrate   Cyclic hemiacetal

Figure 3.17   Monomeric forms of glutaraldehyde

(a)

(b)

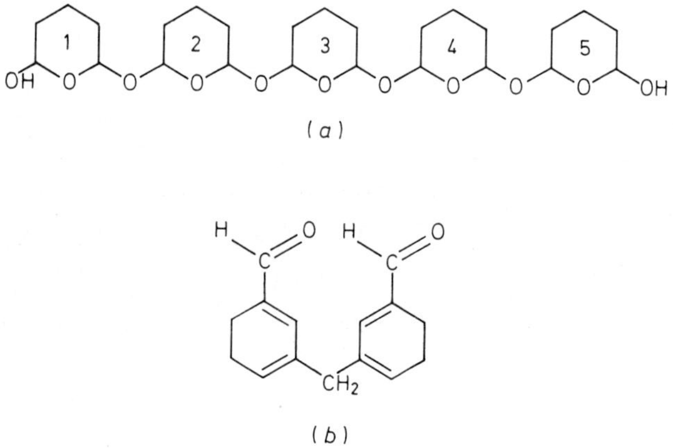

Figure 3.18   Polymeric forms of glutaraldehyde. (*a*) Hemiacetal polymeric glutaraldehyde; and (*b*) Aldol condensate of glutaraldehyde

glutaraldehyde to yield aldol condensates (*Figure 3.18b*). This reaction increases exponentially with increased pH, temperature and concentration. Aqueous solubility decreases with increasing molecular weight[46,47]. A third reaction takes place between hemiacetal and aldol condensate polymers to form higher molecular weight polymers. This occurs less frequently than the former two reactions.

Glutaraldehyde–protein interactions

Two basic reactions most likely account for the unique structural stability of connective tissue treated with glutaraldehyde[56]. The free aldehydes of monomeric and/or polymeric (aldol condensates or hydrated cyclic aldehydes) glutaraldehyde react with the primary amines of lysine, hydroxylysine or N-terminal amino acid residues present in the protein to form a Schiff base. The Schiff base is then reduced to form a secondary amine linkage which is extremely stable at physiological temperature and pH (*Figure 3.19*). The second type of stable glutaraldehyde–protein cross-link is the substituted pyridinium salt which is formed by the reaction between monomeric glutaraldehyde and a primary amine (*Figure 3.20*).

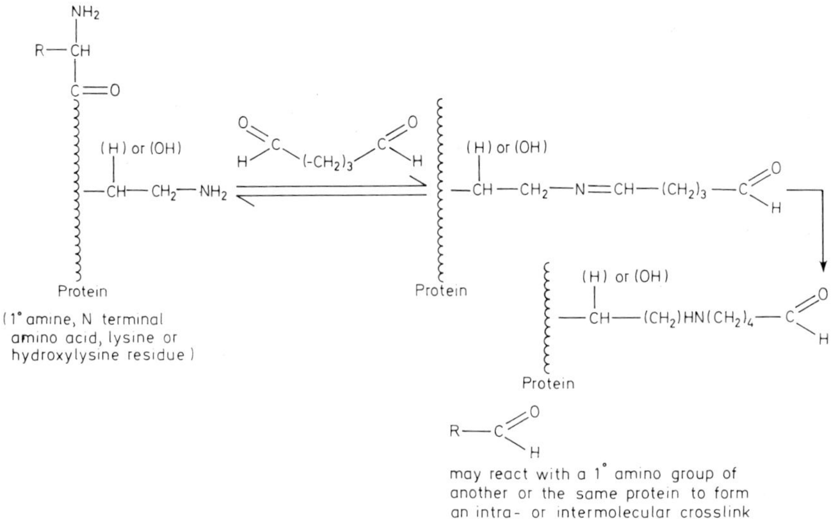

Figure 3.19 A secondary amine. (Reproduced as *Figure 3.5*)

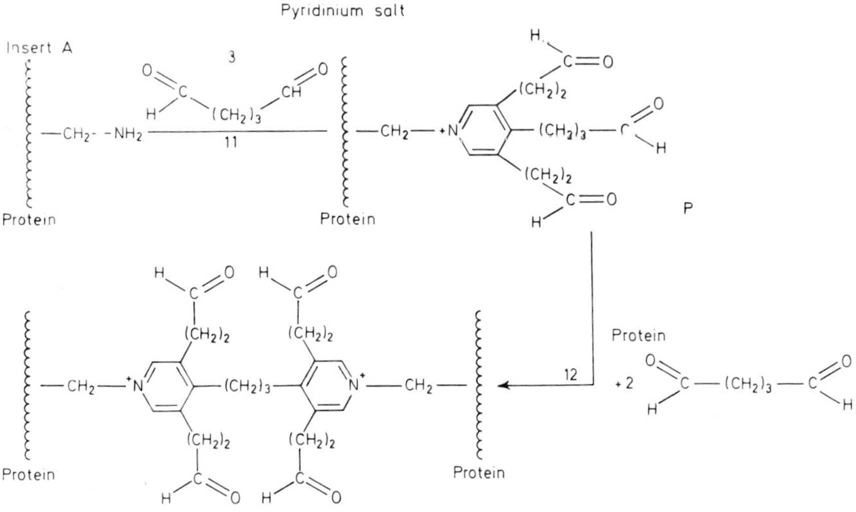

Figure 3.20 Substituted pyridinium salt. (Reproduced as *Figure 3.5*)

Flexibility of glutaraldehyde treated tissue

Preliminary experiments have shown that there is no difference in the flexibility of tissue samples exposed for prolonged periods of time to glutaraldehyde concentrations of 0.2, 0.5 and 0.67 per cent. However, under similar conditions, solutions with concentrations greater than 1 per cent glutaraldehyde produce grossly stiff valves with high gradients at low pressures. Initial studies measuring the temperature of tissue shrinkage which is proportional to the cross-link density indicate that the optimal glutaraldehyde concentration for achieving tissue thermal stability does not necessarily imply superior *in vivo* durability. This is evident from the proportionally higher thermal stability of tissue treated with a corresponding concentration of formaldehyde which has shown inferior *in vivo* durability when compared with the glutaraldehyde treated tissue.

Glutaraldehyde sterilizing ability and sterility testing

In addition to providing increased structural stability, glutaraldehyde has also proved to be an excellent sterilizing agent. In general, the efficacy of these solutions in killing bacterial, fungal and viral micro-organisms is a function of the glutaraldehyde concentration, monomer versus polymer composition, temperature and time of exposure and the pH. The sterilizing ability of glutaraldehyde is improved as each of these parameters is increased[40]. The bactericidal action of glutaraldehyde on organisms present on valve surfaces is similar to its mechanism of tanning mammalian collagen. This effect results from the reaction of free aldehyde groups with the primary amino acid residues in the microorganism to form stable secondary amines which render the organism non-viable. In general, this reaction is most rapidly and completely effective against the bacterial vegetative forms and less effective against those organisms with high lipid content, thus more resistant cell walls such as the *Bacillus subtilis* spore and mycobacteria. The most difficult and perhaps the most important parameter to control in the sterilizing technique is that of glutaraldehyde polymerization. Excessive polymerization serves to reduce the number of active aldehyde groups, thereby effectively decreasing the concentration of the active sterilizing component. With the use of an initial, brief exposure to 5.0 per cent purified glutaraldehyde* followed by storage in a 0.5 per cent solution, we have had only 13 positive cultures in the first 1000 clinically processed valves[50]. Re-exposure of these valves resulted in negative cultures, and in no instance are we aware of a positive culture at the time of surgery in the more than 273 valves which have been implanted in our experience.

As it is essential to obtain and guarantee absolute valve sterility following exposure to glutaraldehyde, it is necessary to have an adequate if not infallible technique of determining sterility. As mentioned earlier, it was not until O'Brien, who pioneered the work with formalin valves, suggested Millipore filtration of valve-containing solutions, that we were able to eliminate the problem of iatrogenic infection encountered with the fresh allografts. Millipore or membrane filtration of the valve solution with its macro-and microscopic particles, including minced tissue coupons, has the benefit of concentrating the viable organisms present both in the solution and attached to or embedded in tissue particles and also of removing all traces of inhibitory aqueous soluble bactericidal and bacteriostatic agents. The possibility that filtration of the solution alone was not representative, and that some organisms remained on the valve even after vigorous rinsing, was examined by comparing the results of culturing 50 whole valves with cultures of just their solutions. We found that the solutions alone provided an excellent sample of any viable organisms present, and believe this to be the procedure of choice for the sterility assurance of commercially produced tissue valves.

*Shiley Laboratories, Inc., Irvine, California

Clinical results

Analysis of our clinical series is presented as actuarially calculated morbidity and mortality. The actuarial method followed that of Berkson and Gage[18] from the Mayo Clinic and the technique more recently reported by Anderson *et al.*[2] from the University of Oregon. The differences are as noted below:

(1) No patients were removed for cause.

(2) Patients were followed up to an adequate percentage (96.8 per cent) so that no significant effect was experienced by those lost to follow-up. All patients lost were treated as having experienced the same percentage of survival as the patients known to follow-up in that same interval.
   Note: Patients lost to follow-up are difficult to analyse. Anderson's group follows these patients for one half the subsequent interval and calls them alive at the end of that interval. As previously stated we minimize the effect of this by adequate follow-up in all groups. We found that approximately 10 per cent of patients who are lost for one year or less are alive when finally traced, and that 85 per cent of the patients lost for greater than one year are found to be dead. In order to be most impartial, we felt that those patients lost to follow-up should be counted as either dead or alive at the end of some interval. One half of the subsequent interval was, therefore, taken and the actuarial survival at that point was used to determine the percentage of patient mortality in the group lost to follow-up.

(3) All patient morbidity and mortality was classified as *known* valve-related, *presumed* valve-related or *non* valve-related. The reported *valve* related morbidity and mortality includes patients from both the *known* and *presumed* categories.

(4) All deaths within 30 days of surgery or related to events within the first 30 days were determined to be *operative* deaths.

(5) All sudden, unknown or unexplained deaths were *presumed* to be valve-related.

(6) All cerebral vascular accidents were *presumed* valve-related.

(7) All haemorrhages which occurred in patients treated with anticoagulants for the valve were *presumed* valve-related.

(8) All re-operations were determined to be *known* valve-related complications.

(9) All cases of infective endocarditis were *presumed* valve-related.

(10) Significant regurgitation or stenosis as determined by clinical and catheterization methods, were determined to be *known* valve-related complications.

(11) Questionable murmurs or haemodynamically insignificant regurgitation were termed *non* valve-related.

(12) Hepatitis was determined to be *non* valve-related.

Figures 3.21 and *3.22* show the five years' actuarial results obtained with the Angell–Shiley glutaraldehyde tanned xenograft implanted in 249 patients. The combined valve-related morbidity and mortality for the aortic and mitral groups is encouragingly low at 21 per cent and 18 per cent respectively (*Figure 3.21*). When both the aortic and mitral patient groups are combined, the valve-related mortality for the entire series is 13 per cent (*Figure 3.22*).

The significance of these results becomes more striking when they are compared to our experience with both the fresh aortic allograft and the Starr-

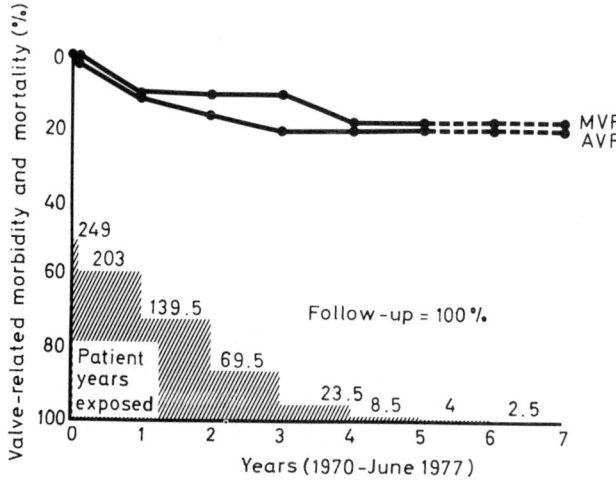

Figure 3.21 Actuarial presentation of valve related morbidity and mortality in patients having mitral valve replacement and aortic valve replacement with the Angell–Shiley glutaraldehyde treated xenograft. (Reproduced as *Figure 3.5*)

Edwards Model 1260 aortic and 6120 mitral prostheses over a similar follow-up interval of five years. With aortic valve replacement (*Figure 3.23*), the five-year combined valve-related morbidity and mortality associated with the fresh aortic allograft and the glutaraldehyde preserved xenograft are acceptable albeit statistically disparate. By contrast, the prosthetic valve curve shows that 49 per cent of patients with aortic valve replacement have experienced death or compli-

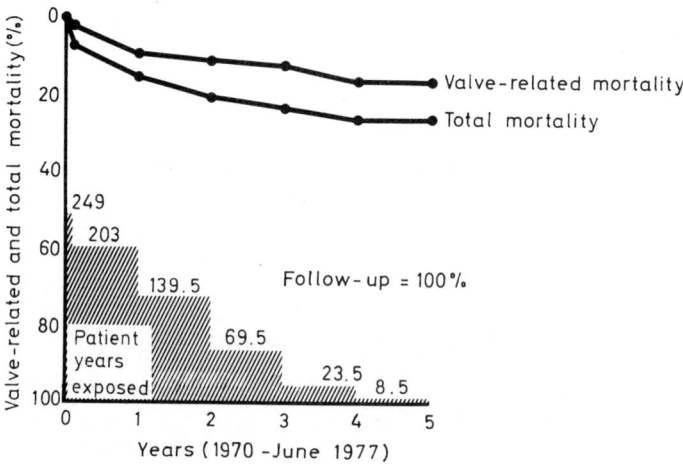

Figure 3.22 Actuarial presentation of both valve related mortality and total mortality in the combined groups of patients having aortic and mitral valve replacement with the Angell–Shiley glutaraldehyde treated xenograft. (Reproduced as *Figure 3.5*)

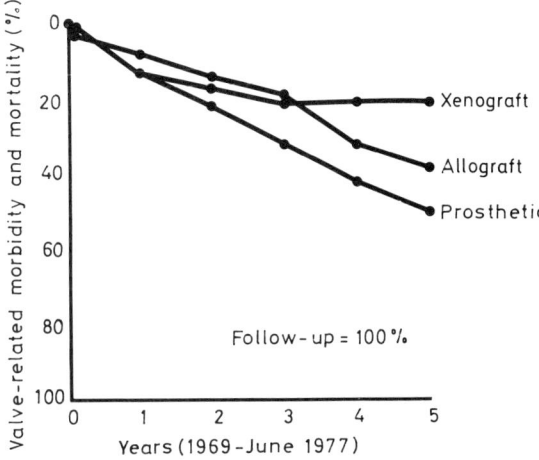

Figure 3.23 Actuarial curves for valve related morbidity and mortality in three groups of patients having aortic valve replacement with glutaraldehyde treated xenografts, fresh aortic allografts and mechanical prostheses respectively. (Reproduced as *Figure 3.5*)

cations related to the valve. A comparison of these three types of valve substitutes inserted in the mitral position shows the glutaraldehyde xenograft valve to be superior (*Figure 3.24*). When valve related mortality, including both patients with aortic and patients with mitral valve replacement, is compared between the xenograft, allograft and Starr–Edwards prosthesis series, there is no statistical difference (*Figure 3.25*).

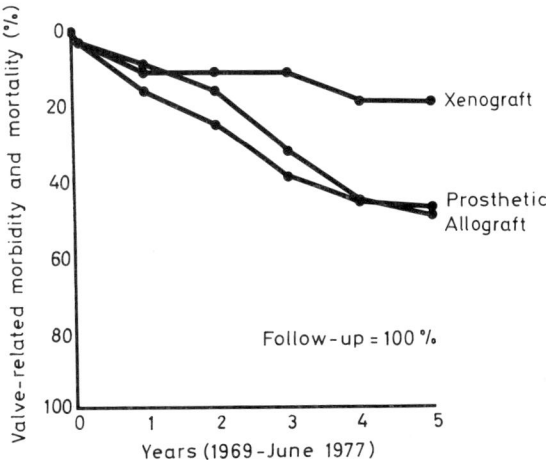

Figure 3.24 Actuarial curves for valve related morbidity and mortality in three groups of patients having mitral valve replacement with glutaraldehyde treated xenografts, fresh aortic allografts and mechanical prostheses respectively. (Reproduced as *Figure 3.5*)

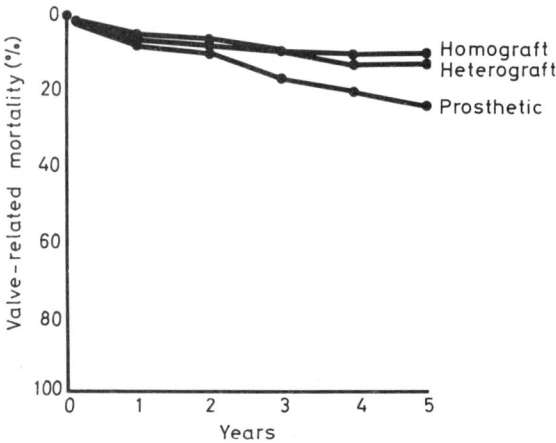

Figure 3.25 Actuarial curves for valve related mortality in three groups of patients having heart valve replacement with glutaraldehyde treated xenografts, fresh aortic allografts and mechanical prostheses respectively. The mitral valve replacement and the aortic valve replacement groups were combined for this calculation. (Reproduced as *Figure 3.5*)

Antigenicity and host reactivity

The morphology of glutaraldehyde treated tissue correlates well with the concept of a stabilized tissue of low antigenicity and reactivity. This is supported by light and electron microscopy, as well as by *in vivo* test systems which show a reduction in antigenicity by a factor of 100-fold when glutaraldehyde cross-linked tissue is compared with fresh tissue against bovine serum albumin (BSA) controls. The mechanism by which glutaraldehyde is thought to reduce connective tissue antigenicity is through conversion of tissue proteins into insoluble cross-linked structures with greatly enhanced resistance to proteolytic degradation and through masking of antigenic sites[53,54,55].

While not biologically inert, histology suggests that the magnitude of host reactivity to glutaraldehyde treated tissue is less than that observed in other types of tissue valves (*Figure 3.26*). These host cell responses are seen to be both beneficial and deleterious. Central fibrous replacement of a single cusp was observed in one valve removed at 27 months following implantation. However, in no instance has host replacement been of functional significance. By contrast, host sheathing is virtually always present as an overgrowth onto the cusp or aortic cuff (*Figure 3.27*). This is seen to form a pseudoendothelium over these otherwise irregular surfaces and, in addition, serves to anchor the valve suture line. The functional significance of this sheath, which is seen to extend 5-7 mm onto the cusp surface, is in its potential ability to reduce, to some degree, cusp flexibility and effective flow orifice during the first few months of implantation.

All of the valves, whether clinical or experimental, are also seen to have scattered, very small fibrinous thrombi. While most of them are invisible at light microscopy, they can be easily demonstrated by scanning electron microscopy (*Figures 3.28a* and *b*) as windrow-like deposits. In addition host macrophages are

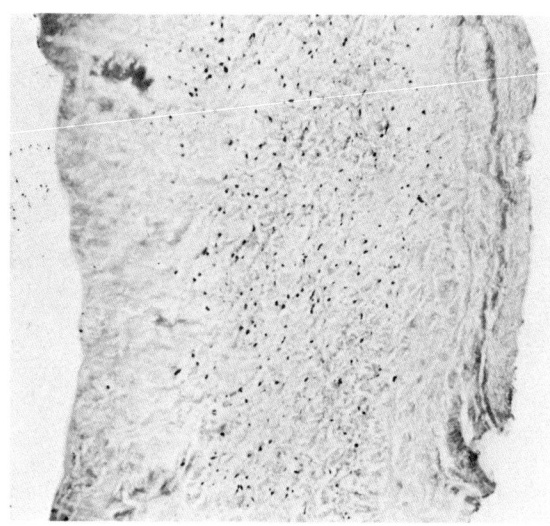

Figure 3.26 Microscopic appearance of a xenogeneic valve cusp treated with glutaraldehyde. There is evidence of low grade host reactivity. Haematoxylin and eosin stain × 50, reduced by 20 per cent in printing

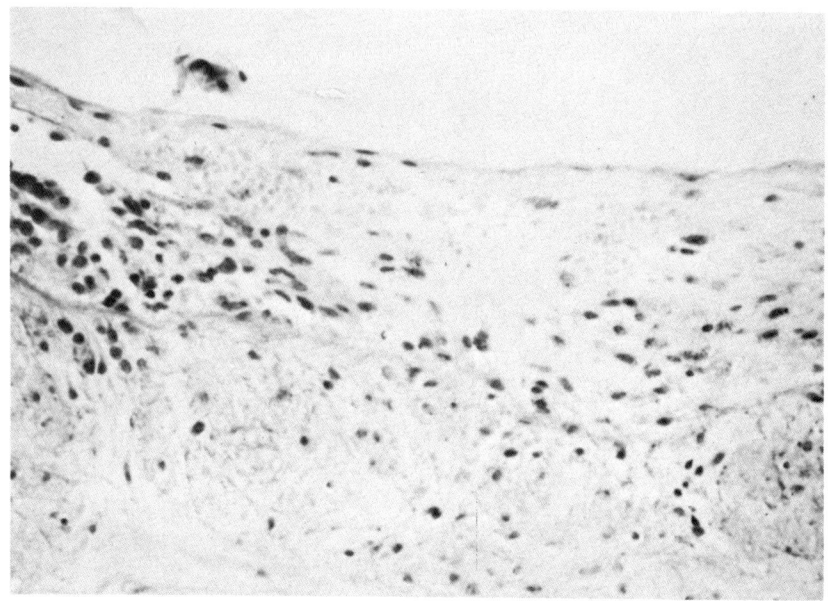

Figure 3.27 Microscopic aspect of the host sheath along the base of a glutaraldehyde treated porcine xenograft. Haematoxylin and eosin stain × 100, reduced by $\frac{1}{3}$ in printing

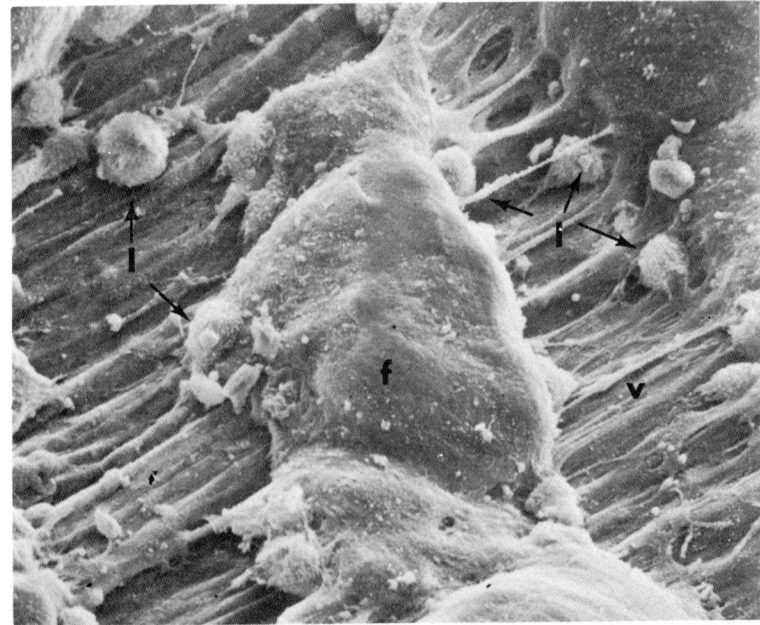

(a)

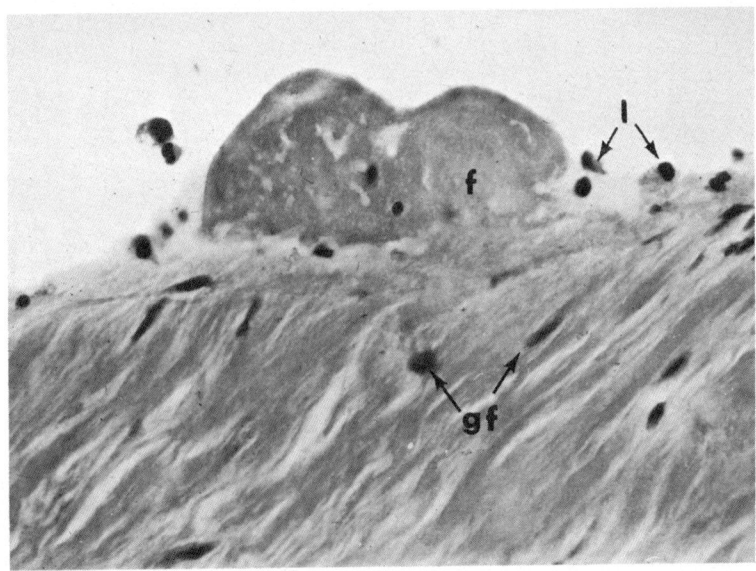

(b)

Figure 3.28 (a) Aortic surface of porcine aortic valve leaflet, glutaraldehyde fixed in orthotopic position in canine heart for one month. f = fibrin thrombi, v = ridge of valve intima,
  1 = leucocytes. Scanning EM × 400, haematoxylin and eosin stain
  (b) Same surface in cross-section. gf = glutaraldehyde fixed leaflet fibrocytes. Scanning
EM × 400, haematoxylin and eosin stain

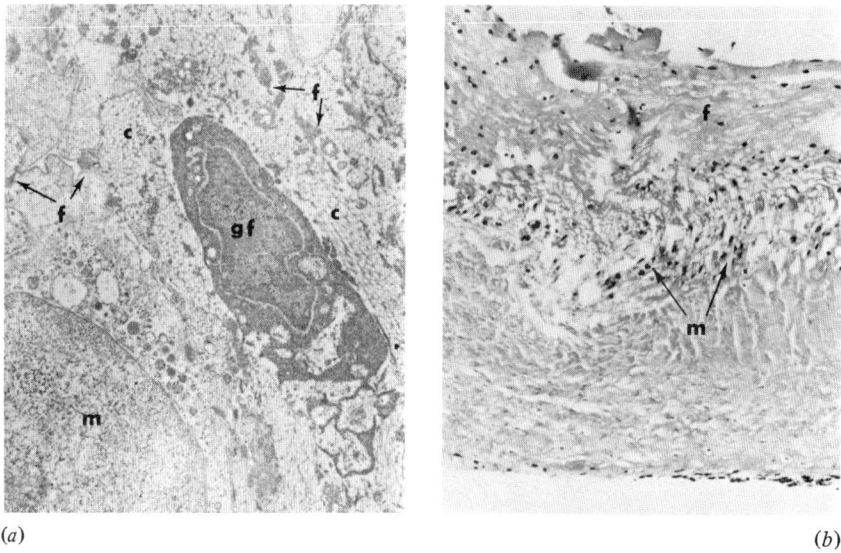

(a)   (b)

Figure 3.29 (*a*) Porcine aortic valve leaflet, glutaraldehyde fixed and in orthotopic position in canine heart for three months. Note host macrophage (m) at lower left partly encompassing glutaraldehyde fixed fibrocyte (gf), collagen (c) and fibrin (f). Transmitting EM × 400, haematoxylin and eosin stain, reduced by $\frac{1}{3}$ in printing
(*b*) Porcine aortic valve leaflet, glutaraldehyde fixed and in orthotopic position for nine months. Note thick fibrin layer on aortic surface above, host macrophage infiltration of valve leaflet and focal decrease in valve thickness. Leaflet structure is otherwise well preserved. Fibrocytic nuclei no longer stainable with haematoxylin. Haematoxylin and eosin stain × 50, reduced by $\frac{1}{3}$ in printing

present focally on the surface and penetrating the substance of the valve cusps. In none are they deeper than one-fourth of the cusp thickness, and in no case are they as extensive as those seen in the formalin-tanned xenografts. These cells show phagocytosis of the graft cellular residua and collagen (*Figures 3.29a* and *b*).

More serious are the structural changes resulting in focal calcification of the glutaraldehyde preserved valve. This has been a rare phenomenon in our experience, having been observed in only one of the 273 glutaraldehyde xenograft valves implanted. Whereas the primary cause of calcium deposition may well be due to complex, abnormal metabolic behaviour of individual patients, the influence of valve construction, the original character of the tissue and the *in vivo* flow turbulence cannot be disregarded. The histological studies of many long-term valves suggest that in some, there is a gradual loss of architectural integrity and a slow lamination of the cusp which is often associated with the insinuation of blood into the valve substance (*Figure 3.30*). In our single observed case, calcification apparently developed in such a lesion and resulted in valvular stenosis.

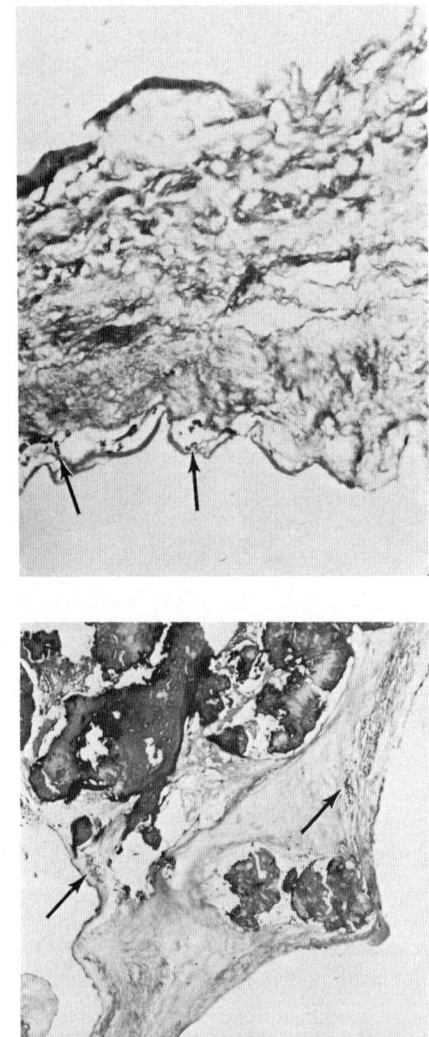

(a)

(b)

Figure 3.30 Microscopic aspects of glutaraldehyde treated porcine aortic xenografts.
(a) The valve was obtained at post-mortem examination performed 32 months following
valve insertion (the death of the patient was not related to the valve which was functionally
intact). There is a loss of skeletal integrity with apparent lamination and dissection by red
blood cells within the valve (arrows). Haematoxylin and eosin, magnification × 250,
reduced by $\frac{1}{3}$ in printing. (b) A similarly treated aortic xenograft obtained for examination
at 50 months following its insertion. There is lamination, red blood cell dissection (arrows)
and associated dense calcific deposits. Haematoxylin and eosin, original magnification × 75,
reduced by $\frac{1}{3}$ in printing. (Reproduced as *Figure 3.5*)

Glutaraldehyde toxicity

The only serious complication which we have encountered with the glutaraldehyde preserved xenograft valve was due to the presence of insoluble glutaraldehyde polymers in valve storage solutions. The free aldehyde groups of these
insoluble polymers remaining on the implanted valve resulted in sterile necrotic
destruction of the host annulus and led to perivalvular leak in 13 patients.
Standardization and purification of glutaraldehyde solutions has resulted in
avoidance of those conditions which lead to excessive polymer formation. This,
in combination with a rigid rinse protocol prior to implantation has virtually
eliminated the problem.

Haemodynamic function

In our experience, the most significant clinical problem associated with the use
of the frame mounted xenograft valve is the gradient measured across the valves
with small annulus diameter. *Figure 3.31* illustrates the pressure drop across the
Angell–Shiley glutaraldehyde preserved xenograft under conditions of steady
flow. Peak flows of 15 and 20 ℓ/min are not uncommon clinically, and with the
small size aortic valves this can result in significant transvalvular pressure gradients
of 20 mmHg or greater. The primary solution to this problem lies in reducing the
internal (tissue) diameter to external (implantation) diameter ratio (ID/OD).

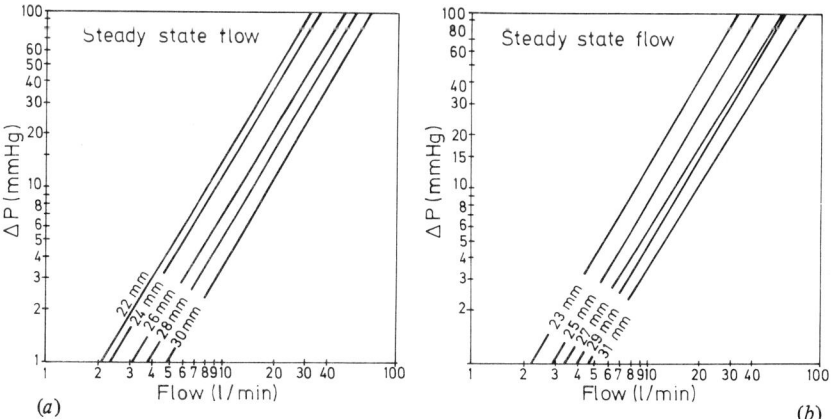

(a) (b)

Figure 3.31 Pressure gradients recorded across Angell–Shiley porcine aortic xenografts
under conditions of steady flow. (*a*) Valves with implantation (annulus) diameter of 22 to
30 mm. (*b*) Valves with implantation diameter of 23 to 31 mm. (Reproduced as *Figure 3.5*)

Potentially, this can be accomplished in several ways:

(1) alteration in stent dimension and configuration;
(2) exclusion of aortic roots with excessive angulation or protrusion of the right
    coronary cusp base into the inflow tract;
(3) finer trimming of the tissue prior to mounting and;
(4) excision of the non-coronary cusp and construction of the valves as a com-

posite of three cusps taken from different valves as used by O'Brien for the original formalin treated xenografts and reported by Buch *et al.*[23] as an experimental triple cusp valve testing preparation.

Our efforts have centred around the first three methods, as we feel that radical modifications in valve design should be viewed with caution because of their potential significant effect on durability.

In addition to the effect of reducing the ID to OD ratio of the valve, data from Wright[57] indicates that valve gradients can be decreased by creating an ideal angle of flow in the compound curve of the ascending aorta. This is accomplished by altering the implantation technique. Placement of the implantation flange and outflow valve support struts well below the left coronary orifice causes the wider stent area supporting the right coronary cusp to be seated above rather than below the host annulus (*Figure 3.32*). This angled, supra-annular seating of the valve in combination with a larger flow orifice valve promises to reduce significantly gradients with the small aortic valves.

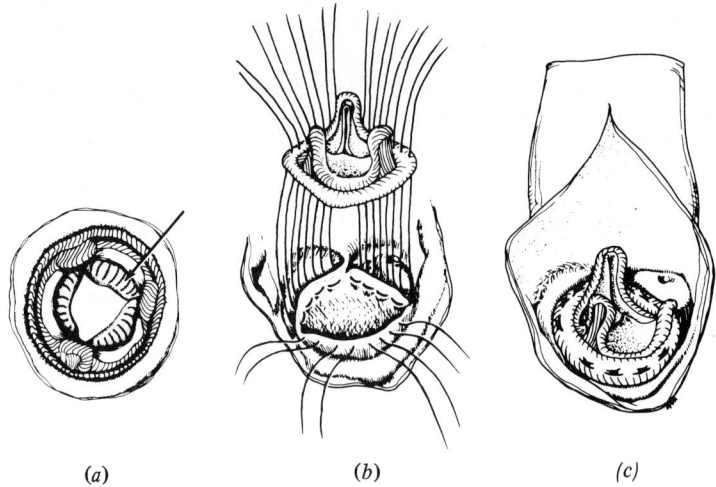

(a)　　　　　　　　(b)　　　　　　　　(c)

Figure 3.32 Schematic drawing showing the supra-annulus implantation technique for aortic valve replacement. From left: The subvalvular obstruction created by the aortic annulus and the ventricular muscle tissue resulting from previous implantation technique; two stages of the supra-annular implantation technique

Thromboembolism and anticoagulation

The incidence of thromboembolism in this series is 1.1 per cent. Two of these three patients died of left ventricular failure in a low cardiac output state. Examination of their valves showed fibrin deposition and immobility of one significantly smaller cusp in each of these two large and very asymmetric valves. Valves with gross cusp size asymmetry are no longer available. This reduced occurrence of thromboembolic complications overall is attributed both to the decreased thrombogenicity of tissue valves in general when compared to the mechanical prostheses, and to the institution of a post-operative short-term anticoagulation regimen which minimizes thromboembolic complications.

Our initial experience with the tissue valve revealed a 2.3 per cent incidence of thromboembolism, half of which was observed to occur at the time of abrupt discontinuation of the anticoagulant treatment. Two per cent of patients who were not anticoagulated had occlusion of the mitral valve, saddle embolus, or thrombus formation on suture lines and on prosthetic surfaces within one week of surgery. These data provided the impetus for an improved anticoagulation regimen which has now been used in 397 patients who received tissue valves with a resultant incidence of thromboembolic complications of 0.26 per cent. This currently used technique begins 24 h post-operatively with the administration of heparin (100 units/kg, twice daily, subcutaneously) plus warfarin sodium until the prothrombin time reaches 20–25 per cent. This range is maintained for three months, and thereafter warfarin is gradually discontinued over a 10-week period.

It is postulated that this early anticoagulation with heparin will prevent thrombus formation and organization and thus fibrosis and pannus growth which can have a deleterious effect on both leaflet mobility and the effective valve flow orifice. Obviously, patients with atrial fibrillation, thrombus in the left atrium at the time of surgery, a history of thromboembolism or with low cardiac output, remain a high risk for thromboembolism, and in these patients chronic anticoagulation should be considered. Contrarily, chronic anticoagulation, using the above described technique does not seem necessary for direct protection of the patient from valve-related thrombus and subsequent emboli when using the glutaraldehyde tanned xenograft.

CONCLUSIONS

The clinical results of valve replacement surgery are, for the most part, determined by the characteristics of the chosen valve substitute. Analysis of our clinical series continues to suggest that the tissue valve provides the greatest safety to the patient in terms of both valve-related morbidity and mortality, and this supports the general trend toward the use of this type of valve. While the reported valve-related mortality alone, for variously prepared tissue valves and mechanical prostheses, is statistically quite similar, the inclusion of valve-related morbidity, particularly for mitral valve replacement, shows the glutaraldehyde tanning of xenografts to be a superior method of tissue valve preparation.

Fresh human tissue valves are reported to remain functional for 10 to 20 years following implantation in the aortic position. However, at five years' follow-up these valves can be expected to result in a 63 per cent incidence of valve-related morbidity and mortality when used for aortic valve replacement, while only 50 per cent of patients with such valves in the mitral position are alive without complications at the end of this interval. The clinical failure of the majority of these fresh valves is a result of structural deterioration of valve collagen presumably due to a combination of traumatic preparation techniques, host reactivity and, in the case of mounted valves, the abnormal haemodynamic stress.

By contrast, collagen cross-linking of xenograft valves using glutaraldehyde markedly increases valve leaflet integrity and tensile strength while maintaining near normal cusp flexibility. This treatment has produced a valve which has proved consistently functional in all intracardiac positions for up to eight years. Mounting on an anatomically configured stent is considered to have reduced the abnormal haemodynamic stress and thus contribute to increased functional longevity. Transvalvular pressure gradients are sub-optimal and evidence of some persistent reactivity, morphological alteration and calcification does exist. In our experience, the combined valve-related morbidity and mortality with this type of valve is 13 per cent at five years' follow-up, and more important, we have encountered no instance of valve failure due to tissue deterioration in more than 287 implanted valves. The other problems associated with the use of tissue valves such as, ready availability of adequate numbers of properly sized valves with guaranteed sterility, thrombogenicity, reactivity and propensity for endocarditis seem to be solved, and therefore, the glutaraldehyde xenograft valve appears to be superior to any other type of tissue valve preparation.

REFERENCES

[1] Albright, J. F., Makinoda, T. and Mazur, P. 'Preservation of antibody producing cells at low temperatures: A method of storage that allows complete recovery of activity', *Proceedings of the Society of experimental Biology and Medicine,* 114, 489 (1963)

[2] Anderson, R. P., Bonchek, L. I., Grunkemeier, G. L., Lambert, L. E. and Starr, A. 'The analysis and presentation of surgical results by actuarial methods', *Journal of surgical Research,* 16, 244 (1974)

[3] Angell, W. W., Angell, J. D. and Sywak, A. 'The tissue valve as a superior cardiac valve replacement', *Surgery,* 82, 875 (1977)

[4] Angell, W. W., Buch, W. S. and Shumway, N. W. 'The viable aortic homograft'. In *Biological Tissue in Heart Valve Replacement*. Ed. by M. I. Ionescu, D. N. Ross and G. H. Wooler, p. 543. London; Butterworths (1972)

[5] Angell, W. W., de Lanerolle, P. and Shumway, N. E. 'Valve replacement: Present status of homograft valves', *Progress in cardiovascular Disease,* 15, 589 (1973)

[6] Angell, W. W., Grehl, T. M., Buch, W. S. and Wuerflein, R. D. 'Mounted fresh homografts for aortic valve replacement', *Medical Journal of Australia, (Suppl. 2)* 74 (1972)

[7] Angell, J. D., Christopher, B. S., Hawtrey, C. O. and Angell, W. W. 'A fresh, viable human heart valve bank; sterilization, sterility testing, and cryogenic preservation', *Transplantation Proceedings,* 8 *(Suppl. 1)* 139 (1976)

[8] Angell, W. W., Iben, A. B., Gianelly, R. E. and Shumway, N. E. 'Aortic homograft valves for mitral valve replacement', *Circulation,* 39 *(Suppl.)* 39 (1969)

[9] Angell, W. W., Iben, A. B. and Shumway, N. E. 'Fresh aortic homografts for multiple valve replacement', *Archives of Surgery,* 97, 826 (1968)

[10] Angell, W. W., Pillsbury, R. C. and Shumway, N. E. 'Storage and function of the canine aortic valve homograft', *Archives of Surgery,* 99, 92 (1969)

[11] Angell, W. W., Shumway, N. E. and Kosek, J. E. 'A five-year study of the viable aortic valve homograft', *Journal of thoracic and cardiovascular Surgery,* 64, 329 (1972)

[12] Angell, W. W., Wuerflein, R. D. and Shumway, N. E. 'Mitral valve replacement with the fresh aortic valve homograft: Experimental results and clinical application', *Surgery,* 62, 807 (1967)

[13] Angell, W. W., Wuerflein, R. D. and Shumway, N. E. 'Long-term results following mitral valve replacement with fresh aortic homografts', *Advances in Cardiology,* 7, 99 (1972)

[14] Barratt-Boyes, B. G. 'Homograft aortic valve replacement in aortic incompetence and stenosis', *Thorax,* 19, 133 (1964)

[15] Barratt-Boyes, B. G., Roche, A., Agnew, T. M., Cole, D., Kerr, A., Monro, J. L., Lowe, J. B. and Brandt, P. W. T. 'Homograft valves', *Medical Journal of Australia, (Suppl. 2)* 38 (1972)

[16] Barratt-Boyes, B. G., Roche, A. H. and Whitlock, R. M. 'Six-year review of results of free-hand aortic valve replacement using an antibiotic sterilized homograft valve', *Circulation,* 55, 353 (1977)

[17] Baue, A. E., Donawick, W. J. and Blakemore, W. S. 'The immunologic response to heterotopic allovital aortic valve transplants in pre-sensitized and non-sensitized recipients', *Journal of thoracic and cardiovascular Surgery*, **56**, 775 (1968)

[18] Berkson, J. and Gage, R. P. 'Calculation of survival rates of cancer', *Proceedings of the staff meeting of the Mayo Clinic*, **25**, 270 (1950)

[19] Bigelow, W. G., Yao, J. K., Aldridge, H. E., Heimbacker, R. O. and Marray, G. D. 'Clinical homograft valve transplantation', *Journal of thoracic and cardiovascular Surgery*, **48**, 333 (1964)

[20] Binet, J. P., Duran, C. G., Carpentier, A. and Langlois, J. 'Heterologous aortic valve transplantation', *Lancet*, **2**, 1275 (1965)

[21] Bolooki, H., Rubinson, R. M., Prochazka, J. and Jude, J. R. 'A simple method of aortic homograft valve sterilization and preservation', *Journal of thoracic and cardiovascular Surgery*, **63**, 249 (1972)

[22] Bondoc, C. C. and Burke, J. F. 'Clinical experience with viable frozen human skin and frozen skin bank', *Annals of Surgery*, **174**, 371 (1971)

[23] Buch, W. S., Kosek, J., Angell, W. W. and Shumway, N. E. 'Deterioration of formalin treated aortic valve heterografts', *Journal of thoracic and cardiovascular Surgery*, **60**, 673 (1970)

[24] Buch, W. S, Kosek, J. C., Angell, W. W. and Shumway, N. E. 'The role of rejection and mechanical trauma on valve graft viability', *Journal of thoracic and cardiovascular Surgery*, **62**, 696 (1971)

[25] Carpentier, A., Deloche, A., Relland, J., Fabiani, J. N., Forman, J., Camilleri, J. P., Soyer, R. and Dubost, C. 'Six-year follow-up of glutaraldehyde preserved heterografts', *Journal of thoracic and cardiovascular Surgery*, **68**, 771 (1974)

[26] Duran, C. G. and Gunning, A. J. 'Methods for placing a total homologous aortic valve in the sub-coronary position', *Lancet*, **2**, 488 (1962)

[27] Gallucci, V., Cevese, P. G., Morea, M., Dalla Volta, F. and Casarotto, D. 'Hancock bioprosthesis: analysis of long-term results (six years)', *Circulation*, **54** (*Suppl. 2*), 149 (1976)

[28] Gianelly, R. E., Angell, W. W., Stinson, E. B., Shumway, N. E. and Harrison, D. C. 'Homograft replacement of the mitral valve', *Circulation*, **28**, 664 (1968)

[29] Heimbecker, R. O. Personal communication (1976)

[30] Hoeksema, T. D., Titus, J. L., Giullani, E. R. and Kirklin, J. W. 'Early results of the use of homografts for replacement of the aortic valve', *Circulation*, **35**, 1 (1967)

[31] Kaufman, H. E. and Capella, J. A. 'Transplantation of frozen tissues', *Journal of Cryosurgery*, **1**, 125 (1968)

[32] Kosek, J. C., Iben, A. B., Shumway, N. E. and Angell, W. W. 'Morphology of fresh heart valve homografts', *Surgery*, **66**, 269 (1969)

[33] Kwong, K. H., Paton, B. C. and Hill, R. B. 'Experimental use of immunosuppression in aortic valve homografts and heterografts', *Journal of thoracic and cardiovascular Surgery*, **54**, 199 (1967)

[34] Lam, C. R., Aram, H. H. and Munnell, E. R. 'An experimental study of the aortic valve homografts', *Surgery, Gynecology and Obstetrics*, **94**, 129 (1952)

[35] Leibo, S. P., Farrant, J., Mazur, P., Hanna, M. G. and Smith L. H. 'Effects of freezing on marrow stem cell suspensions: interactions of cooling and warming rates in the presence of PVP, sucrose, or glycerol', *Cryobiology*, **6**, 315 (1970)

[36] Lovelock, J. E. 'Heat mechanism of the protective action of glycerol against haemolysis by freezing and thawing', *Biochemica et Biophysica Acta*, **11**, 28 (1953)

[37] Lower, R. R., Stofer, R. C. and Shumway, N. E. 'A study of pulmonary valve autotransplantation', *Surgery*, **48**, 1090 (1960)

[38] Malm, M. R., Bowman, F. O., Harris, P. D. and Kowalik, A. T. 'An evaluation of aortic valve homografts sterilized by electron beam energy', *Journal of thoracic and cardiovascular Surgery*, **54**, 471 (1967)

[39] Mazur, P., Leibo, S. P., Farrant, J., Chu, E. H. Y., Hanna, M. G. and Smith, L. H. 'Interactions of cooling rate, warming rate and protective additive on the survival of frozen mammalian cells'. In *The Frozen Cell*. Ed. by G. E. W. Wolstenholm and M. O'Connor, p. 69. London; Churchill (1970)

[40] McDowell, J. Personal communication. Arbrook Inc., Arlington, Texas (1976)

[41] Mohri, H., Reichenbach, P. D., Barner, R. W., Nelson, R. J. and Merendino, K. A. 'Studies of antigenicity of the homologous aortic valve', *Journal of thoracic and cardiovascular Surgery*, **54**, 564 (1967)

[42] Mohri, H., Reichenbach, P. D., Nelson, R. J., Barnes, R. W. and Merendino, K. A. 'Preparation and preservation of aortic valve grafts with special attention to problem areas', *Journal of thoracic and cardiovascular Surgery, 56*, 546 (1968)

[43] Murray, G. 'Homologous aortic valve segment transplant as surgical treatment for aortic and mitral insufficiency', *Angiology, 7*, 466 (1956)

[44] O'Brien, M. F. and Clarebrough, J. K. 'Heterograft aortic valve transplantation for human valve disease', *Medical Journal of Australia, 2*, 228 (1966)

[45] Polge, C., Smith, A. U. and Parkes, A. S. 'Revival of spermatozoa after virification and dehydration at low temperatures', *Nature, 164*, 666 (1949)

[46] Richards, F. M. and Knowles, J. R. 'Letters to the Editor. (Glutaraldehyde as a protein cross-linking reagent)', *Journal of molecular Biology, 37*, 231 (1968)

[47] Robertson, E. A. and Schultz, R. L. 'The impurities in commercial glutaraldehyde and their effect on the fixation of brain', *Journal of Ultrastructure Research, 30*, 275 (1970)

[48] Ross, D. N. 'Homograft replacement of the aortic valve', *Lancet, 2*, 488 (1962)

[49] Ross, D. N. Personal communication. National Heart Hospital, London, England (1975)

[50] Shiley Laboratories, Inc., Irvine, California. Personal communication (1978)

[51] Stinson, E. B., Angell, W. W., Iben, A. B. and Shumway, N. E. 'Aortic valve replacement with fresh valve homograft', *American Journal of Surgery, 116*, 204 (1968)

[52] Stinson, E. B., Angell, W. W. and Shumway, N. E. 'Triple valve replacement with aortic homografts', *Journal of american medical Association, 204*, 67 (1968)

[53] Tavis, M. J., Thornton, J. H., Harney, J. H., Woodroof, E. A. and Bartlett, R. H. 'Adherence to de-epithelialized surface: A comparative study', *Surgical Forum, 25*, 39 (1974)

[54] Tavis, M. J., Thornton, J. H., Harney, J. H., Woodroof, E. A. and Bartlett, R. H. 'Modified collagen membrane as a skin substitute: preliminary studies', *Journal of biomedical Material Research, 9*, 285 (1975)

[55] Tavis, M. J., Thornton, J. H., Harney, J. H., Woodroof, E. A. and Bartlett, R. H. 'Graft adherence to de-epithelialized surfaces: A comparative study', *Annals of Surgery, 184*, 549 (1976)

[56] Woodroof, E. A. 'The chemistry and biology of aldehyde treated tissue heart valve xenografts'. In *Tissue Heart Valves*. Ed. by M. I. Ionescu. London; Butterworths (1979)

[57] Wright, J. T. M. '*In vitro* comparison between the hydrodynamic characteristics of the Hancock 250 (modified orifice) xenograft and the Björk–Shiley aortic valve prosthesis', *Presented at the 23rd ASAIO meeting*, April 21, 1977, Montreal, Quebec, Canada (1977)

[58] Zuhdi, N., Hawley, W., Voehl, V., Hancock, W., Carey, J. and Greer, A. 'Porcine aortic valves as replacement for human heart valves', *Annals of thoracic Surgery, 17*, 479 (1974)

4

Allograft and Autograft Valves used for Aortic Valve Replacement

Donald N. Ross
Valentino Martelli
and William H. Wain

Le temps est le plus sage de tous les conseillers.

Périclès (495–429 av. J.C.)

INTRODUCTION

Allograft valves, formerly called homograft valves, are usually aortic valves taken from human cadavers. When allograft valves are used to replace diseased aortic valves the important advantages are that the valve is identical in design and structure with the valve being replaced. Therefore, not surprisingly, such allograft valves which have a central non-obstructive flow are free from thromboembolism and haemolysis. The major disadvantage of the allografts has been the ultimate failure of the valve due to degenerative changes. These have included cusp rupture, thinning, retraction and calcification. The methods of sterilization and storage of the allograft valves can affect the incidence and rate of the degenerative process. In spite of such changes the allograft valves remain non-living structures but do function well for long periods of time.

An alternative approach to the problem has been to seek an autogenous living substitute which would not require sterilization and which would last indefinitely. Such a valve is the pulmonary autograft valve, which is transferred from the pulmonary to the aortic area and is replaced in turn by an allograft or xenograft valve. In the low pressure pulmonary position it is assumed that a replacement allograft valve should last for a longer time than in the high pressure aortic area. Even if the allograft fails as a pulmonary valve, the right side of the heart can easily tolerate such a malfunction, in a similar way to surgical correction of pulmonary stenosis in Fallot's tetralogy.

Our clinical experience of biological aortic valve replacement began in July 1962, when an aortic valve taken from a cadaver (allograft aortic valve), was inserted in the sub-coronary position[26]. This procedure was initially adopted world-wide and since that time allograft aortic valves have also been used in the pulmonary, tricuspid and mitral positions. We have continued to expand and modify the techniques and in 1966 introduced the concept of right ventricular reconstruction with a valved conduit[29] and did the first pulmonary autograft operation in 1967[27].

Despite unfavourable reports from several centres which have discontinued the use of allograft valves[6,34], we have continued to alter and improve the procedure. We have, however, discontinued the use of frame mounted valves in the mitral position following their poor performance[31]. After 15 years' experience with 476 isolated allograft aortic valves and ten years with 188 autografts we are convinced that the use of such valves is a valid procedure in current cardiac surgery. The results for 664 aortic valve replacements with allograft or autograft valves are presented in support of this conviction.

STRUCTURE OF THE VALVES

The aortic and pulmonary valves are similar in appearance, both having three semilunar cusps. Each cusp is attached by two commissures to the artery wall, merging with an inferior attachment to the annulus fibrosus. There is a small fibrocartilaginous nodule, the corpus arantii in the centre of the superior, free margin of each cusp. The thin border, the lunula, extends along the free edge and is frequently perforated by congenital lacunae. Radiating from the corpus arantii over the belly of the cusp are several fibrous thickenings. During diastole the free edges of the cusp meet over an area of apposition which is several millimetres deep. This generous overlap is produced by the shape of the cusps which allows the central part to reach the centre of the valvular orifice. Each cusp is formed of a fold of connective tissue inserted in the annulus fibrosus and covered with endothelium. Collagen fibres predominate in the connective tissue on the arterial side of the cusp, and elastic fibres are more common on the proximal, ventricular side.

Changes in the collagen or elastic fibre structure or in the mucopolysaccharide ground substance may affect the long-term function of the cusps. The preservation of the intact viable endothelial cells is probably essential for the continued viability of the cusps of an autograft pulmonary valve.

Two of the sinuses of Valsalva of the aortic valve have ostia for the right and left coronary arteries.

PROCURING, PROCESSING AND PRESERVING ALLOGRAFT VALVES

The first 16 allograft valves used by Barratt-Boyes in 1962 were collected under sterile conditions within a few hours of death[7]. Such valves are difficult to obtain. In practice our valves are collected under non-sterile, routine post-mortem conditions. Providing the body has been refrigerated the valves may be collected within 48 h of death. Young donors are preferred, but older valves may be accepted. Details are recorded of the age and sex of the donor, and the date and cause of death. The ideal donors are those that had died accidentally (e.g. car accident, suicide or drug overdose) rather than those whose death was caused by a pathological disease process, but valves can be used from any patients except those with serum hepatitis, tuberculosis, venereal disease, primary carcinoma of the heart and septicaemia.

The valves are scrutinized in the laboratory and those having defects such as extensive atheroma and calcification are discarded. The technician, wearing gown, gloves and mask then dissects suitable valves in a safety cabinet, using sterile instruments to reduce cross-infection between the valves, while washing the valves frequently in physiological solution to keep them moist.

The ventricular muscle is dissected away from the aortic valve leaving a ring of myocardium and also the anterior mitral leaflet (*Figure 4.1*). The aorta, after removal of loose fascia, is left as long as possible and four segments of the aortic wall are removed for microbiological testing. The length of the aorta is measured and the diameter of the valve and of the aorta are gauged with a set of obturators to within 1 mm.

The next step is to destroy the contaminating micro-organisms and to prevent autolytic destruction of the valve tissue. These processes may conveniently be termed 'sterilization' and 'preservation'.

Fixatives such as formaldehyde and beta-propriolactone are no longer used as sterilizing agents as they are now thought to cause degenerative changes in the valves[30,17]. Between 1964 and 1969 a simple antibiotic mixture of penicillin, streptomycin and nystatin followed by treatment with 10 per cent ethylene oxide in 90 per cent carbon dioxide was used at the National Heart Hospital[18]. Gamma irradiation with 2 Mrad for 5 s at $-70\,^{\circ}$C has also been used as described by Malm *et al.*[20]. These sterilization methods were followed either by freeze-drying or deep freezing for preservation and storage of the valves. The freeze-drying process was found to be associated with tissue damage[17] and has, therefore, been abandoned.

Following the early work of Barratt-Boyes with sterile grafts and the introduction of the living pulmonary autograft[27], Stinson *et al.*[33] used a technique for the preservation of sterile valves in a tissue culture medium. This was extended by Barratt-Boyes and Roche[8] who sterilized contaminated valves in an antibiotic mixture in Hanks balanced salt solution. There have been many subsequent formulations of antibiotic mixtures[35]. The concept of tissue viability, and allograft maintenance and repair prompted the substitution of Hanks balanced salt solution with a nutrient medium[4]. Between 1972 and 1976, at the National Heart Hospital, a fragment of the mitral leaflet, removed from each allograft at the time of valve insertion, was tested for viability using autoradiography of incorporated tritiated thymidine[2].

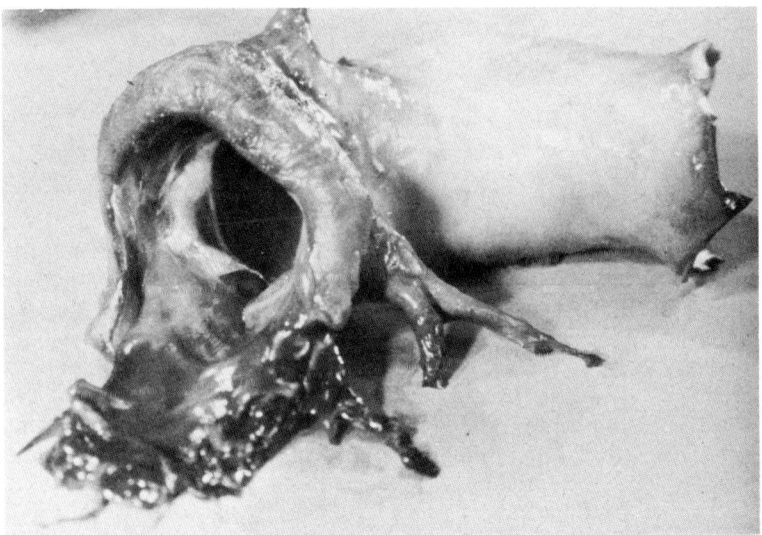

Figure 4.1   Allograft aortic valve dissected and prepared for storage. Trimming for surgery is shown in *Figures 4.12* to *4.14*

The procedure which we use at present for preserving the allograft valve and for preventing the growth of contaminating micro-organisms is as follows:

The prepared valve is placed in a wide-necked jar which is filled with 200 ml of a nutrient medium–antibiotic mixture. The same nutrient medium–antibiotic mixture is used for the preservation of the four pieces of ascending aorta kept for microbiological testing. These pieces are placed in universal bottles containing 30 ml each of the solution. The nutrient medium–antibiotic mixture is formulated from Tissue Culture Medium 199 (Gibco Biocult) containing 7 per cent heat-activated newborn calf serum buffered to pH 7.4 with 4.4 per cent sodium bicarbonate. The antibiotics are dissolved in this medium in the following concentrations per litre (quantity for five valves):

cephaloridine	0.04	g
carbenicillin	10.0	g
neomycin sulphate	1.0	g
polymyxin B	0.7	g

This solution retains its effectiveness for seven days at $4\,^\circ$C in the dark. The antifungal agent, nystatin, being less stable, is added to the mixture just before the valve is placed in the jar. The nystatin concentration is 0.5 g/ℓ, or 100 mg (500 000 units)/200 ml for each valve.

The valve and the four pieces for microbiological testing are kept in the mixture at room temperature for 24 h, to allow the growth-dependent antibiotics such as penicillin, to be effective. The valve is then stored at $4\,^\circ$C until the microbiological tests on three tissue pieces have failed to grow any aerobic or anaerobic bacteria or any fungi during a five-day period. The valve is then released for surgical use. The fourth piece of tissue is tested for *Mycobacteria* species over an eight-week period. The culture report is attached to the valve documentation.

VIABILITY

The introduction of tissue culture media for allograft valve preservation[4,33], was associated with the concept of allograft viability. It was hoped that the fresh valves would retain their viability and be incorporated by the host and so maintain the valve structure indefinitely.

Cell viability declines as cell death follows clinical death, and the various parameters which may be monitored as indices of cell viability include cell proliferation, DNA synthesis, RNA synthesis, protein synthesis and enzyme activity. The enzyme activity may be assessed specifically as substrate utilization or product formation or as a general reaction as in vital staining, or dye exclusion methods. The particular parameter chosen to monitor viability should reflect the practical problem of the situation as well as the theoretical concepts of viability.

Thus the rapid decreases in protein synthesis and oxidative enzyme activity during the first few hours *post mortem*[19] do not reflect the tissues' ability to proliferate. We have chosen to measure the ability of the allograft nuclei to incorporate thymidine into DNA on the assumption that nuclei which can incorporate thymidine into DNA will subsequently divide as part of a population of proliferating cells. It is difficult to quantify cell proliferation in tissue culture to assess cell viability but by using autoradiography to locate tritium-labelled thymidine in nuclei of allograft valves it is possible to make a quantitative assessment of the viability of the tissue in terms of the proportion of labelled nuclei[4].

Method

Small pieces (5 × 5 mm) of aortic wall or mitral valve leaflet, trimmed from the allograft valve at the time of its surgical insertion, were incubated at $37\,^\circ$C for 48 h in 2 ml tissue culture medium 199 with 7 per cent fetal calf serum buffered to pH 7.4, which contained penicillin and streptomycin. At the start of the incubation, 0.01 mCi of tritiated methyl thymidine was added to each 2 ml of incubation medium. The tissue was rinsed in the medium 199 after 48 h incubation and cultured for 5–6 h in the absence of any radioactive thymidine. At the end of the incubation period the tissue was fixed in formol–saline. Following conventional embedding, 7 μm sections were coated with nuclear emulsion (Ilford type K2) and exposed at 4 °C in the dark for seven days. After developing the emulsion the sections were stained with haematoxylin and eosin or Geimsa and mounted. Microscopic investigation detected silver grains over stained nuclei and where more than four grains/nucleus were found the nucleus was designated as 'viable'. For any one valve between 100 and 200 nuclei were counted in five to ten microscope fields from two sections on two slides, examining both the central and peripheral nuclei. Viability was scored as the percentage of observed nuclei which were 'viable' in terms of detected silver grains.

Results

The decline in viability during experimental storage described by Al-Janabi *et al.*[4], has been observed in the allograft valves stored for different periods before clinical use (*Figure 4.2*). There has also been a variation in viability due to the use of different antibiotic mixtures and this is shown in *Figure 4.3*.

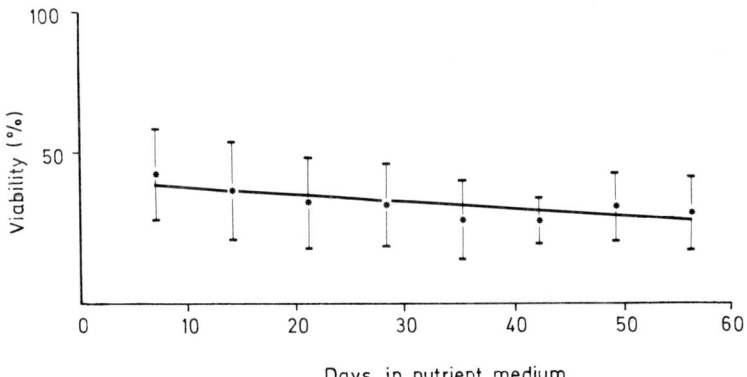

Days in nutrient medium

Figure 4.2 Graphic presentation of viability of 250 'aortic' allograft valves stored for varying periods of time, for clinical use, in Mixture B nutrient medium. Fragments of unused aortic wall and anterior mitral leaflet were obtained from the allograft at the time of valve insertion and were exposed to radioactive thymidine for 48 h immediately following the valve replacement operation. The percentage of viability was obtained from the proportion of stained nuclei which had incorporated the radioactive thymidine. Each point on the graph represents the mean (and standard deviation) of one week's accumulated total. (Reproduced from Lockey, E., Al-Janabi, N., Gonzalez-Lavin, L. and Ross, D. N. 'A method of sterilizing and preserving fresh allograft heart valves, *Thorax*, **27**, 398 (1972))

Viability studies have also been made on allograft valves removed from eight patients after periods of implantation ranging from 8 to 1292 days and these demonstrated a decline in viability during the period of time the valve was inserted in the patient (*Figure 4.4*). The histological appearance of the valves removed from patients will be discussed later in this chapter but the paucity of

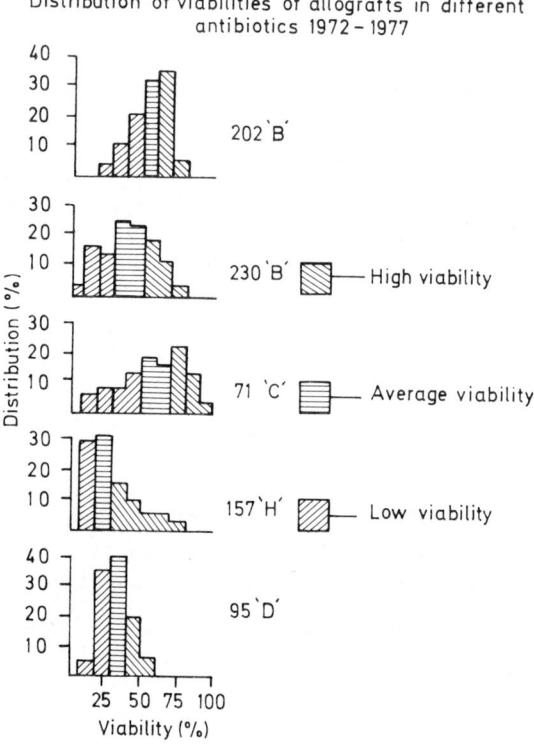

Figure 4.3 Percentage distribution of viability of fresh aortic allografts studied between 1972 and 1977. The histograms show the variation in the distribution of viability for the different antibiotic mixtures used for the preservation of fresh allografts. The numbers represent results obtained from all the allografts used clinically, for either isolated aortic valve replacement or for multiple valve replacement procedures.

'B' Reproduced from Lockey, E., Al-Janabi, N., Gonzalez-Lavin, L. and Ross, D. N. 'A method of sterilizing and preserving fresh allograft heart valves', *Thorax*, 27, 398 (1972)

'C' Reproduced from Waterworth, P. M., Lockey, E., Berry, E. M. and Pearce, H. M. 'A critical investigation into the antibiotic sterilization of heart valve homografts', *Thorax*, 29, 432 (1974)

'H' Reproduced from Yacoub, M., Knight, E. J. and Towers, M. 'Aortic valve replacement using fresh unstented homografts', *Thoraxchirurgie*, 21, 451 (1973)

'D' Reproduced from Wain, W. H., Pearce, Helen, M., Riddell, R. W. and Ross, D. N. 'A re-evaluation of antibiotic sterilization of heart valve allografts', *Thorax*, 32, 740 (1977)

Shaded areas: Low viability on the left, high viability on the right

nuclei observed in these tissues obviously affected the recorded viability. The low numbers of nuclei also affected attempts to determine the sex of the tissues. It had been hoped that by inserting male allografts into female patients, and vice versa, it would be possible to determine the extent of graft incorporation, but despite the use of a range of special techniques this has not been possible.

The decline in viability, together with the problems of nuclear sexing and the degenerative changes seen in some of the allograft valves removed has suggested that the concept of allograft valve incorporation as a living tissue capable of cellular proliferation, tissue maintenance and repair is not a valid one.

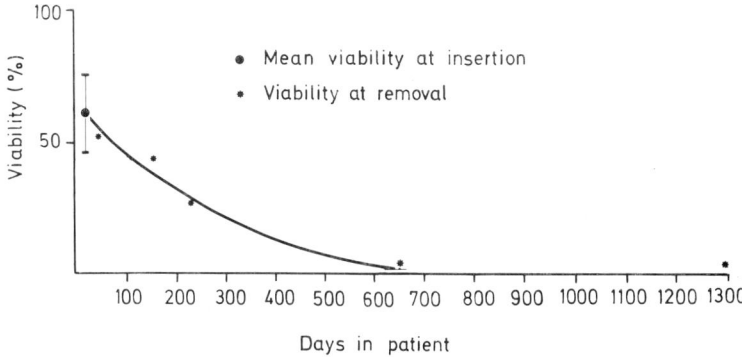

Figure 4.4 Graphic presentation of tissue viability of allograft aortic valve cusps removed from patients after varying periods of time of implantation. The valve cusps were exposed to radioactive thymidine for 48 h following their removal. The tissue viability after removal (*) is related to the viability at insertion (•) expressed as mean value ± standard error of the mean at time zero

After four years of investigation of the viability of more than 800 implanted allograft valves, we may conclude that viability estimated by the autoradiography of incorporated tritiated thymidine is an indication of the quality of the valve. It reflects a combination of the deleterious effects of post-mortem autolysis, delays in collection and in preparation of the valves and the different methods of tissue sterilization and preservation.

The more recent work with protein synthesis on canine allograft valves has shown that valves harvested under ideal experimental conditions are viable[36]. However, such viable valves were shown to shrink and to malfunction, possibly due to acute rejection, within eight weeks of implantation, in contrast to valves which had been shown to be non-viable by protein synthesis tests. Wheatley and McGregor[36] have suggested that very few of the valves used in clinical practice were viable, in terms of protein synthesis or cell proliferation. It is difficult to compare studies made with two different techniques, but it is probably correct to say that the clinical allograft valves which have been used would have been non-viable according to the criteria of Wheatley and McGregor. However, this does not affect the viability values we obtained by thymidine studies, providing they are used to describe the state of the valve rather than any growth potential within the host.

Testing of new procedures

Experimental testing of new techniques for processing and preserving allograft valves should bear some relationship to the eventual function of the valve following its implantation. Viability studies on 800 allograft valves have been extended as a test procedure for alternative preservation methods such as deep-freeze storage[3] and antibiotic mixtures[23]. In this way a cytotoxic antibiotic may be seen to affect the metabolic function of the allograft tissue. The viability test has been interpreted by us as correlating high viabilities with relatively undamaged valves (*Figure 4.5*). Since these viability tests involve histological techniques, the changes in tissue architecture have also been examined during

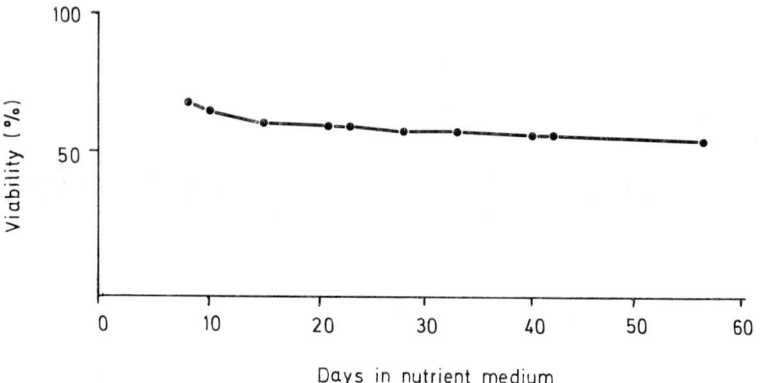

Figure 4.5 Graphic presentation of experimental results of tissue viability. Aortic valve allografts were stored in Mixture B nutrient medium[1] for predetermined periods of time, following which they were exposed to radioactive thymidine for 48 h. (Data from Al-Janabi, N. and Ross, D. N. 'Enhanced viability of fresh aortic homografts stored in nutrient medium', *Cardiovascular Research,* **8**, 817 (1973))

[1] Lockey, E., Al-Janabi, N., Gonzalez-Lavin, L. and Ross, D. N. 'A method of sterilizing and preserving fresh allograft heart valves', *Thorax,* **27**, 398 (1972)

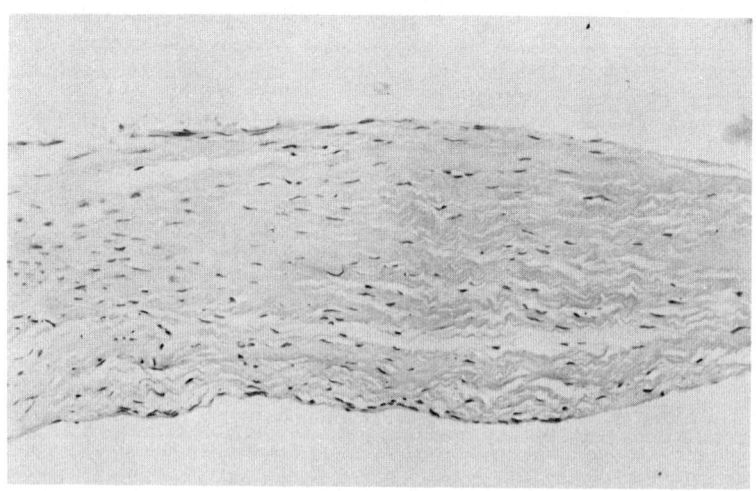

Figure 4.6 Microscopic appearance of an aortic allograft valve cusp after one month's storage in antibiotic nutrient medium mixture. The retention of nuclei and the normal tissue architecture are demonstrated. Haematoxylin and eosin, magnification × 125, reduced by 40 per cent in printing

the tests for new processing and preserving methods[2,23]. Degeneration of collagen and loss of elastic fibres increase with prolonged or damaging storage (*Figure 4.6*). The decline in nuclearity mirrors the decrease in viability, although the viability tests measure only the nuclei which can be seen. These tests, of viability and microstructure, allow evaluation of the state of the tissue.

The allografts processed between 1964 and 1968 were subjected to a 'tear-out-strength' test[18]. Another technique, which measured valve cusp function rather

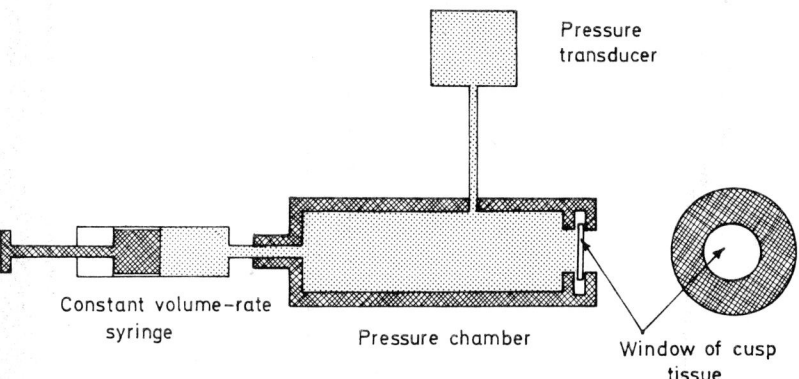

Figure 4.7 Apparatus for measuring elastic properties of valve cusps. The pressure changes are monitored as the volume is decreased at a constant rate by the motor-driven syringe. Bulging of the cusp window is an expression of the elastic property of the cusp and is reflected in the transducer recording

than the ability of the artery wall to tolerate strains after stitching, is that of pressure responses of stretched cusps. The elastic properties of the cusp were tested by a stress/strain technique, where physiological pressures were applied to a 'window' of a cusp in a steel chamber (*Figure 4.7*)[38]. As the valves deteriorate the tissue becomes stiffer and less compliant and there is a smaller volume change associated with a given pressure (*Figure 4.8*). Such a decrease in the elastic property of the cusps was associated with a deterioration of the tissue[22]. In general, an adverse histological change, a decrease in viability and a decrease in elastic property are all, individually and in combination, associated with undesirable changes in the allograft valve[23]. Examining the elastic properties of the valve is thus another prospective testing procedure applicable to allograft valves and used to evaluate novel preparation or preservation procedures[23].

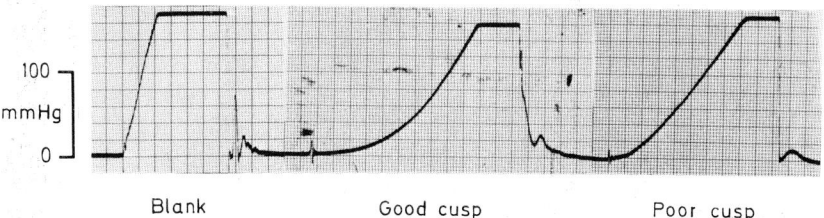

Figure 4.8 Pressure–volume traces from valve cusps. This figure shows the straight line response from a brass blanking plate, and the curved line responses from aortic valve cusps

OPERATIVE TECHNIQUES

Surgical insertion of allograft valves

The technique of insertion of allograft valves has varied over the years. Initially, the technique as described by Duran and Gunning[12] was used and the valve was inserted with a single continuous suture line. This resulted in a high incidence of

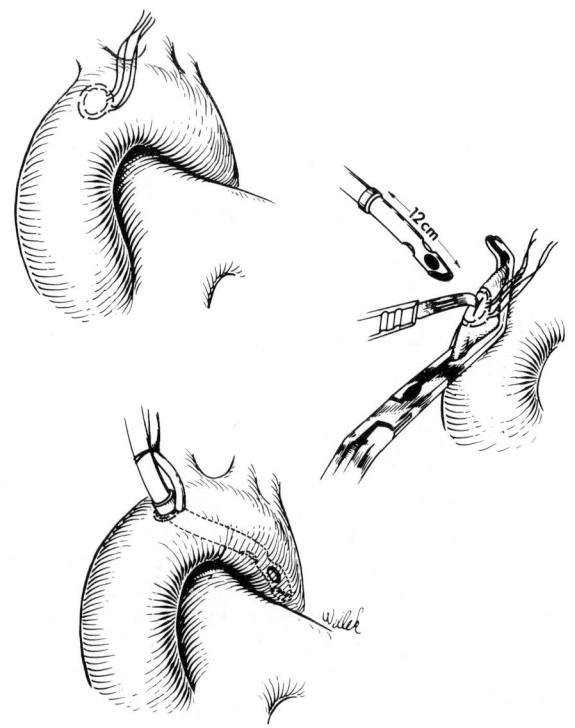

Figure 4.9 Technique for cannulation of the ascending aorta. Note that the perfusion cannula was advanced into the descending aorta

aortic regurgitation. It is now well established that two suture lines are required for the insertion of a competent allograft aortic valve and a description of our technique follows.

The heart is approached through a midline sternotomy and a vertical incision of the pericardial sac. Cannulation of the ascending aorta and the right atrium is performed routinely (*Figure 4.9*). Hypothermic, high flow, cardiopulmonary bypass is established using a bubble oxygenator and haemodilution. After cross-clamping the aorta as high as possible, a vent is placed in the left ventricle and the aorta is opened with a long oblique incision carried well down in the non-coronary sinus (*Figure 4.10*). This approach provides the best exposure for allograft aortic valve replacement. Bilateral coronary perfusion is established and continued throughout the open heart procedure. The diseased valve is excised down to the base of the cusps and calcium is meticulously removed leaving the base of the excised valve clearly defined (*Figure 4.11*). During these manoeuvres the left ventricular cavity is obliterated with a small 5 × 5 cm cylinder of foam rubber to prevent small calcific particles from dropping into the cavity. In cases of aortic regurgitation, the cusps are trimmed close to their origins leaving a 5 mm margin to hold sutures, but this is trimmed completely flat at the points of excision at the commissures. The aortic annulus is then measured with a set of cylindrical obturators while the heart is beating and has a normal tone. The obturator of the correct size should be held rather than be allowed to fall into the left ventricle. The correctly sized allograft should have an internal diameter

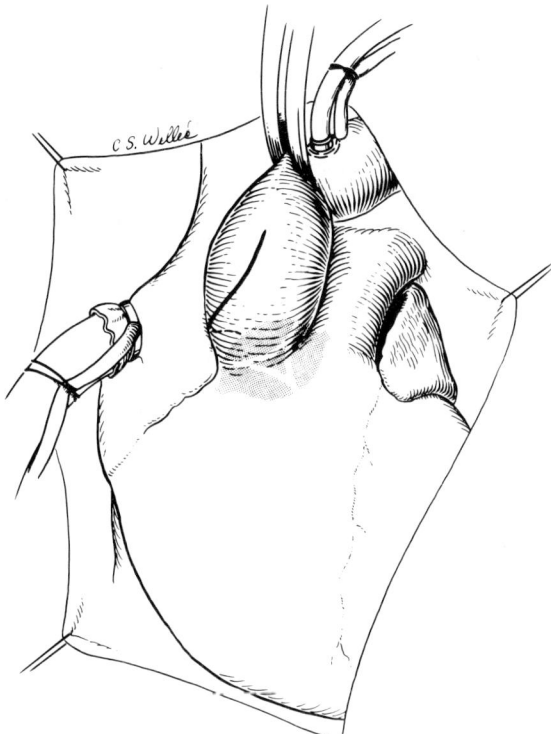

Figure 4.10 The ascending aorta is opened through an oblique incision carried downwards into the non-coronary sinus of Valsalva

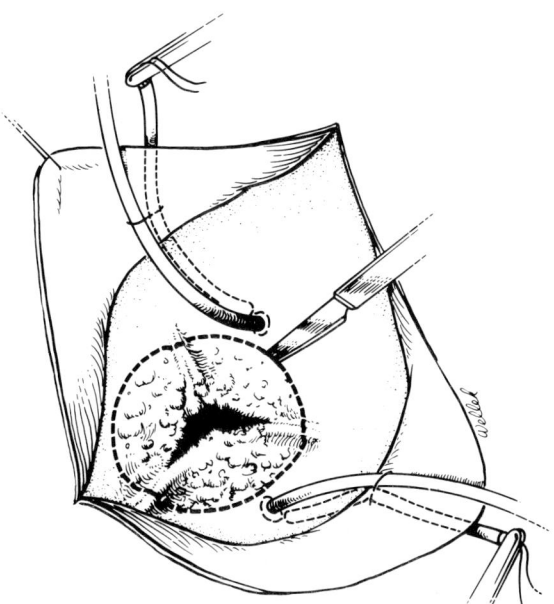

Figure 4.11 Following cannulation of both coronary ostia, the aortic valve is exposed. The excision of the valve is carried out, in most instances, with a knife

similar to the aortic root. The 2–3 mm thickness of the aortic wall of the graft ensures slight excess of the cusp tissue.

Varying degrees of muscular hypertrophic sub-aortic stenosis are encountered and ought to be taken into consideration. This hypertrophic muscle may obstruct the outflow tract and in such cases a myotomy was often carried out before insertion of the allograft.

The lower margin of the selected allograft valve is trimmed to within 1 mm of the cusp attachments. This requires the removal of all soft muscle and leaves a tough sewing margin adjacent to the cusp. In the conventional method of insertion the upper margin of the graft is trimmed by excision of the aortic wall of the sinuses including both coronary orifices. Only 3 mm of aortic wall are left adjacent to the cusps. The non-coronary sinus is left intact (*Figure 4.12*).

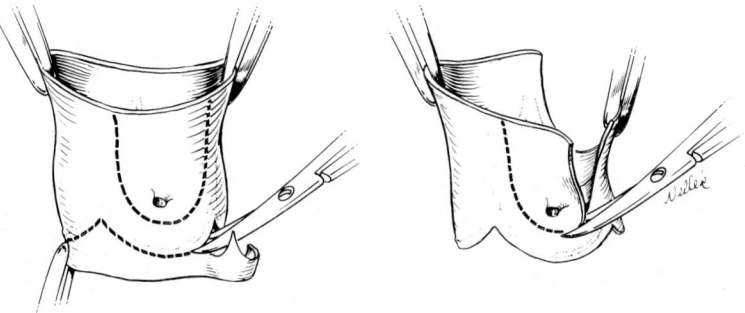

Figure 4.12 Trimming of the aortic allograft valve prior to its surgical insertion

Three key stitches are placed in the recipient aortic ring using 4–0 double-armed Prolene sutures which pick up a deep bite at the mid-point of the base of each sinus. These three sutures are then brought through the corresponding parts of the lower margin of the allograft and held with rubber-shod haemostats. This divides the lower margin of the allograft into six sub-segments separated by the three sutures plus the three commissures. In to each of these six sub-segments seven closely and evenly spaced 4–0 single sutures are placed, first in the aortic annulus and then in the lower margin of the allograft (*Figure 4.13a*). After all the sutures are in place, the graft is gently slid down into position. The sutures are then tied down and the lower suture line is completed.

To support the graft commissures three double-armed 2–0 Mersilene sutures are now placed through the entire thickness of the graft just above the point of attachment of the commissures and through the whole thickness of the recipient aortic wall. This positions the graft about 5 mm above the normal location of the commissure under slight tension.

A double-armed 4–0 Mersilene suture is then placed at the mid-point of the left aortic sinus of the allograft and subsequently through the host aortic wall just below the left coronary ostium. It is tied and run as an over-and-over suture in each direction along the upper border of the allograft attaching the graft to the host's sinus of Valsalva (*Figure 4.13b*). The same manoeuvre is performed for the right coronary sinus.

After completion of the upper suture line, along the unexcised non-coronary sinus, the competence of the valve is tested by filling the aorta with saline. The

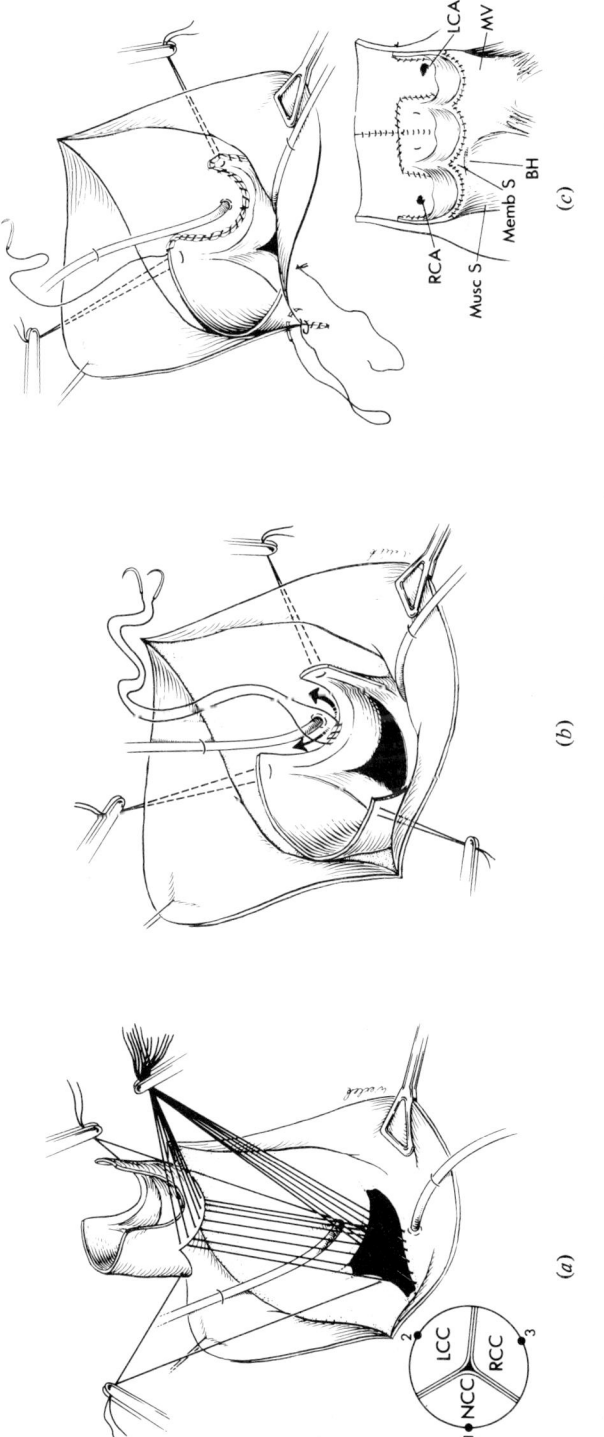

Figure 4.13 Schematic drawings illustrating the operative technique for aortic valve replacement with an aortic allograft: (*a*) Three key stitches were placed in the recipient aortic ring using 4–0 double-armed Mersilene sutures (see insert). Approximately 12, evenly spaced, interrupted sutures are placed for each third of the aortic annulus; (*b*) The upper suture line is started at the midpoint of the left aortic sinus, just below the left coronary ostium. An over-and-over suture is run in each direction; (*c*) The non-coronary sinus of the allograft is incorporated into the aortic suture line. The lower diagram shows the proximity of the lower suture line to the conduction bundle (RCA = right coronary artery ostium; LCA = left coronary artery ostium; Musc S = muscular septum; Memb S = membranous septum; MV = mitral valve; BH = bundle of His)

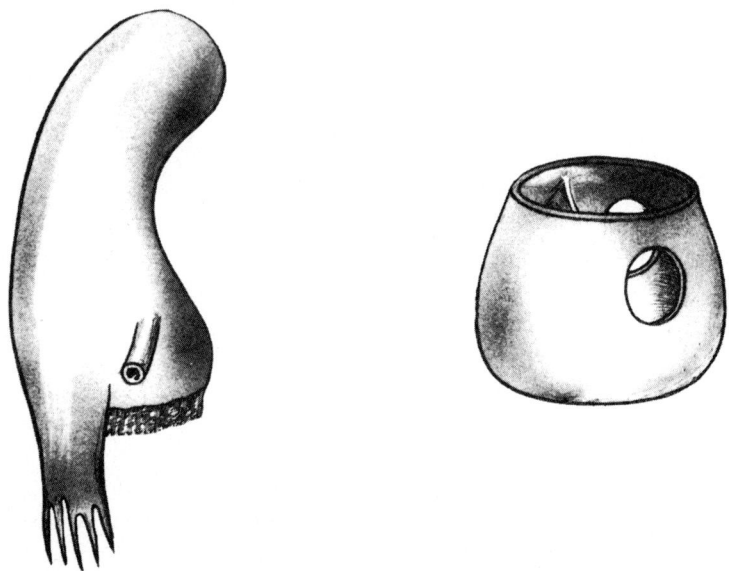

Figure 4.14 Preparation of the aortic allograft as a cylinder for the *in toto* technique
of insertion

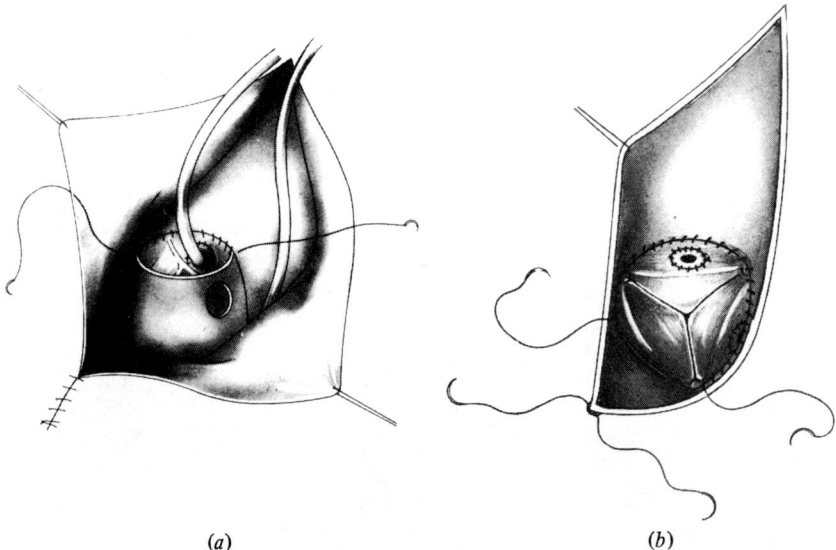

(*a*)   (*b*)

Figure 4.15 Schematic drawings illustrating the operative steps followed for the insertion
of an aortic allograft using the *in toto* technique. (*a*) A continuous circular suture line is
made at the upper margin of the allograft. (*b*) The coronary orifices are attached side-to-
side to the windows cut in the allograft cylinder at the approximate location of the host
coronary ostia

aortic incision is closed with a running 3–0 Mersilene suture incorporating the non-coronary sinus of the allograft into the suture line (*Figure 4.13c*).

More recently, in an endeavour to improve the competence of the valve, the allograft has been inserted as an integral cylinder of aorta including the valve (*Figure 4.14*). This technique involves a continuous circular suture line of the upper margin of the graft (*Figure 4.15a*). The coronary orifices are attached side-to-side using 6–0 Prolene sutures, to appropriate windows cut in the side of the allograft cylinder. These windows should be well clear of the true coronary orifices (*Figure 4.15b*). Alternatively, where there is distortion and hypoplasia of the aortic valve ring and supra-valvular region (tunnel stenosis), the whole valve root is excised down to the mitral cusp below, leaving the coronary arteries free but attached to a small 3 mm cuff of recipient aorta. The lower margin of the allograft cylinder is then sewn in using multiple interrupted sutures. The two coronary orifices of the host are anastomosed side-to-side to the enlarged coronary orifices of the allograft. Finally, the upper margin of the graft is anastomosed end-to-end to the ascending aorta (*Figure 4.16*). The difference between the two techniques is that in the first one the allograft is inserted within the aorta of the host whereas in the second the aortic root has been excised leaving the allograft unsupported.

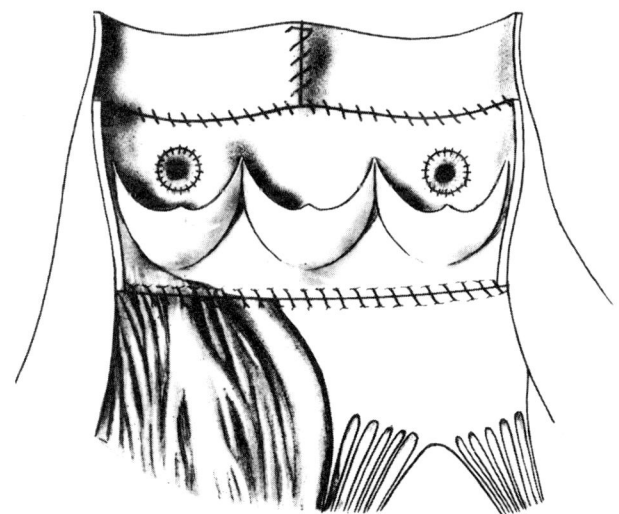

Figure 4.16 In cases of complete excision of the aortic valve and annulus, down to the anterior mitral cusp, the *in toto* technique is used. Schematic drawings show surgical insertion of a cylinder of aortic valve allograft. The graft is secured in position with two continuous end-to-end suture lines, above to the ascending aorta and below to the aortic root. As shown in *Figure 4.15b* the coronary ostia are attached to the windows made in the graft cylinder

In the presence of a rather small aortic annulus, an elliptical Dacron gusset is incorporated within the aortic suture line well into the non-coronary sinus in order to enlarge the sinus and to avoid the prolapse of the non-coronary cusp (*Figure 4.17*).

Air is expelled from the heart and cardiopulmonary bypass discontinued allowing the heart to take over the load of the circulation (*Figure 4.18*). When

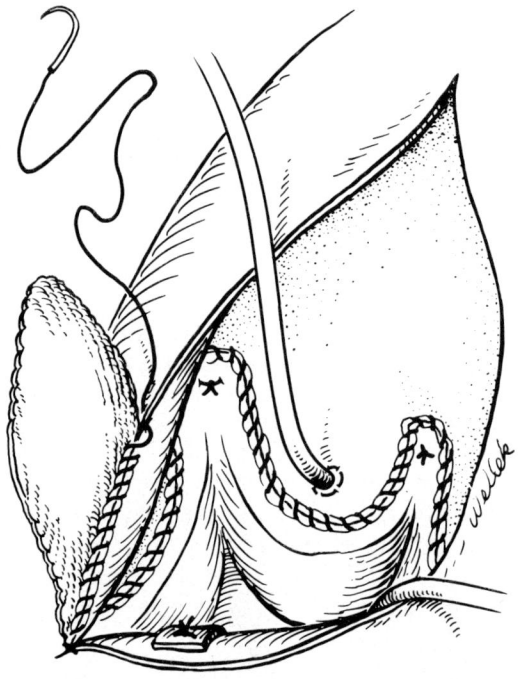

Figure 4.17 In the presence of a rather small aortic annulus, an oval Dacron gusset is incorporated into the aortic suture line in order to enlarge the non-coronary sinus and to avoid the possible prolapse of that cusp

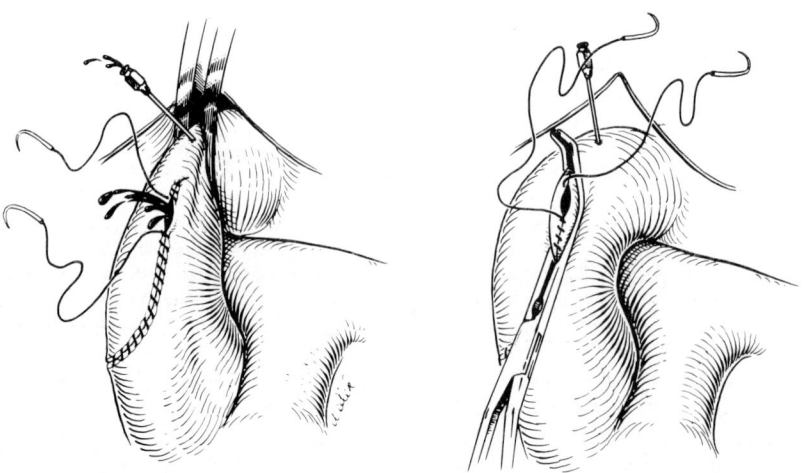

Figure 4.18 Schematic drawings showing the authors' preferred method for expelling air from the left heart

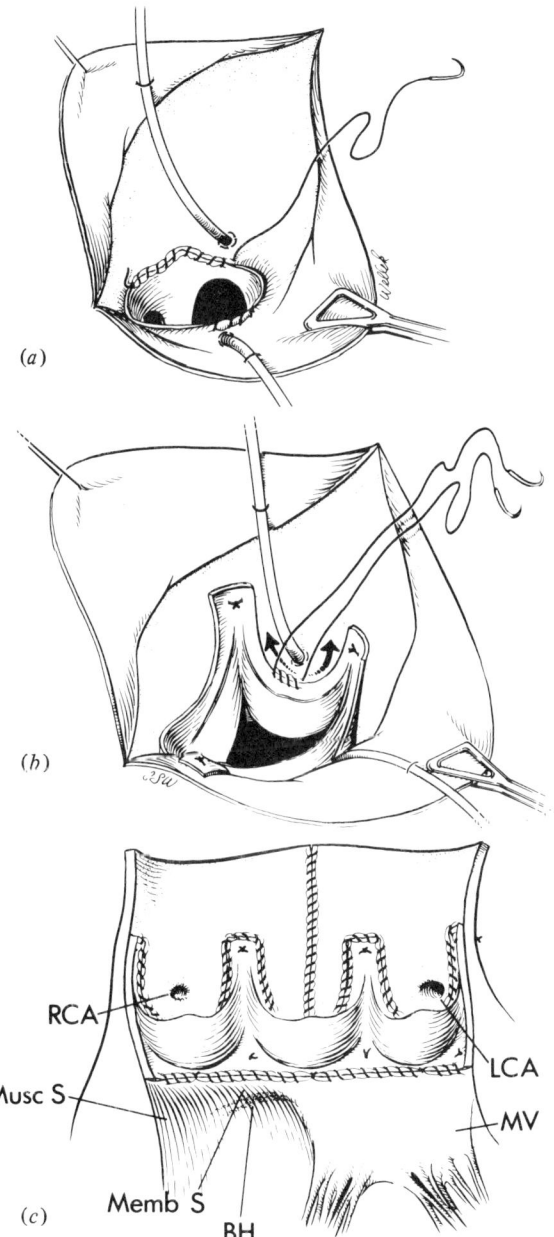

RCA

LCA

Musc S

MV

Memb S

BH

(c)

Figure 4.19 Schematic drawings illustrating Barratt-Boyes technique for aortic allograft valve replacement. (*a*) The allograft was turned inside out and placed inside the left ventricular cavity. The lower suture line is made with a continuous running 3–0 silk suture; (*b*) The upper suture line is made with a running suture. The non-coronary sinus of the allograft is removed as shown in the drawing; (*c*) Diagram showing the completed insertion of the allograft valve using the Barratt-Boyes technique with the two suture lines placed with a running stitch and three sub-commissural interrupted sutures inserted in order to obliterate the dead space between the allograft valve and the host aorta. (RCA = right coronary artery, LCA = left coronary artery, Musc S = muscular septum, Memb S = membranous septum, MV = mitral valve, BH = bundle of His)

the heart maintains a stable systolic pressure and venous pressure, the cannulae are removed. A competent valve can be judged by the absence of a fall in the by-pass line pressure and, on discontinuing the heart–lung bypass, by the easily felt closing shock of the valve and the absence of a diastolic thrill in the root of the aorta. A normal left atrial pressure is considered as confirmatory evidence of a well-functioning aortic valve allograft. After haemostasis is obtained, the chest is closed in layers.

In patients with multivalvular disease both venae cavae are cannulated. The mitral valve is examined and dealt with before the aortic valve. Anoxic arrest of up to 15 min is used in these cases or if a longer operative time is envisaged, coronary perfusion is instituted.

A slightly different principle in preparing and inserting an aortic allograft valve has been used by Barratt-Boyes[7]. In his technique the lower suture line is placed with a continuous running stitch of 3–0 silk (*Figure 4.19a*). The upper suture line is made with a running stitch of 3–0 silk starting at the bottom of the left coronary sinus (*Figure 4.19b*). Barratt-Boyes has made two major modifications in his technique: (1) the aortic root is tailored by excision of an elliptical piece of the non-coronary sinus when there is a gross disparity between the aortic annulus and the available grafts[9]; (2) a vertical mattress suture is placed in each commissural region in order to obliterate the dead space between the graft and the aortic wall (*Figure 4.19c*)[14]. Post-operative angiographic studies[10] have shown a definite decrease and almost disappearance of important peripheral leaks after the introduction of these innovations.

Surgical insertion of autograft valves

In the case of an autograft replacement of the aortic valve a general assessment is first made of the outside diameter of the aortic root and pulmonary artery.

Figure 4.20 Schematic presentation of the surgical technique used for aortic valve replacement with the pulmonary autograft. (*a*) The first step in this operation is the excision of the diseased aortic valve. This is followed by careful and exacting removal of the pulmonary valve. The arrow indicates the point at which the transection of the pulmonary artery begins. (*b*) The lower part of the pulmonary artery is freed by entering a plane of dissection near to the aorta. The dissection is continued around the base of the pulmonary artery until it is cleaned of adventitia. (*c*) The right ventricle is opened just below the pulmonary valve by incising at the base of the anterior commissure. (*d*) the enucleation of the pulmonary valve is almost completed. At this stage care must be taken to avoid injury to the septal branches of the left anterior descending coronary artery. (*e*) The pulmonary valve is completely excised. The first septal branch of the left anterior descending coronary artery is indicated as it branches off just below the incision separating the valve from the right ventricle. (*f*) An aortic allograft valve is used to replace the excised pulmonary valve. The sutures are made in such a way as to place the sinuses of the allograft into their appropriate positions. (*g*) Insertion of the pulmonary autograft valve into the aortic position, using the same technique as for the insertion of an aortic allograft. (*h*) The lower suture line was completed and the commissural sutures were passed through the aortic wall. The arrows indicate the direction of tension exerted on the valve while scalloping it around the left coronary ostium. (*i*) The insertion of the pulmonary autograft valve is completed by attaching the upper margin of the graft to the host aorta. Each series of continuous sutures begins at the centre of a sinus. (Figures (*a*) (*d*) (*e*) and (*f*) reproduced from Gonzalez-Lavin, L., Geens, M. and Ross, D. N.[15]. Figure (*b*) (*c*) (*g*) (*h*) and (*i*) reproduced from Ross, D. N. and Geens, M. 'Heart valve replacement with pulmonary autografts'. In *Biological Tissue in Heart Valve Replacement*. Ed. by M. I. Ionescu, D. N. Ross and G. H. Wooler, pp. 575–599. London; Butterworths (1972)

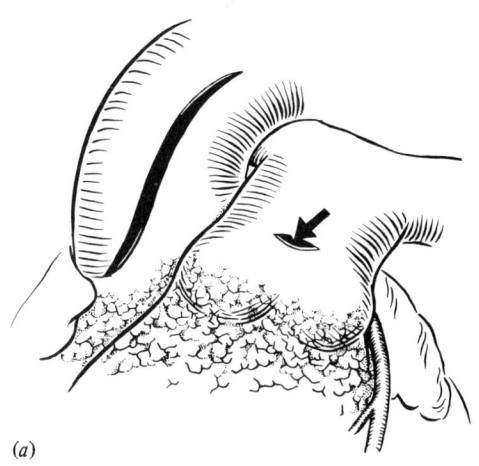

(a)

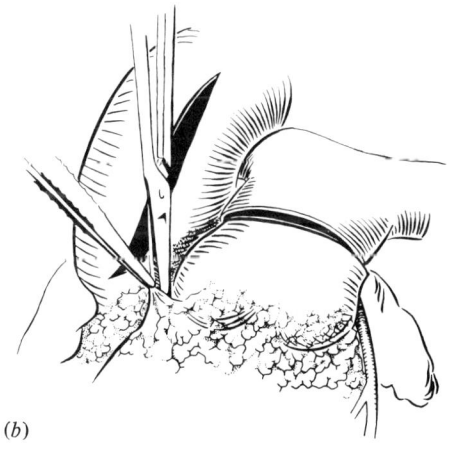

(b)

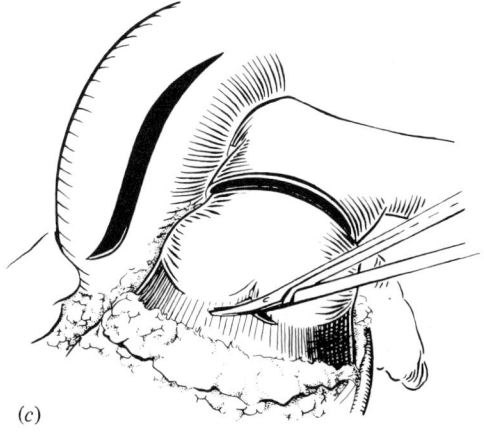

(c)

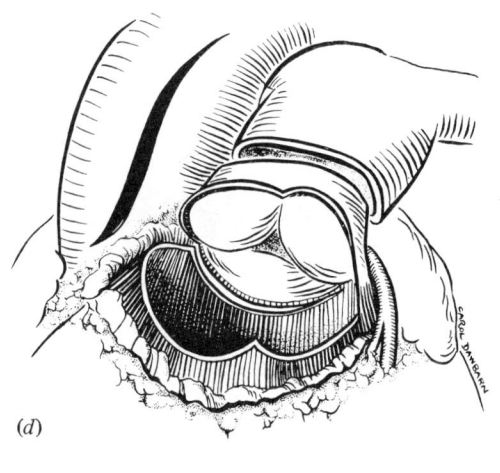

(d)

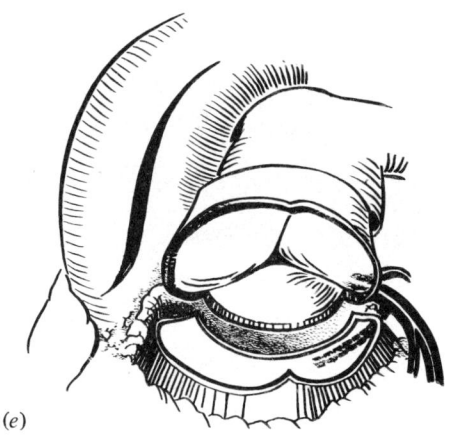

(e)

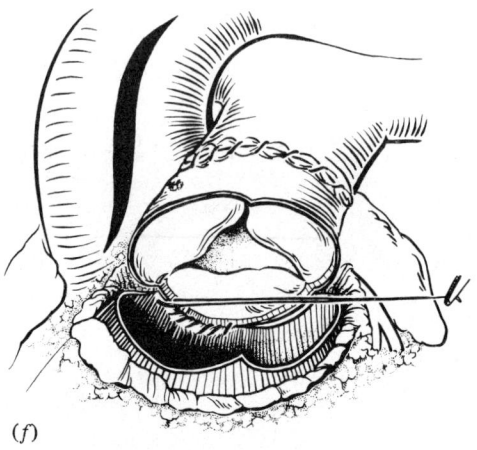

(f)

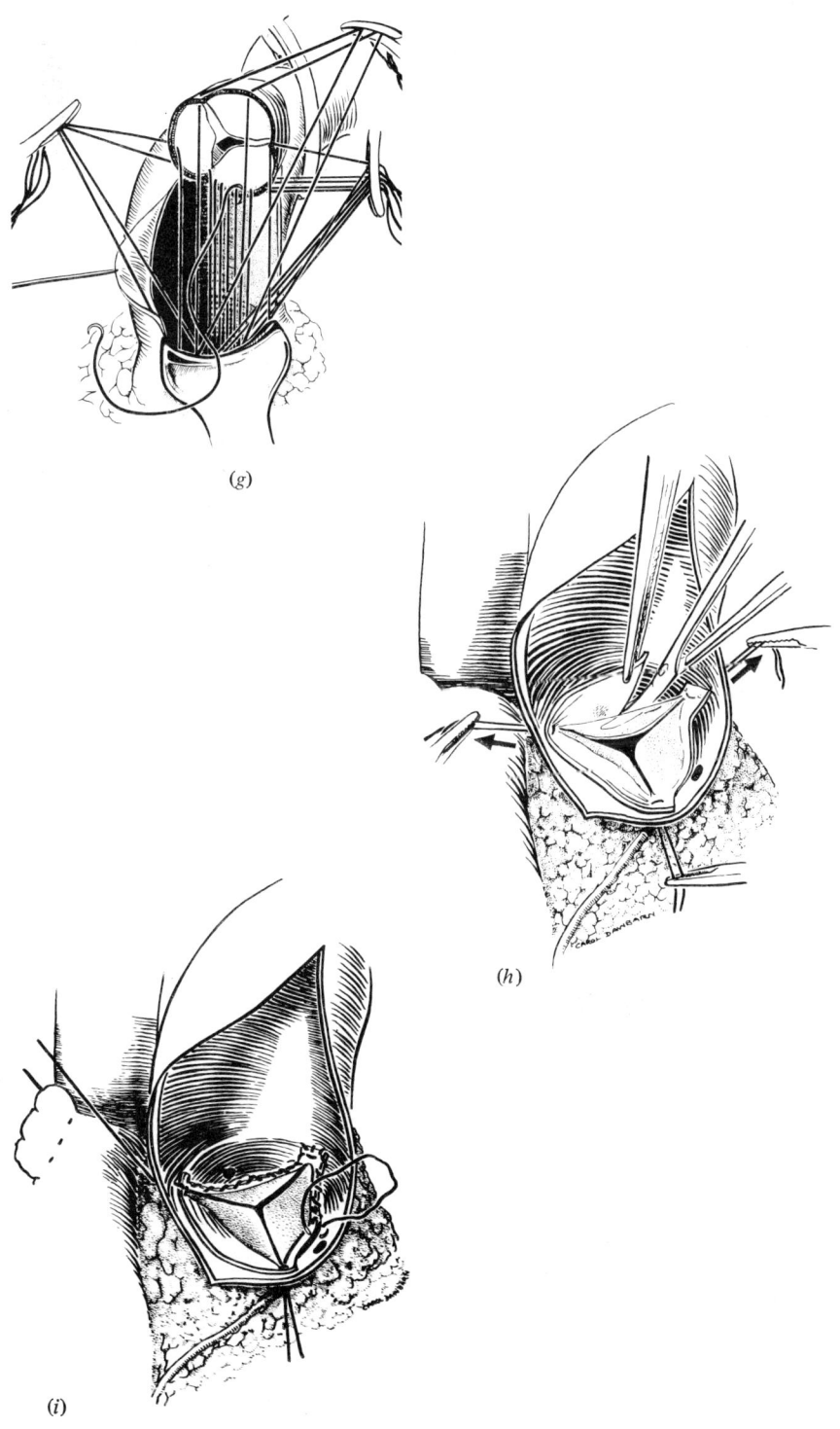

(g)

(h)

(i)

Since equal volumes of blood flow through both, there is seldom much discrepancy. If there is a considerable disproportion an alternative valve replacement technique is used.

Once heart–lung bypass has been established the aorta is opened and bilateral coronary perfusion commenced since the replacement involves about 2 h of extracorporeal circulation. The aortic valve is excised and attention is then directed to the pulmonary valve (*Figure 4.20a*).

A transverse incision is made in the pulmonary artery, well above the commissures, and the valve is inspected, following which the pulmonary artery is transected. It is then dissected from above downwards towards the right ventricle keeping close to the pulmonary artery well until muscle is encountered in the base of the sinuses (*Figure 4.20c*) and to enucleate the valve cusps with virtually no muscle from within the right ventricle (*Figure 4.20d*). In this way a scalloped muscular defect is left in the outflow of the right ventricle and danger of damage to the adjacent septal branches of the left anterior descending coronary artery is avoided (*Figure 4.20e*)[15].

The pulmonary valve is then replaced with a suitable aortic allograft[27,15]. This is attached first to the distal pulmonary artery incorporating the loose adventitia of the pulmonary artery in the 4-0 suture for added strength.

The proximal anastomosis of the allograft to the right ventricular outflow is usually completed with small bites of 4-0 continuous suture and with the heart relaxed in temporary ischaemic arrest to avoid the sutures tearing out during contractions of the heart muscle (*Figure 4.20f*).

Once continuity of right ventricular outflow has been re-established, coronary perfusion is resumed and attention directed to the aortic valve replacement. During the preceding period the excised pulmonary valve autograft is generally allowed to lie in the pool of blood in the pericardial cavity.

The autograft is now trimmed of all excess muscle up to within about 1 mm of the cusp insertions and any loose adventitia are dissected from the pulmonary artery wall.

Insertion of the autograft is performed in exactly the same way as insertion of an allograft[28]. Multiple interrupted 4-0 sutures are used along the lower margin in order to match the sinuses of the graft to the corresponding areas of the excised valve ring as accurately as possible. The sutures are passed close to the actual cusp insertions where the tissue is tough (*Figure 4.20g*). It is usual to delay scalloping of the pulmonary artery wall around the coronary orifices until the commissural fixation sutures have been placed through the aortic wall. By holding adjacent fixation sutures under tension, the scalloping could be carried out accurately (*Figure 4.20h*). The upper margin of the graft is then sewn to the aortic wall with 4-0 continuous sutures which start at the centre of each sinus and end at the commissures. These sutures are tied to the through-and-through commissural suspending sutures (*Figure 4.20i*).

After testing the valve for competence with saline during left ventricular suction, the aortotomy is closed with a running 3-0 suture. Further evidence of a competent valve is obtained from palpation of the closing shock of the valve and the absence of a diastolic murmur and thrill on direct auscultation.

RESULTS

Between 1964 and 1977, 664 patients underwent isolated aortic valve replacement with either allograft or autograft valves. This chapter details the results obtained in this series of patients. The term isolated valve replacement is being used in this chapter to denote that only the aortic valve was replaced but that other cardiac surgical procedures could have been performed at the same time. *Tables 4.1* and *4.2* show that 172 patients underwent associated surgical operations such as mitral valvotomy or repair, closure of septal defects of direct myocardial revascularization with saphenous vein-coronary artery bypass grafts.

TABLE 4.1
Additional surgical procedures performed at the time of
aortic valve replacement with allograft valves in 476 patients

Concomitant surgical procedure	*Number of patients*
Closure of atrial septal defect	2
Closure of ventricular septal defect	10
Mitral valvotomy	76
Mitral annuloplasty	41
Tricuspid annuloplasty	1
Aorta to coronary artery saphenous vein bypass graft	9
Total	139

TABLE 4.2
Additional surgical procedures performed at the time of
aortic valve replacement with autograft valves in 188 patients

Concomitant surgical procedure	*Number of patients*
Mitral valvotomy	15
Left ventricular myotomy	13
Closure of atrial or ventricular septal defect, and/or aorta to coronary artery saphenous vein bypass graft	5
Total	33

TABLE 4.3
Type and number of valve grafts inserted according to the
period of time of their clinical use

Period of time of valve graft usage	*Type of valve graft (mode of sterilization)*	*Number*
1964–1967	Freeze-dried allografts (ethylene oxide)	184
1968–1969	Frozen allografts (ethylene oxide or gamma rays)	31
1971–1977	Fresh allografts (antibiotics)	261
1967–1977	Pulmonary valve autografts	188
1964–1977	Total	664

Of the total of 664 patients, 188 received a pulmonary autograft while 476 patients received an allograft valve, as shown in *Table 4.3* which gives details of the methods of preparation and preservation used for allograft valves during this period of time.

The average age of the allograft valve recipients was 40 years, whilst that for the pulmonary autograft patients was 30 years. In the allograft valve replacement group there were 360 males and 116 females, whereas of the 188 patients who received pulmonary autograft valves 154 were males and 34 females. Of the 664 patients, 32 per cent presented with aortic stenosis, 37 per cent with aortic regurgitation, 19 per cent with mixed stenosis and insufficiency and 6 per cent with sequelae of infective endocarditis. A further 6 per cent required re-operation for failure of previously inserted valves.

The average hospital mortality for the last five years has been 5.4 per cent for the allograft insertions and 4.6 per cent for the pulmonary autograft insertions (*Figures 4.21* and *4.22*).

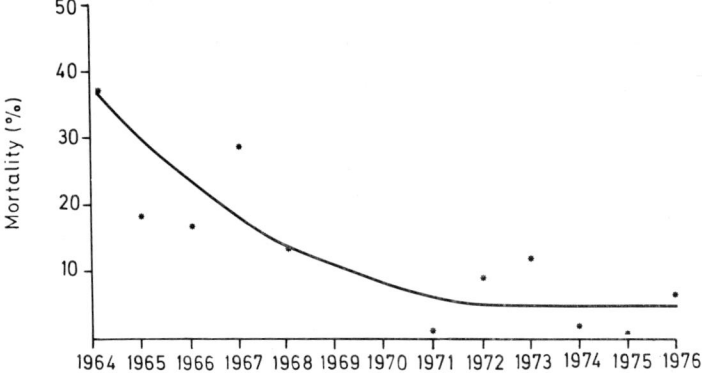

Figure 4.21 Graphic presentation of annual hospital mortality for patients having aortic valve replacement with allograft valves

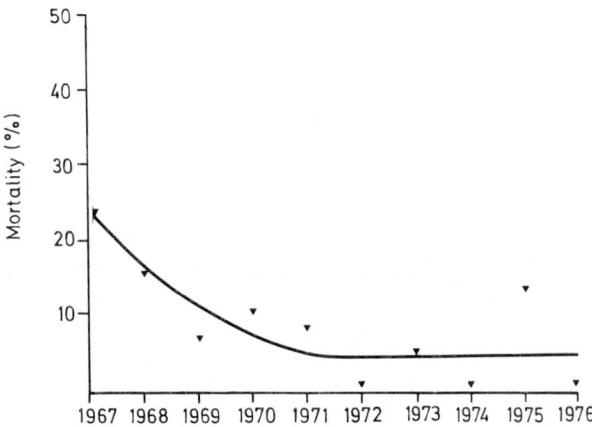

Figure 4.22 Graphic presentation of annual hospital mortality for patients having aortic valve replacement with autograft pulmonary valves

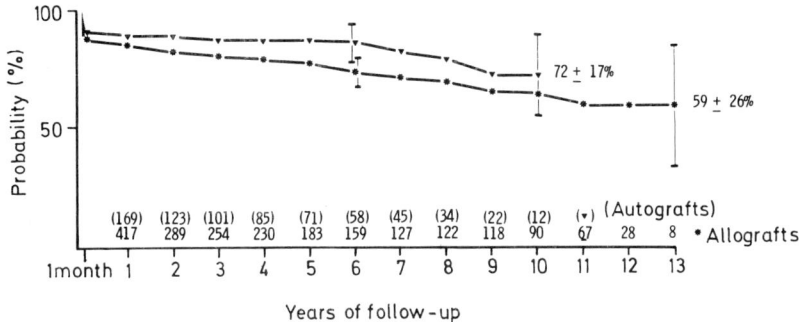

Figure 4.23 Actuarial analysis of survival rate for patients having aortic valve replacement with either allograft or autograft valves. The figures along the abcissa represent the number of valves entering each year of follow-up*, patients with allografts; △, patients with autografts. The survival rate is expressed in per cent ± standard error. The hospital mortality is included. (From Anderson *et al.*[5])

The long-term results for the two groups of patients with allograft and autograft valves are presented in an actuarial manner calculated according to the method of Anderson *et al.*[5], including the hospital mortality (*Figure 4.23*). This shows that patients who received an allograft valve had a 59 per cent probability of survival at 13 years from the time of their operation. Similarly, the patients who received an autograft valve had a 72 per cent probability of survival at ten years. When the same date was analysed with special reference to the type of allograft valve preparation (*Figure 4.24*), a slightly different picture emerged. There was a considerable difference in the probability of survival of patients who received freeze-dried allograft valves when compared with patients who received allografts prepared in other different ways. It became immediately apparent that the main difference was due to the higher hospital mortality of patients with freeze-dried allograft valves. As shown in *Figure 4.21*, the hospital mortality between 1964 and 1967 was high and freeze-dried allografts were inserted during that period of time (*Table 4.3*). The reduced hospital mortality

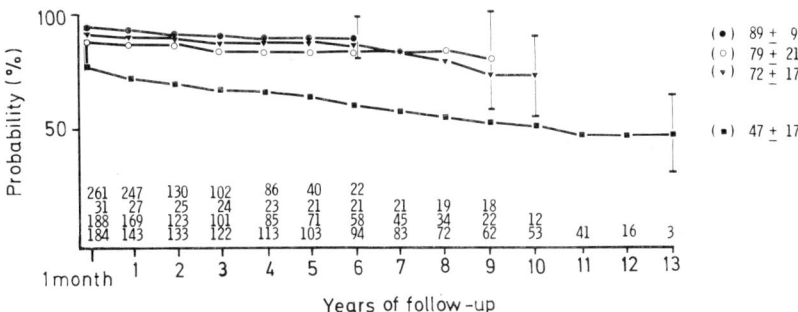

Figure 4.24 Actuarial analysis of survival rate for patients with aortic valve replacement. Individual curves are presented for the four groups of patients receiving respectively: fresh allografts (●); frozen allografts (○); pulmonary autografts (△); and freeze-dried allografts (□). The figures along the abcissa represent the number of valves entering each year of follow-up. The survival rate is expressed in per cent ± standard error. The hospital mortality is included. * = coincidental points. (From Anderson *et al.*[5])

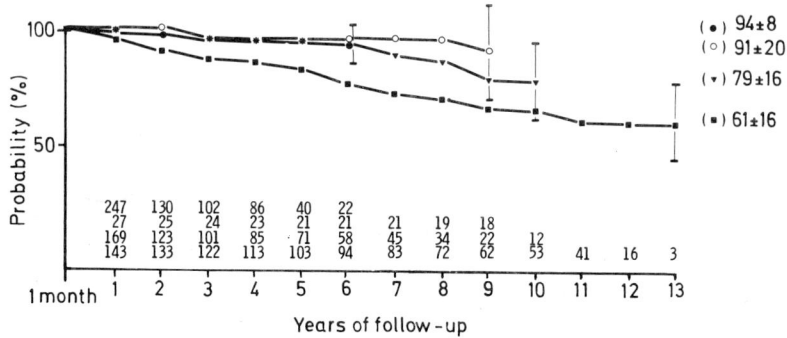

Figure 4.25 Actuarial analysis of survival rate for patients with aortic valve replacement. The presentation and symbols are identical to those in *Figure 4.24* except that the hospital mortality was excluded from the analysis. (From Anderson *et al.*[5])

in the last five years is due to improvement in surgical technique and not related to the method of allograft valve preparation. For this reason it is considered appropriate to exclude the hospital mortality from the subsequent results, as in *Figure 4.25*. As it is necessary to know what has happened to each of the four groups of valves, as well as the patients, this method of presentation allows a fair comparison of the long-term follow-up.

The comparison of patient survival shown in *Figure 4.25* uses the same technique of presentation as described by Anderson *et al.*[5], but excludes the hospital mortality. The probability of survival at 13 years becomes therefore, 61 per cent for the groups of patients who received a freeze-dried allograft. There is still a difference between these freeze-dried allograft recipients and those receiving the other valves but this is not as striking as in *Figure 4.24*. Examination of *Figures 4.21, 4.22* and *4.25* together shows that a patient who received an autograft or an allograft valve, other than a freeze-dried one, has an operative risk of 5 per cent and a 94 per cent probability of surviving for six years following the operation.

Long-term follow-up data provide information about patients' survival and valve failures. Valve failure is defined as a valve related complication which results in the death of the patients or the need to re-operate and replace or repair the valve. In order to present this detailed information we have used the cumulative curves based on a hierarchy of importance described by Grunkemeier *et al.*[16] and applied them to the patient groups in *Table 4.3* for each year of analysis. During the analysis year the patient may die or incur a valve failure, fatal or not, and these three consequences are sequential in importance. The results, excluding the hospital mortality, are calculated on an actuarial patient basis, referring death, fatal valve failures and non-fatal valve failures in one year to the number of patients entering that year of follow-up. In this way, as in the description of Grunkemeier *et al.*[16], the breakdown of the population at any one time adds up to 100 per cent.

Using this method, the results of the freeze-dried allograft valves presented in *Figure 4.26* show that of the 143 patients operated upon between 1964 and 1967, and who survived the operation, the probability of survival at 13 years was 59 per cent, although only 38 per cent survived with the original valve graft. In

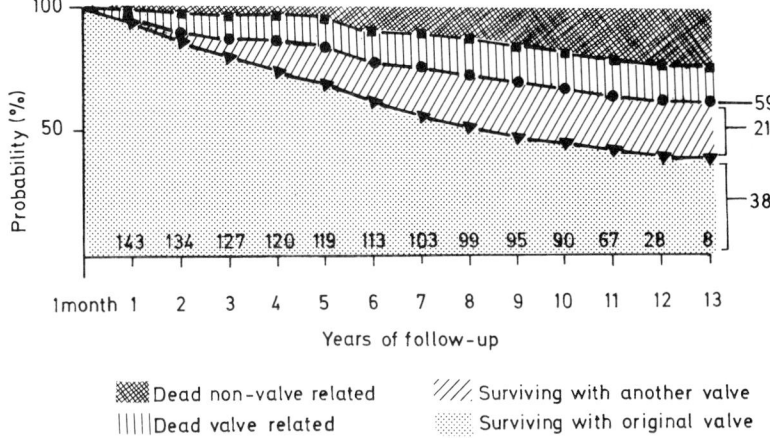

Figure 4.26 Actuarial analysis of patients having aortic valve replacement with freeze-dried allograft valves. The individual cumulative curves represent, from above, downwards: deaths not related to the allograft valve (25 per cent); valve related deaths (16 per cent); patients surviving with another valve, following re-operation for valve related complications (21 per cent); and patients surviving with the original allograft (38 per cent). The figures along the abcissa represent the number of patients entering each year of follow-up. The hospital mortality was not included in the analysis

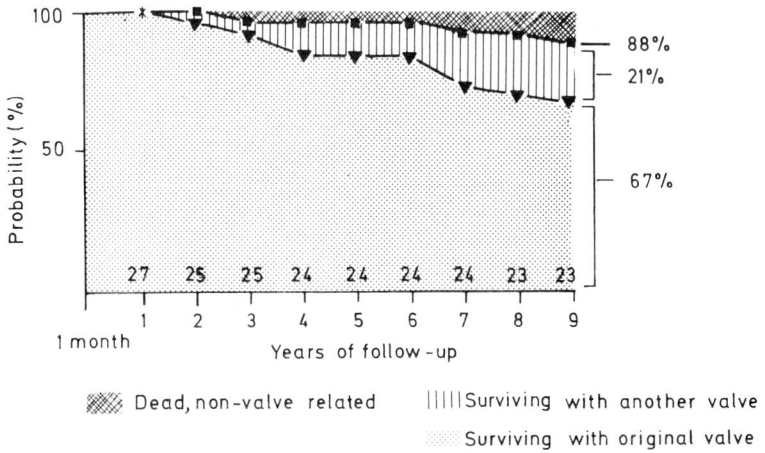

Figure 4.27 Actuarial analysis of patients having aortic valve replacement with frozen allograft valves. The individual cumulative curves represent from the top downwards: deaths not related to the allograft valve (12 per cent); patients surviving with another valve, following re-operation for valve related complications (21 per cent); and patients surviving with the original allograft (67 per cent). The figures along the abcissa denote the number of patients entering each year of follow-up. The hospital mortality was not included in the analysis

other words, 21 per cent had a second successful operation following a valve complication.

Similarly, of the 27 patients who survived an operation to insert a frozen allograft valve between 1968 and 1969 (*Figure 4.27*), the probability of survival at nine years was 88 per cent whereas only 67 per cent had a probability of surviving with the original valve graft and 21 per cent therefore had survived a re-operation to replace or repair a failed valve. There have been no late deaths associated with valve complications in this cohort of 27 patients, who had a 12 per cent probability of non-valve related death over the nine-year period of follow-up.

The 247 patients who received a fresh allograft valve between 1971 and 1977 and who survived the operation are presented in *Figure 4.28*. There was a 93 per cent probability of survival at six years and 84 per cent probability of surviving with the original fresh allograft valve, 9 per cent surviving a re-operation to repair or replace a failing valve.

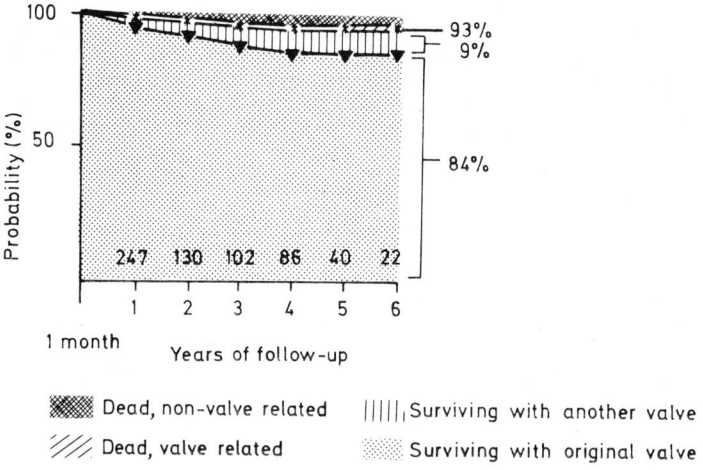

Figure 4.28 Actuarial analysis of patients having aortic valve replacement with fresh allograft valves. The individual cumulative curves represent, from the top downwards: deaths not related to the allograft valve (6 per cent); valve related death (1 per cent); patients surviving with another valve, following re-operation for valve related complications (9 per cent); and patients surviving with the original allograft (84 per cent). The figures along the abcissa denote the number of patients entering each year of follow-up. The hospital mortality was not included in the analysis

Between 1967 and 1977 there were 169 patients who survived an operation to insert a pulmonary autograft valve and these are presented in *Figure 4.29*. There was a probability that 78 per cent of these patients would survive for ten years, 70 per cent with the original autograft valve and the remaining 8 per cent with another valve inserted at a re-operation to repair or replace the original valve.

The actuarial analyses only present probability of survival and valve failure. In order to compare the actual results of the different groups of valves shown in *Table 4.3* we have chosen to analyse cohorts of patients who have been followed-

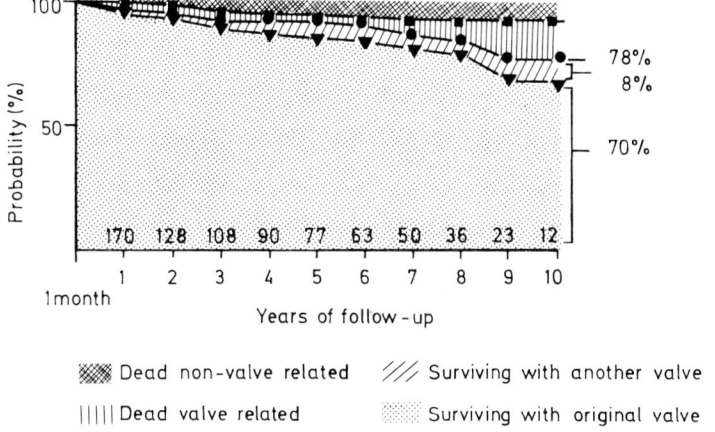

Dead non-valve related   Surviving with another valve

Dead valve related   Surviving with original valve

Figure 4.29 Actuarial analysis of patients having aortic valve replacement with pulmonary autograft valves. The individual cumulative curves represent, from the top downwards: deaths not related to the autograft valve (7 per cent); valve related deaths (15 per cent); patients surviving with another valve, following re-operation for valve related complications (8 per cent); and patients surviving with the original pulmonary autograft (70 per cent). The figures along the abcissa indicate the number of patients entering each year of follow-up. The hospital mortality was not included in the analysis. The difference in the number of patients with autograft valves analysed in this figure and in *Figure 4.24* is due to the fact that two patients had their autograft valve removed during the first 30 post-operative days

up, each one of them, for at least five years, or at least nine years. Unlike the actuarial analyses, the patients with less than five or less than nine years follow-up have been excluded from the cohort analyses and these results permit an unbiased comparison of the groups at five- and nine-year follow-up. The intervals of five and nine years were selected in order to have large enough numbers in each group to make the comparisons valid. The numbers of patients in each cohort, for each type of valve, are presented in *Table 4.4*. Only 47 of the 261 patients who received a fresh allograft valve between 1971 and 1977 have been followed-up for at least five years, and none for nine years. Similarly, 82 of the 188 patients receiving a pulmonary autograft between 1967 and 1977 have been followed-up for at least nine years. The frozen allografts were inserted during the

TABLE 4.4

Groups of patients according to the type of valve graft inserted, studied by cohorts in order to compare the results at five and nine years follow-up

Period of time of valve graft usage	Type of valve graft	Number of patients	
		5-year cohort	*9-year cohort*
1964–1967	Freeze-dried allografts	137	135
1968–1969	Frozen allografts	25	25
1971–1977	Fresh allografts	47	0
1967–1977	Pulmonary autografts	82	27

years 1968 to 1969 and so form a single cohort of 25 patients at both five and nine years of follow-up.

The analysis of data at five years shows clearly that there has been an improvement in results since 1967 when the freeze-dried allograft valve was abandoned (*Figure 4.30*). Survival with the original valve has increased with both frozen and fresh allografts and autografts whilst the proportion of failures has decreased.

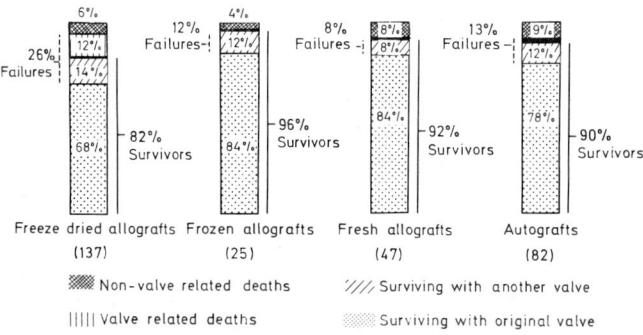

Figure 4.30 Graphic presentation of comparative analysis of cohorts of patients having aortic valve replacement with allografts and autografts and who were observed for at least a period of five years. Figures in parentheses denote the number of patients in each cohort

The mortality from failure of the valve has almost disappeared in these three groups when compared with the 12 per cent for freeze-dried allograft valves.

So far there is no significant difference between the frozen or fresh allografts and the autografts. By following the patients for nine years (*Figure 4.31*), the differences between the freeze-dried allografts and the other groups is emphasized, but some new information emerges. The failure rate of freeze-dried allografts increased from 26 per cent at five years to 51 per cent at nine years and this incidence of failure is higher than that for the frozen allograft valves.

Although the freeze-dried allograft has a high record of failure, it is clear at nine years that, with the improvements in surgical technique, many more patients

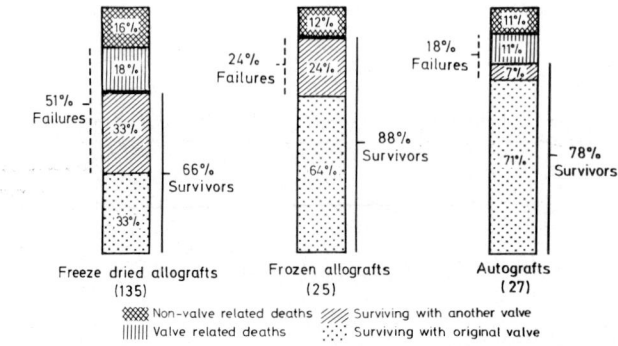

Figure 4.31 Graphic presentation of comparative analysis of cohorts of patients having aortic valve replacement with allografts and autografts and who were observed for at least a period of nine years. Figures in parentheses denote the number of patients in each cohort

survived re-operation required for valve failure. At five years (*Figure 4.30*), the freeze-dried group shows that approximately half the failures resulted in death of the patients (14 per cent as compared to 12 per cent of valve failure with survival of the patients). At nine years however, only one-third of the valve failures resulted in death (18 per cent), whereas two-thirds (33 per cent) of the patients had a valve failure which was successfully re-operated upon (*Figure 4.31*).

The other important observation from *Figure 4.31* is that all the patients with failed frozen valves survived re-operation (24 per cent), whereas in the case of the autografts more than half of the failures (11 per cent out of 18 per cent) resulted in death of the patients.

The analyses in *Figures 4.26* to *4.31* have examined patient survival in order to assess the long-term function of biological valves such as allografts and autografts. It is recognized that these valves are all liable to late onset degenerative processes. We have, therefore, examined all valve failures, fatal or non-fatal, in order to assess the time of failure related to the time of operation. A comparison of allograft and autograft valve failures (*Figure 4.32*), at ten years shows that there is no statistically significant difference between the two types of valve grafts.

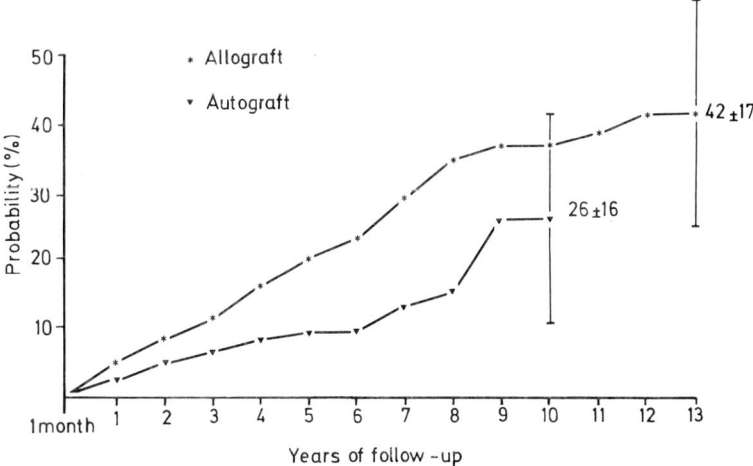

Figure 4.32 Actuarial probability of allograft (all preparations) and autograft valve failure at 13 and 10 years' follow-up respectively ± standard error

Analysis of the four groups of valves (*Table 4.3* and *Figure 4.33*) shows that the freeze-dried group has a higher incidence of valve failure whilst the other three groups are comparable. Furthermore, in the first four years of follow-up the failures in the freeze-dried group show an increasing rate, not seen in the other groups. Thereafter the freeze-dried failure curve tends to flatten off.

The causes of valve failure may be separated conveniently into three divisions; technical, infective and degenerative. Technical failures occur during the first four post-operative years and are usually due to malpositioning of the valve, damage to the valve at the time of insertion or dehiscence of one or more sutures.

Infective failures are associated with either a primary infection of the allograft manifesting itself during the first three months post-operatively or a

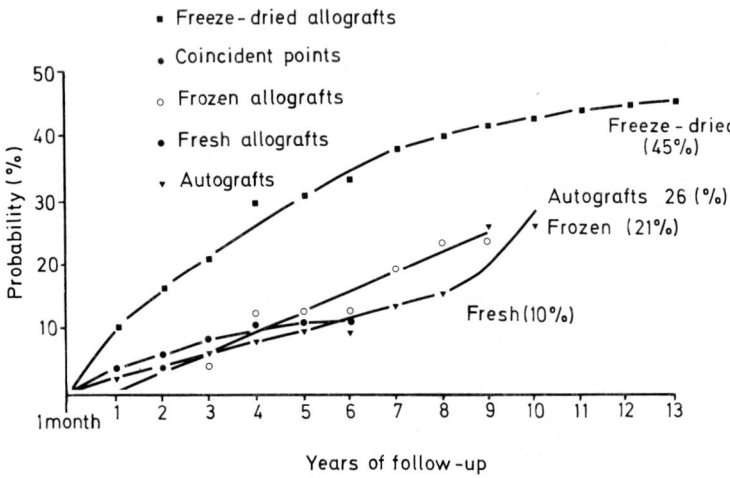

Figure 4.33 Actuarial probability of valve graft failure for allografts (freeze-dried, frozen or fresh) and autografts

TABLE 4.5
Incidence of valve graft failure due to technical, infective and degenerative causes

Time since the operation	Allograft valves									Autograft valves		
	Freeze-dried– 143 patients			Frozen– 27 patients			Fresh– 247 patients			169 patients		
	T	I	D	T	I	D	T	I	D	T	I	D
months												
1–3	–	1(1)	–	–	–	–	–	1(1)	–	–	–	–
4–12	4(3)	1(1)	–	–	–	–	9(2)	–	–	4	–	–
years												
2	7(3)	2(1)	1(1)	1	–	–	2	–	–	2	–	–
3	3(1)	2(1)	1	–	–	–	–	1	2	2(1)	–	–
4	3(1)	1	5	–	1	1	1	1	–	–	1	1
5	–	3(1)	4(2)	–	–	–	–	–	–	–	1	–
6	–	2(1)	4(1)	–	–	–	–	–	–	–	–	–
7	–	1	8(2)	–	–	2				–	1(1)	1(1)
8	–	3	5(2)	–	–	1				–	1(1)	–
9	–	1	3	–	–	–				–	1(1)	2(1)
10	–	–	1(1)							–	–	–
11	–	–	2(1)									
12	–	–	1									
13	–	–	–									
Total	17(8)	17(6)	35(10) (10)	1	1	4	12(2)	3(1)	2	8(1)	5(3)	4(2)

Causes of valve graft failure: T = technical errors at the time of valve graft insertion; I = infection of the valve graft; D = primary tissue degeneration of the valve graft

Figures in parentheses denote failure-related deaths. Hospital mortality not included.

secondary infection which can occur at any time. Degenerative failure may become manifest within four years of valve insertion and can present with calcification or with attenuation or perforation of the cusps. Histological examination often shows degenerative collagen fibres, absence of nuclei and destruction of the tissue architecture.

Table 4.5 presents all the valve failures, relating them to the time since insertion, their valve group and the type of valve failure. This table enables detailed comparisons to be made between the four groups of valves. In general it is clear that the number of technical failures, which was high in the freeze-dried group (12 per cent probability after four years), has declined to a probability of only 6 per cent at four years for the other three groups which were inserted after 1967.

The probability of freedom from infective endocarditis is shown in *Figure 4.34*. There is no significant difference between allografts and autografts at ten years' follow-up. It is not necessary to compare actuarial curves for the individual groups of allograft valves as they are similar (*Table 4.5*). The mean probability of

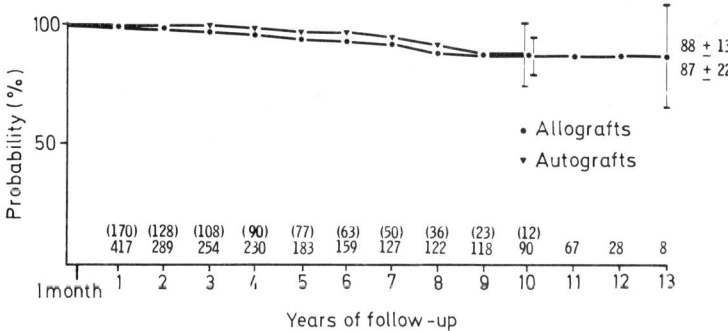

Figure 4.34 Actuarial probability (± standard error) of freedom from infective endocarditis amongst patients with allograft and autograft valves. Figures along the abcissa represent the number of patients entering each year of follow-up (autografts in parentheses)

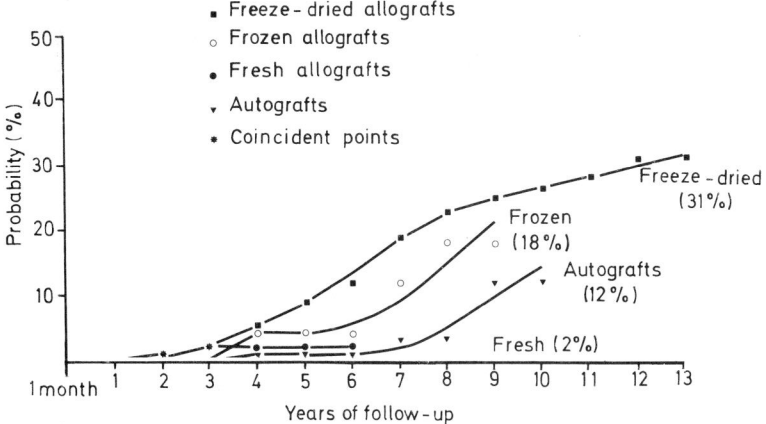

Figure 4.35 Actuarial probability of tissue degeneration resulting in valve graft failure for allografts (freeze-dried, frozen or fresh) and autografts

infective endocarditis over a period of 13 years is 12 per cent, an infection rate of 0.92 per cent/year.

For many years the major disadvantage of allograft valve replacement has been considered to be the degenerative processes which have resulted in valve failure. However, even in what is regarded as the worst group, the freeze-dried valves, there is only an actuarial probability of 31 per cent of degenerative failure of the valve after 13 years of implantation. This is in contrast with the widely-held opinion[21].

In the freeze-dried group the degenerative failures tend to occur after three to four years following insertion, whereas the frozen allografts only show an increase in degenerative failure after six years (*Figure 4.35*). The autograft valves show a similar increase in the probability of degenerative valve failure after seven to eight years and, so far, there has been no such increase in the fresh allograft valves after six years. We therefore feel that a minimum follow-up period of six to eight years is necessary before assessing the biological valves prospects.

Another important fact, not shown in *Figure 4.35*, is the observation that the degeneration of freeze-dried valves seen at four years has been characterized by the finding of compact foci of calcification. Any calcification seen in fresh and frozen allografts presents as loose, friable deposits and the more usual picture of degenerative failure in these valves is of thinned-out atrophic tissue, with attenuated cusp structure and without calcification.

Another feature which causes concern and is specifically associated with allograft and autograft valves is the presence of an early post-operative diastolic murmur. Of the 664 patients in this study, 424 have been followed-up particularly in order to assess the significance of this murmur. In this group of 424 patients, 318 had an allograft valve and 106 had an autograft valve. From

TABLE 4.6

Relationship between the incidence of early post-operative aortic diastolic murmur and the occurrence of valve graft failure in patients with allograft and autograft aortic valve replacement*

	Early post-operative EDM present		*Early post-operative EDM absent*	
Valve graft related event	*Allograft valves* number (per cent)	*Autograft valves* number (per cent)	*Allograft valves* number (per cent)	*Autograft valves* number (per cent)
Event-free	50 (53)	22 (88)	178 (80)	70 (86)
Valve failure caused by infection	5 (5)	1 (4)	17 (8)	3 (4)
Valve failure caused by non-infective processes†	41 (42)	2 (8)	27 (12)	8 (10)
Total	96	25	222	81

EDM = early diastolic murmur

*The 98 operative deaths, as well as the 142 patients who were either lost to follow-up or were followed for only one year or less, were not included in this table.

†Denotes valve failure caused by either surgical technical problems or primary tissue degeneration

Table 4.6 it can be seen that 121 patients developed an early post-operative diastolic murmur whilst 303 did not. The two groups, with and without murmur, have been analysed separately for both allograft and autograft valve replacement with respect to the occurrence of valve graft failure. Three groups of patients were identified: those without valve failure, those with valve failure caused by infection and finally patients with valve failure due to technical or degenerative causes grouped together as non-infective failures.

Table 4.6 shows that there is no correlation between infective valve failure and an early diastolic murmur. There was an incidence of 4–8 per cent of infective endocarditis in all groups, both with and without a diastolic murmur. In the group of patients who received allograft valves, the incidence of non-infective failure (42 per cent), was much higher in patients with an early diastolic murmur than in the group of patients with an allograft valve and without murmur (12 per cent). There is a statistically significant difference between these two groups ($p < 0.0001$).

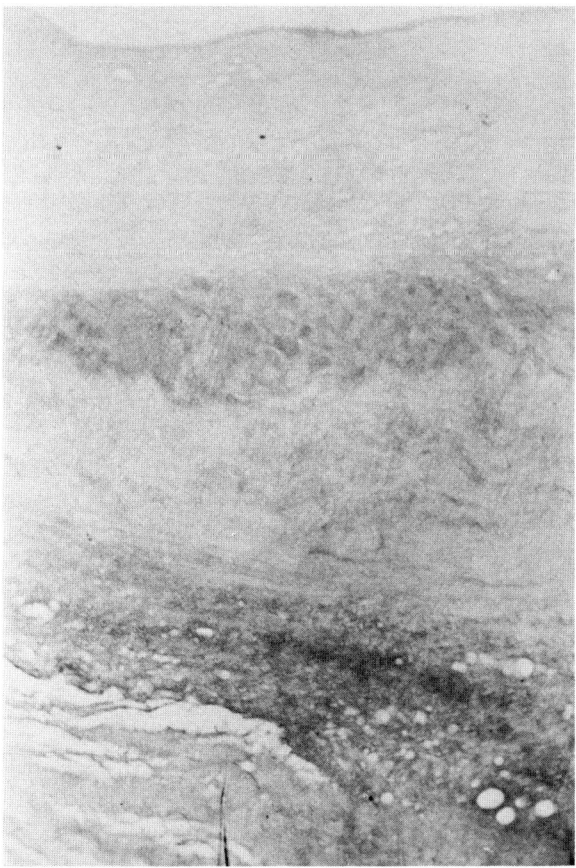

Figure 4.36 Microscopic appearance of a fresh allograft valve removed from a patient three years following its insertion. This shows absence of nuclei and loss of tissue architecture. Haematoxylin and eosin, magnification $\times$ 500, reduced by $\frac{1}{3}$ in printing

Examination of removed valves

The viability studies performed on allograft valves removed from patients have shown a fall in viability to zero within two to three years of insertion (*Figure 4.4*). The histological appearance of the removed valves correlates with the viability changes, and shows a decrease in nuclear content. *Figure 4.36* shows a fresh allograft valve removed after three years, and *Figure 4.37* shows a freeze-dried allograft valve removed after nine years. Microscopic examination of these valves removed at three and nine years following their insertion showed absent nuclei and a marked loss of tissue architecture with degeneration of the collagen and elastic fibres. Detailed histological reports have been received from 20 valves removed more than four years after insertion. This group of 20 valves does not include reports made on valves removed because of technical failure, and the results are summarized in *Table 4.7*. This table only presents the information on the 20 valves for which detailed histological information is available. In other cases of failure or death outside the hospital, no such detailed information was available.

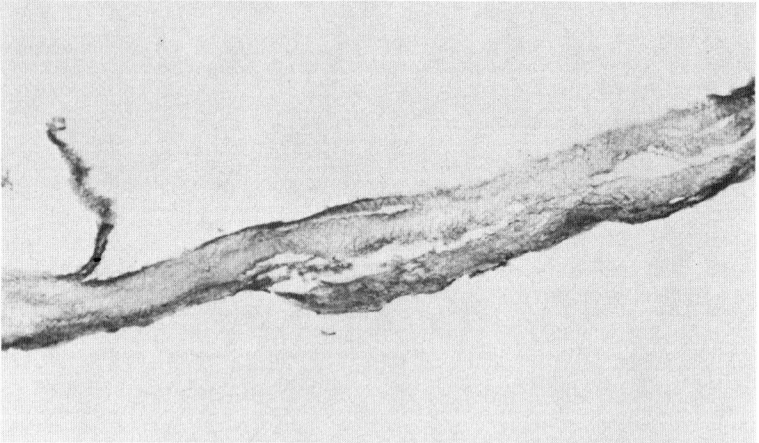

Figure 4.37 Microscopic appearance of a freeze-dried allograft valve removed from a patient nine years following its insertion. The main features are the absence of nuclei and degeneration of collagen fibres. Haematoxylin and eosin, magnification × 125, reduced by 40 per cent in printing

The overall impression from these results is that the valves with late, degenerative failure do not contain visible nuclei, but show degeneration of collagen fibres, frequently with foci of calcification, and a loss of tissue architecture. This is clearly demonstrated in *Figures 4.36* and *4.37*. The macroscopic appearance of the valves removed at surgery suggests that late degenerative failure of frozen and fresh allografts is an atrophic thinning of the cusps, a process of attenuation or wearing out, sometimes with loose friable calcification (*Figure 4.38*). This is in contrast with the degenerative failure of the freeze-dried valves, which is characterized by thickening of the cusps and the formation of nodules of calcium incorporated within the substance of the cusps and the adjacent aortic wall (*Figure 4.39*).

TABLE 4.7
Summary of microscopy findings in 20 valve grafts removed from patients more than four years following insertion

| | Type and number of valve grafts examined | | | |
| | Allografts | | | Autografts |
	Freeze-dried (12)	Frozen (4)	Fresh (2)	(2)
Nuclei				
Normal	—	—	—	—
Few	1	—	1	2
Absent	11	3	—	—
Collagen				
Normal	—	—	1	—
Degenerate	8	3	1	1
Elastin				
Normal	1	1	—	—
Degenerate	2	—	—	—
Calcium				
Absent	1	—	—	—
Present	6	3	2	—
Tissue architecture				
Normal	6	—	—	1
Abnormal	3	1	1	1
Perforations and tears	2	—	1	—
Cusp thickening	5	1	1	2

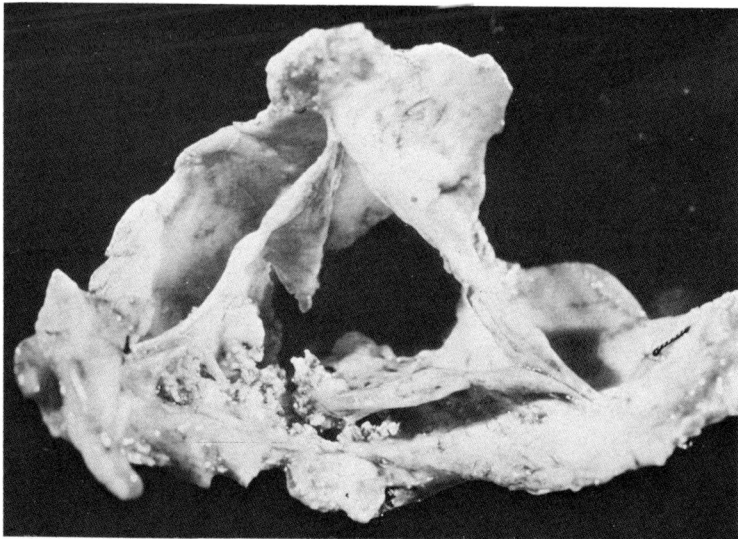

Figure 4.38 Macroscopic appearance of a fresh allograft valve removed from a patient five years following its insertion. The cusps are generally attenuated and thinned. The calcification at the commissure and in the cusps is friable and loose

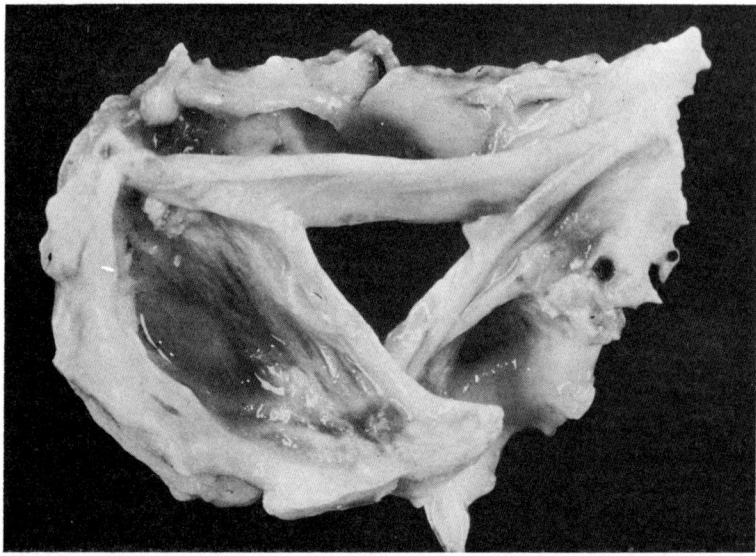

Figure 4.39 Macroscopic appearance of a freeze-dried allograft valve removed from a patient ten years following its insertion. Hard, compact foci of calcification are present in the substance of the valve

DISCUSSION

The results presented so far attempt to show what the surgeon or the patient may expect in terms of survival, based on actuarial analyses of past experience. The comparisons which will be made between these results and those published by contemporary authors using other types of aortic valve replacements, prosthetic or biological, do not adequately reflect the improvement in the quality of life associated with allograft valve replacement since this is a subjective phenomenon. This is most readily appreciated in negative terms. Unlike prosthetic valves, there is no risk of associated thromboembolism, and in consequence no need for anticoagulant therapy, and therefore there is no risk of anticoagulant-associated bleeding. A further advantage of the allograft and autograft valves, not reflected in this survey, is the fact that when degenerative changes occur, the process of valve graft failure is a slow and gradual one. This offers the prospect of safe elective re-replacement surgery. This factor, together with the progressively decreasing hospital mortality contributed to a greater overall survival rate of these patients. In fact, in the cohort of 27 patients receiving frozen allografts in 1968, all of the eight patients who required re-operation for a second valve replacement survived the operative procedure (*Figure 4.27* and *Table 4.5*).

The hospital mortality (*Figures 4.21* and *4.22*) has averaged 5 per cent during the past five years. These figures may be compared with data published from other insitutions. For example Cevese *et al.*[11] report a hospital mortality of 10.7 per cent for a group of 102 patients with porcine xenografts operated upon between 1970 and 1976. Gerbeaux *et al.*[13] report a hospital mortality of 12 per cent for patients receiving six different types of aortic prostheses between 1970 and 1973. The recently published results of Starr *et al.*[32] show the hospital mortality for 81 aortic valve replacements with the 2400 composite-track Starr–Edwards prosthesis to be 3 per cent. This series specifically excluded the patients with associated cardiac operations such as aorta to coronary artery saphenous vein bypass grafts. Hospital mortality will obviously vary from centre to centre depending on the selection criteria. In general, the 664 patients in this study reflect an atypical distribution in that the National Heart Hospital receives patients from all regions of the United Kingdom, including cases referred from the regional cardiac centres. The average hospital mortality of 5 per cent (*Figures 4.21* and *4.22*) is thus comparable with most other reported aortic valve replacement series.

Late results (*Figure 4.23*) have shown that allografts and autografts have similar actuarial survival curves over a ten-year period of follow-up. The long-term survival rate of 59 per cent at 13 years predicts a 61 per cent survival at ten years. Since there are few such long-term surveys extending for ten years[32] it is perhaps more meaningful to compare results over a six-year period. In this way the overall figure for allografts at six years' follow-up shows a 73 per cent survival (inclusive of hospital mortality) (*Figure 4.23*). This compares with the six years' survival rate of 60 per cent for several types of prosthetic valves[13] and 57 per cent for Hancock porcine xenografts[11]. These overall values include the poor results from older surgical techniques and valve models and also the higher hospital mortality experienced during the early years (*Figures 4.21* and *4.22*). A more appropriate comparison may be obtained by excluding the hospital mortality and by only considering the most recent technique or model which has been used over the past six years. For allograft valves this will be the fresh allograft, for which the operative survivors have six years' actuarial probability of survival of 94 per cent (*Figure 4.25*). This compares with the value of 84 per cent at six years for the S.M. Cutter valve[13] and with 78 per cent at six years for Model 1200/1260 Starr–Edwards prosthetic valve[32].

A further comparison which may be made between the allograft valves and published information about other valve substitutes is that of event-free survival. In the case of allograft valves an event is defined as re-replacement or a further operation to repair the valve. There have been no other non-fatal valve events or complications. *Figure 4.28* shows at six years' follow-up an event-free survival of 84 per cent for patients with fresh allografts. This figure could be compared with the value of 60 per cent for patients with the cloth-covered Starr–Edwards prosthesis series 2310/2320[32]. From these three comparisons (survival rate including hospital mortality, the most recent valves with six years' follow-up, and event-free survival) it is clear that allograft replacement of the aortic valve is comparable with, or better than any current alternatives.

The main criticism of the biological valve is based on the assumed eventuality of degeneration of the cusp tissue. McGoon[21], Pluth and McGoon[24] and Angell, DeLanerolle and Shumway[6] have all reported degenerative valve failure at five to six years' follow-up. As a result of such reported failures the majority of cardiac surgical centres in the USA have discontinued allograft valve replacement in the widespread belief that all allograft valves will fail. The data in *Table 4.5* show that from a total of 586 operative survivors 45 valves have presented with degenerative failure over a 13-year period (7.6 per cent). Actuarial analysis shows that the probability of degenerative failure at six years is only 2 per cent for fresh allografts and autografts (*Figure 4.35*).

The results for the three main storage varieties of allograft valves (*Table 4.4*) have been presented independently (*Figures 4.26* to *4.29*) since it was hoped that this would provide information concerning the best sterilization and storage technique and would elucidate the importance of tissue viability. In retrospect, the results in *Figure 4.25* have shown that there is no difference between the various groups except between the early, freeze-dried valves and the others. There is no significant difference between frozen allografts, fresh allograft and autograft valves in terms of either survival or event-free survival rate (*Figures 4.25* to *4.29*). Although the freeze-dried allografts are different from the other allografts used (*Figures 4.24* and *4.25*), this is mainly because of two, interconnected reasons; the high hospital mortality for the early, freeze-dried valves and the improvement in surgical technique which has benefited the later frozen and fresh valves. There is one additional difference between the freeze-dried valves and the others which cannot be explained by improvements in surgical technique. This is the onset of degeneration as a cause of valve failure at 4–6 years following implantation of the freeze-dried valves whereas degeneration in frozen allograft and autografts has only become apparent after 6–8 years (*Figure 4.35*). This suggests that seven years is a crucial period in the life of an allograft valve. While the fresh allograft valves have shown only a 2 per cent probability of degenerative failure at six years (*Figure 4.35*), this may be misleading since their greatest risk period is still ahead.

One may go further and assume that in support of this hypothesis, any biological valve will eventually fail, and the histological appearance of removed allograft valves (*Figures 4.36* and *4.37*) is very similar to that of removed porcine xenografts[1]. Foci of calcification are frequently associated with degenerative failure (*Table 4.7*) and these have also been seen in xenografts[1].

Improvements in surgical technique and in methods of valve preparation are intended to facilitate correct positioning of the valve and to ensure a completely competent valve. Although the experience with fresh allograft valves has shown a probability of survival of 94 per cent at six years (*Figure 4.25*) it is possible that an improved surgical technique, and a lower incidence of diastolic murmurs will produce still better results.

The diastolic murmur, which is a serious feature of allograft and autograft valve replacement, may present, usually within three months of the operation, as an early post-operative diastolic murmur. *Table 4.6* shows that 121 of 424 valves have presented with such a murmur (27 per cent). Undoubtedly the main cause of this diastolic murmur is an imperfect positioning or size-matching of the inserted valve. Occasionally it may be due to a poorly selected malfunctioning valve. The presence of this early post-operative murmur is not an absolute indication of early valve failure, since 53 per cent of the patients with the murmur still have their original valve and 12 per cent of the patients without this murmur have had their valve replaced (*Table 4.6*). The late onset of a diastolic murmur has a very definite significance however and heralds the onset of degenerative valve changes or impending failure.

The late failure of correctly implanted valves may be seen as an inevitable consequence of the insertion of non-living valves, and may apply to all biological tissue valves. However, this late failure or degeneration occurs with a lower incidence and over a longer period of time in correctly seated valves than in those with an early diastolic murmur. Thus in the group of allograft valves with an early post-operative diastolic murmur the 42 per cent incidence of failure is significantly greater than the 12 per cent incidence seen in the murmur-free patients (*Table 4.6*).

One complication of allograft and autograft valves which has no correlation with the presence of an early diastolic murmur is infective endocarditis. In this series its occurrence was sporadic over the 13 years studied (*Table 4.5*). The annual rate of infective endocarditis was 0.92 per cent throughout the period of observation of 13 years (*Figure 4.34*) and this may be compared with 0.98 per cent for 4760 prosthetic heart valves inserted during a period of ten years[37]. The incidence of infective endocarditis is higher in patients with valve replacement than in those without operation[25], presumably due to disturbed haemodynamics associated with valve replacement surgery. The incidence of infection amongst patients with allograft and autograft valves is not higher than in those with any other type of valve replacements.

Between 40 and 50 per cent of degenerative allograft valve cusps contain foci of calcification (*Table 4.7*). The macroscopic appearance of this calcification at the time of surgical removal is generally different in fresh allografts when compared with the freeze-dried valves. The more recent fresh valves present with large masses of friable, loose calcification lightly adherent to the upper surface of the cusps while in the freeze-dried valves the calcification tends to be in more compact foci within the substance of the cusps.

In contrast, none of the autograft valves have presented with calcification. A similar lack of calcification was found in patients with failed autologous fascia lata valves and it is possible that the calcification is a late consequence of an immunological reaction. On this basis the assumed destruction of porcine antigenicity by the glutaraldehyde used to treat xenograft valves should therefore preclude any calcification. Acar *et al.*[1] have refuted this hypothesis by demonstrating calcium in these valves and the calcific reaction may be more subtle than a classic antigen–antibody interaction. The presence of non-viable tissue does not necessarily predispose to calcification since the process occurs naturally even in functioning living valves in the older age group and a number of non-living freeze-dried allografts have been seen as late as ten years following insertion without calcification. On the other hand congenitally bicuspid aortic valves regularly calcify early and therefore turbulence may be considered a significant factor which would apply equally to the malseated allograft valve.

It is hoped that the use of less cytotoxic concentrations of antibiotics[35] for storage and the insertion of totally competent, non-turbulent and wholly flexible valves will improve the long-term survival prospects for allograft valves. At present the autograft valve does not seem to offer significant advantages but its continued evaluation provides an important comparison as a living valve replacement.

SUMMARY

This chapter describes our experience with 664 patients who underwent isolated aortic valve replacement with allograft and autograft valves during the past 13 years. Of this total number 476 patients received allograft valves and 188 received autografts. The average age of the allograft recipients was 40 years and 30 years for those who had an autograft.

The first allograft valves were inserted in July 1962 and the first pulmonary autograft in 1967. Several sterilization and preservation methods have been used for the allografts: ethylene oxide and freeze-drying; ethylene oxide or gamma radiation and deep freezing and antibiotics and tissue culture medium. The current technique is described, together with the results of some experiments on the different methods which have been tried. The surgical procedure has also undergone continuous improvement and modification, and this is described in detail.

In this series 32 per cent of patients had aortic stenosis, 37 per cent aortic regurgitation and 19 per cent mixed stenosis and insufficiency. In 6 per cent the cause of valve disease was infective endocarditis and 6 per cent of patients had previous aortic valve replacement surgery.

The overall hospital mortality was 14.8 per cent, which has fallen over the last five years to 5.4 per cent for allografts and 4.6 per cent for autografts. Of the 476 patients who had received an allograft, 184 had freeze-dried valves, 31 had frozen valves and 261 had fresh allograft valves.

The long-term follow-up evaluation showed that the allograft valves at 13 years and the autograft valves at ten years had actuarial probabilities of survival of 59 per cent and 72 per cent respectively. There was no significant difference between the two groups at six or at ten years.

Analysis of the allograft valves with reference to the method of preparation has shown that the freeze-dried allograft valves were significantly worse at six years' follow-up. Due to the small numbers involved the difference at ten years was not significant. It is clear that frozen allograft valves, fresh allograft valves and pulmonary autograft valves have a similar long-term performance in terms of survival. We expect that the ten-year probability of survival of 78 per cent for the autograft valves will also be shown by the frozen allograft valves (which so far have shown an 88 per cent probability of survival at nine years) and by the fresh allograft valves (93 per cent at six years; similar to 92 per cent of the autograft valves at six years).

The freeze-dried allograft valves showed signs of tissue degeneration after 4–6 years' follow-up, while the frozen allograft valves had a later appearance of degeneration after 6–8 years. The fresh allograft valves have not exhibited an appreciable record of tissue degeneration in up to six years of follow-up.

Early post-operative diastolic murmurs occurred in 35 per cent of patients with allograft valves and the incidence of valve dysfunction was significantly higher in the group of patients with an early diastolic murmur (42 per cent) than in the group without a murmur (12 per cent).

Examination of the removed valves has shown a loss of nuclearity and tissue architecture which correlated with the loss of viability. The fresh and frozen allograft valves degenerate after 6–8 years with an atrophic thinning of the cusps, sometimes with loose, friable calcification. This is in contrast with the freeze-dried allograft valves which presented after 4–6 years with thickened cusps and nodules of calcification within the substance of the cusp.

Our results with fresh and frozen allograft valves have been compared with recent reports of allograft valves, xenografts and prosthetic devices, and these comparisons support the conviction that allograft and autograft valves are acceptable replacements for the human aortic valve.

Acknowledgement

We would like to acknowledge our indebtedness to Miss P. Carr for her pains-taking work in the preparation of many of the figures in this chapter.

REFERENCES

[1] Acar, J., Carpentier, A., Chomette, G., Lelguen, C., Geschwind, H. and Starkman, S. 'Evolution stenosante des hétérograffes en position aortique ou mitrale. A propos de deux cas', *Archives des Maladies du Coeur*, 69, 929 (1976)

[2] Al-Janabi, N. and Ross, D. N. 'Enhanced viability of fresh aortic homografts stored in nutrient medium', *Cardiovascular Research*, 7, 817 (1973)

[3] Al-Janabi, N. and Ross, D. N. 'Long-term preservation of fresh viable aortic homografts by freezing', *British Journal of Surgery*, 61, 229 (1974)

[4] Al-Janabi, N., Gonzalez-Lavin, L., Neirotti, R. and Ross, D. N. 'Viability of fresh aortic valve homografts: a quantitative assessment', *Thorax*, 27, 83 (1972)

[5] Anderson, R. P., Bonchek, L. I., Grunkemeier, G. L., Lambert, L. E. and Starr, A. 'The analysis and preparation of surgical results by actuarial methods', *Journal of surgical Research*, 16, 224 (1974)

[6] Angell, W. W., DeLanerolle, P. and Shumway, N. E. 'Valve replacement: present status of homograft valves', *Progress in cardiovascular Diseases*, 15, 589 (1973)

[7] Barratt-Boyes, B. G. 'Homograft aortic valve replacement in aortic incompetence and stenosis', *Thorax*, 19, 131 (1964)

[8] Barratt-Boyes, B. G. and Roche, A. M. G. 'A review of aortic valve homografts over a six-and-one-half year period', *Annals of Surgery*, 170, 483 (1969)

[9] Barratt-Boyes, B. G., Lowe, J. B., Cole, D. S. and Kelly, D. T. 'Homograft valve replacement for aortic valve disease', *Thorax*, 20, 495 (1965)

[10] Brandt, P. W. T., Roche, A. M. G., Barratt-Boyes, B. G. and Lowe, J. B. 'Radiology of homograft aortic valves', *Thorax*, 24, 129 (1969)

[11] Cevese, P. G., Gallucci, V., Morea, M., Dalla Volta, S., Fasoli, G. and Casarotto, D. 'Heart valve replacement with the Hancock bioprosthesis. Analysis of long-term results', *Circulation*, 56 (*Suppl. 2*), 111 (1977)

[12] Duran, C. G. and Gunning, A. J. 'Total homologous aortic valve in the sub-coronary position', *Lancet*, 2, 488 (1962)

[13] Gerbeaux, A., Manania, G., Letterfon, M., Valtry, J., Magnier, S., Penther, P., Bensaid, J., Assouline, S. and Belfante, M. 'Resultats à long terme des remplacements valvulaires aortiques par prosthèse', *Archives des Maladies du Coeur*, 69, 117 (1976)

[14] Gonzalez-Lavin, L. and Barratt-Boyes, B. G. 'Surgical considerations in the treatment of ventricular septal defect associated with aortic valvular incompetence', *Journal of thoracic and cardiovascular Surgery*, 57, 422 (1969)

[15] Gonzalez-Lavin, L., Geens, M. and Ross, D. N. 'Aortic valve replacement with a pulmonary valve autograft: indications and surgical technique', *Surgery*, 68, 450 (1970)

[16] Grunkemeier, G. L., Lambert, L. E., Bonchek, L. I. and Starr, A. 'An improved statistical method for assessing the results of operation', *Annals of thoracic Surgery*, 20, 289 (1975)

[17] Harris, P. D., Kovalik, A. T. W., Marks, J. A. and Malm, J. R. 'Factors modifying aortic homograft structure and function', *Surgery*, 63, 45 (1968)

[18] Longmore, D. B., Lockey, E., Ross, D. N. and Pickering, B. N. 'The preparation of aortic valve homografts', *Lancet*, 2, 463 (1966)

[19] Maginn, R. R. 'A rapid test for tissue viability prior to transplantation', *British Journal of Surgery*, 55, 15 (1968)

[20] Malm, J. R., Bowman, F. O., Jr., Harris, P. D. and Kovalik, A. T. W. 'An evaluation of aortic valve homografts sterilized by electron beam energy', *Journal of thoracic and cardiovascular Surgery*, 54, 471 (1967)

[21] McGoon, D. C. 'On evaluating valves', *Mayo Clinic Proceedings*, 49, 233 (1974)

[22] Parker, R., Nandakumaran, K., Al-Janabi, N. and Ross, D. N. 'Elasticity of frozen aortic valve homografts', *Cardiovascular Research*, 11, 156 (1977)

[23] Parker, R., Randev, R., Wain, W. H. and Ross, D. N. 'Storage of heart valve allografts in glycerol with subsequent antibiotic sterilization', *Thorax*, 33, 638 (1978)

[24] Pluth, J. R. and McGoon, D. C. 'Current status of heart valve replacement', *Modern Concepts of cardiovascular Disease*, 43, 65 (1974)

[25] Quenzer, R. W., Edwards, L. D. and Levin, S. 'A comparative study of 48 host valve and 24 prosthetic valve endocarditis cases', *American Heart Journal*, 92, 15 (1976)

[26] Ross, D. N. 'Homograft replacement of the aortic valve', *Lancet*, 2, 487 (1962)

[27] Ross, D. N. 'Replacement of aortic and mitral valve with a pulmonary autograft', *Lancet*, 2, 959 (1967)

[28] Ross, D. N. 'Homograft replacement of the aortic valve: surgical technique', *Surgery*, 63, 382 (1968)

[29] Ross, D. N. and Somerville, J. 'Correction of pulmonary atresia with a homograft aortic valve', *Lancet,* **2,** 1446 (1966)

[30] Smith, J. C. 'The pathology of human aortic valve homografts'. *Thorax,* **22,** 114 (1967)

[31] Somerville, J., Ross, D. N. and Ross, J. K. 'Mitral valve replacement with stored inverted pulmonary homograft valve', *Thorax,* **27,** 583 (1972)

[32] Starr, A., Grunkemeier, G. L., Lambert, L. E., Thomas, D., Sugimura, S. and Lefrak, E. A. 'Aortic valve replacement: a ten-year follow-up of non-cloth-covered *vs.* cloth-covered caged ball prostheses', *Circulation,* **56** (*Suppl. 2*), 133 (1977)

[33] Stinson, E. B., Angell, W. W., Iben, A. B. and Shumway, N. E. 'Aortic valve replacement with the fresh valve homograft', *American Journal of Surgery,* **116,** 204 (1968)

[34] Stinson, E. B., Griepp, R. B., Bieher, C. P. and Shumway, N. E. 'Aortic valve allografts for mitral valve replacement', *Surgery,* **77,** 861 (1975)

[35] Wain, W. H., Pearce, Helen, M., Riddell, R. W. and Ross, D. N. 'A re-evaluation of the antibiotic sterilization of heart valve allografts', *Thorax,* **32,** 740 (1977)

[36] Wheatley, D. J. and McGregor, C. G. A. 'Influence of viability on canine allograft heart valve structure and function', *Cardiovascular Research,* **11,** 223 (1977)

[37] Wilson, W. R. 'Prosthetic valve endocarditis: incidence, anatomic location, cause, morbidity and mortality'. In *Infections of Prosthetic Heart Valves and Vascular Grafts.* Ed. by R. J. Duma, Baltimore: University Park Press (1977)

[38] Wright, J. E. C. and Ng, Y. L. 'Elasticity of human aortic valve cusps', *Cardiovascular Research,* **8,** 384 (1974)

5

The Glutaraldehyde-Stabilized Porcine Xenograft Valve

Lawrence H. Cohn
and John J. Collins, Jr.

Le temps révèle tout: c'est un bavard qui parle sans être interrogé.
Euripide (480–406 av. J.C.)

INTRODUCTION

The remarkable advances made in the design and application of prosthetic and bioprosthetic heart valves has been one of the most important chapters in medical history. Since 1960, with the development of the ball and cage valve by Harken[22], and the subsequent modification and application by Starr[43], thousands of patients with severely diseased cardiac valves have been restored to a normal life-style. Mechanical valves, particularly the ball and cage and the tilting disc valves, have stood the test of time from a mechanical and haemodynamic point of view. The clinical results obtained with the use of the tilting disc valve are discussed in the first chapters of this book. Concomitant with mechanical valve development, heart valves of biological origin were developed and employed. In 1956, Murray successfully placed fresh, aortic allografts in the descending thoracic aorta of patients with aortic regurgitation[34]. Since that time, a number of differently preserved and fresh tissue valves have been used in the aortic and atrioventricular valve position.

The porcine xenograft valve treated with the stabilized glutaraldehyde process by Hancock Laboratories has been used at the Peter Bent Brigham Hospital since 1972, and has assumed a major role as a valve replacement device at our institution for all valvular cardiac lesions[11-13]. This chapter will deal with the development, biological characteristics, our clinical experience and surgical techniques and pathological examination of dysfunctional valves following valve replacement with the Hancock porcine xenograft. Implications concerning long-term durability, thromboembolic experience and haemodynamic performance will be discussed in detail.

HISTORICAL REVIEW

Xenograft replacement of a human aortic valve was first successfully accomplished in September 1965, at the Centre Chirurgical Marie–Lannelongue, in Paris, by Binet and co-workers[1]. The xenograft valve was taken from a calf, sewn in a free-hand fashion after preservation with a 1 in 5000 solution of an organomercurial salt, Cialit. This clinical case followed the animal experiments of Duran and Gunning[16] in 1965, who had demonstrated good function and tolerance of freeze-dried xenografts inserted in the dog's descending thoracic aorta. Binet and his co-workers performed more than 90 xenograft valve replacements in their original series, the majority preserved with organomercurial salt solution[2]. The results of this clinical series were unacceptable when analysis of the four-year follow-up period showed that only 10 per cent of the valves were functioning normally, indicating that the preservation agent had acted detrimentally on the collagen components of the graft. In the last 26 cases of their original series of 80 patients, a rigid stent of titanium covered with Teflon cloth was used to sew on the graft prior to insertion. The insertion of the stented xenograft valve was then similar to other conventional prosthetic valve replacement devices. The difficulty with valve durability in this initial series promoted the search for other agents to improve reliability of xenogeneic valves.

O'Brien in Australia began a clinical series of formaldehyde-treated xenograft valve replacement in collaboration with Clarebrough in 1966[35]. In his initial clinical series, numbering 23 patients, 4 per cent buffered acid formaldehyde was used as the preservation and sterilization agent of the xenograft valves. The valves were then trimmed and free-sewn into the human aortic root. During 1967–69, these investigators used a tri-leaflet free-sewn xenograft valve constructed from three different non-coronary aortic valve leaflets. In the tri-leaflet valve there were no denuded areas of myocardium and there was optimal haemodynamic performance. Despite initial clinical success in a series of 100 patients operated upon by O'Brien, he reported[36] that by three years of follow-up there was only an 80 per cent graft survival and that 38 per cent of patients had developed severe aortic incompetence. He stated that these grafts treated by the

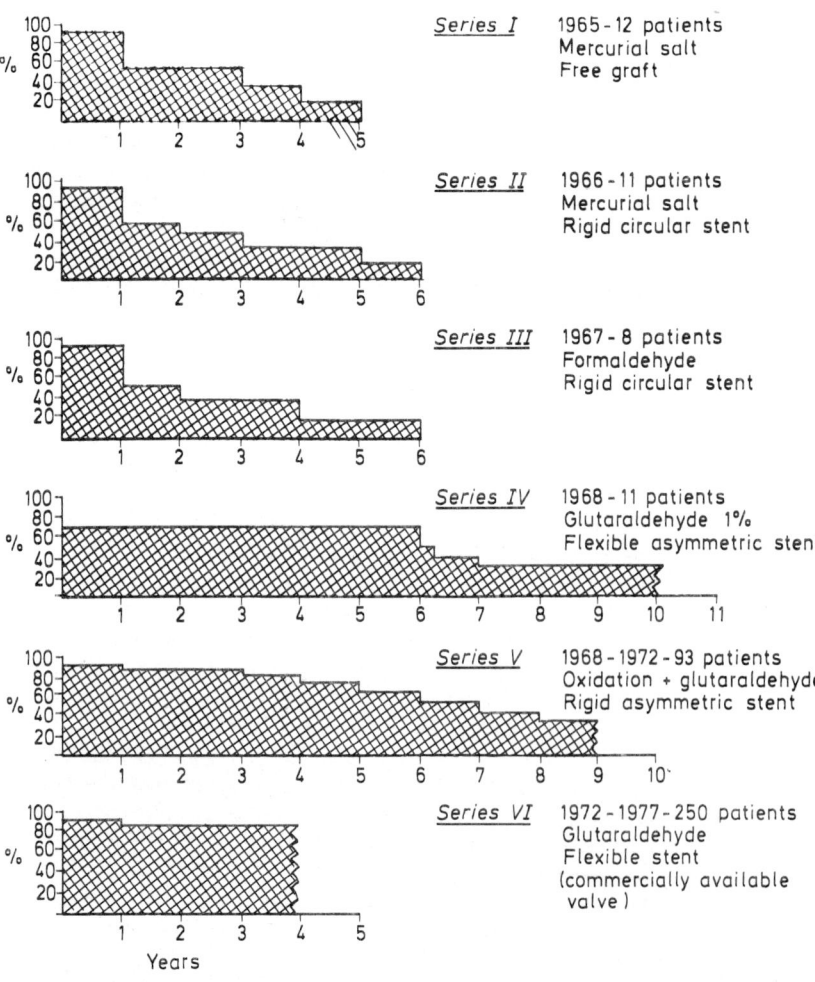

Figure 5.1 Graphic presentation of the experience of Carpentier with xenograft valve replacement utilizing various forms of graft preservation and support frames. (Reproduced with permission of A. Carpentier)

formalin fixation method, were not suitable for long-term clinical usage. This experience was duplicated by Angell and co-workers[5], who also had a high incidence of problems with durability in the formalin-fixed xenograft.

The next agent used to sterilize and treat xenogeneic valves was glutaraldehyde, first advocated by Carpentier at the Hospital Broussais in Paris. After having found dissolution of the cross-linkages of cusp collagen treated with formaldehyde, he then turned to the use of the tanning agent glutaraldehyde to promote cross-linkage stabilization of collagen as well as sterilization. Carpentier found that agents such as formalin and chromic acid were not able to assure the durability of the graft because the intramolecular cross-links were reversible and because all glycoproteins and telopeptides were eliminated. The use of glutaraldehyde was determined by Carpentier to maintain the cross-linkages of collagen[6] and thus form 'bioprostheses'. In an initial series of 28 patients with aortic bioprostheses there were three late deaths and two valve failures during an average follow-up of six years. Actuarial graft survival was 90 per cent at three years and 80 per cent at six years. *Figure 5.1* shows Carpentier's experience over ten years with the xenograft valves preserved and stabilized by a variety of agents.

The fabrication of a semi-flexible valve stent was reported by Reis *et al.* in 1971[39]. The entire stent (the base ring and the struts for commissural support) was made of polypropylene and was reinforced at the base with a thin stellite ring. The whole structure was covered with Dacron cloth. The xenograft aortic valves were mounted onto stents of varying diameters. This development was considered an important advance since it allowed buffering of the pressure load delivered to the valve cusps by causing a slight inward movement of the flexible struts.

Suturing of a porcine aortic valve stabilized with a special glutaraldehyde process by the Hancock Laboratories on the flexible stent resulted in the first

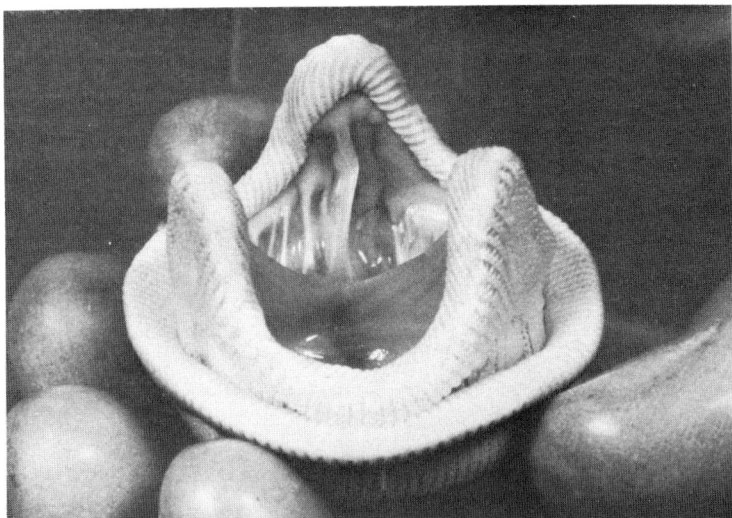

Figure 5.2 The Hancock porcine xenograft treated with the stabilized glutaraldehyde process. Aortic model seen from its outflow aspect

commercially produced, quality controlled tissue valve, the Hancock porcine glutaraldehyde valve (*Figure 5.2*), in clinical use since May 1970. Two new forms of the porcine glutaraldehyde treated valves have been developed, the Carpentier-Edwards valve and the Angell–Shiley valve which will be discussed below.

BIOLOGICAL AND PHYSICAL CHARACTERISTICS OF THE GLUTARALDEHYDE-TREATED PORCINE XENOGRAFTS

The Hancock Valve

Aortic valves of young growing pigs are removed and trimmed under sterile conditions for use as an atrioventricular or aortic valve replacement device depending upon the frame upon which they are placed. The Hancock valve is treated with the Stabilized Glutaraldehyde Process (SGP) which creates cross-links in the porcine valve connective tissue. The primary mode of cross-linking is through amino acid groups normally present in these tissues. Glutaraldehyde, under optimal conditions will form polymers; the polymers span an intermolecular distance twice that of the monomer. Polymerization is critical in determining final physical characteristics such as flexibility and strength of the tissue. This process is controlled with optimal physical, chemical and viscoelastic properties. The cross-links are formed by glutaraldehyde within the collagen fibres and between the fibres in the protein skeleton[20].

Several tests are used to evaluate the efficacy of this process. The first is the resistance of SGP-treated tissue to enzyme digestion by exposure of valves to papain for varying periods of time. Secondly, shrink-temperature was used to assess cross-link stability. In this test, tissue specimens were prepared according to various fixation methods and maintained in a balanced electrolyte solution for up to six years. Small portions of tissue were periodically removed from the specimens and were subjected to increasing temperatures. The temperature at which these tissues suddenly reduce in length was considered the shrink temperature. Change in size of the specimen was related to breaking of added cross-links permitting the fibres to move relative to one another. The higher the shrink temperature of the valve the greater the number of stable collagen cross-linkages. With the SGP treatment of the Hancock valve there was apparently remarkable similarity in the performance of tissues *in vitro* and *in vivo*[20].

The valves were subjected to a number of complicated and prolonged culturing techniques which have been reviewed in view of a recent report of a possible mycobacterial contamination in a small number of valves[30]. The valves are now quarantined for six weeks prior to release. As noted above, the valves are mounted on the Dacron-covered, semi-flexible stent. The 'buffering' ability of the flexible struts has been recently challenged by Thomson and Barratt-Boyes[44] who investigated the Hancock valve in a series of flow experiments and measured the deflection of the tip of each stent post. They found less deflection of the stents than previously thought and, therefore, attributed the excellent durability of the valve to the glutaraldehyde process and to the use of reinforcing layers of Dacron cloth when attaching the valve to the support stent.

The valves range from 19–31 mm annulus (sewing) diameter for the aortic position, and from 25–35 mm annulus (sewing) diameter for the mitral valve position. Newer modifications of the small aortic valves now employ a free leaflet in the area where the previous right coronary cusp and muscular bar were present.

The Carpentier-Edwards Valve

The porcine valve is removed in a similar fashion to the Hancock valve. The preserving solution is 0.625 per cent glutaraldehyde and phosphate buffered saline at pH of 7.4. (The manufacturers claim that lower concentrations of glutaraldehyde (Hancock process) provide a higher shrink temperature than the 0.625 per cent solution but they believe that the degree of difference is not significant[17] and suggest that sterility may be more definitive.)

The frame upon which the valve is sewn has been designed to be totally flexible at the sewing orifice as well as at the commissural struts. Compliance of the commissural supports is intended to reduce the loading shock on the valve cusps similar to the Hancock valve. The flexible orifice is intended to reduce loading shock on the base of the leaflets as well. It is thought that the flexible orifice will allow leaflets to close with a sliding-type apposition at the free margins in a manner similar to that observed in the normal human valve motion and in free-sewn aortic valve allografts[4]. The metal used in the frame is Elgiloy, a corrosion-resistant alloy of cobalt and nickel, chosen because of its high fatigue life, superior strength and bio-compatibility. The metal frame is covered with porous knitted Teflon in such a way as to create a support for the right coronary cusp at the inflow orifice contour. The porous Teflon facilitates tissue ingrowth. The commissural supports are unequally placed around the circumference and are slightly slanted inward to conform to the anatomical shape of the porcine aortic valve. The sewing rim has a silicone rubber insert which is covered with a porous Teflon cloth for easy suturing to the heart valve annulus. Clinical experience with this valve dates from April 1, 1976, and at the time of writing (September, 1977) approximately 4000 valves have been inserted. Haemodynamic data were obtained from patients with larger sizes of Carpentier-Edwards valves and were found to be similar to other porcine and prosthetic valves[17].

The Angell-Shiley Valve

The Angell-Shiley porcine xenograft is similarly produced from a healthy young pig aortic root and is trimmed according to the specific indications which allow for a thin right coronary muscular cusp. After initial fixation in 0.5 per cent glutaraldehyde, the valves are trimmed and mounted in one of 70 different anatomic stent configurations varying in shape and size, produced from precise castings of actual porcine aortic roots. The entire Delrin stent (base and struts) is covered with Dacron cloth. This method of anatomic tailoring provides a xenograft that closely retains the original configuration of the valve, thus providing a natural position and support for the porcine tissue. The resulting annular sewing rim is not circular in shape and therefore the internal diameter of the bare stent is a calculated quantity. Valve sizes are produced from 23–34 mm annulus diameter[41]. Clinical results date from May 1970, and are discussed elsewhere in this book by Angell and his associates.

CLINICAL MATERIAL–PETER BENT BRIGHAM HOSPITAL EXPERIENCE (1972–1977)

The first Hancock porcine xenograft valve was inserted at this institution in January 1972. Up to January 1977 (a 60-month period), 365 Hancock porcine valves have been inserted in 323 patients. This section will detail the clinical characteristics of this patient group consisting of 152 patients who had aortic valve replacement, 131 patients who underwent mitral valve replacement, and 40 patients who had multiple valve replacement.

Aortic valve replacement

In this group, there were 113 males and 39 females, ranging in age from 18–84 years with a mean age of 58 years (*Table 5.1*). Though a number of mixed lesions were found in many patients, the lesion of primary importance was determined to be aortic stenosis in 110 and aortic insufficiency in 42 patients.

TABLE 5.1
Demographic analysis of three groups of patients having Hancock porcine xenograft valve replacement

Valves replaced	Number of patients	Sex		Age (years)	
		Male	*Female*	*Range*	*Mean*
Aortic	152	113	39	18–84	58
Mitral	131	37	94	25–75	54
Multiple valves	40	21	19	19–75	53
Total	323	171	152	18–84	56

There were two patients in functional class II, 76 in class III and 44 in class IV (New York Heart Association (NYHA) classification). In patients with aortic stenosis the pre-operative mean left ventricle to aorta pressure gradient was 84 mmHg (range 30–140 mmHg). The concomitant operative procedures performed in 39 of the 152 patients (25 per cent) are listed in *Table 5.2*. Direct myocardial revascularization with grafts to coronary arteries was required in 25 patients, ascending aorta replacement for aneurysm was performed in six and mitral reconstructive operations in seven patients.

The sizes of valves implanted were as follows: 11 patients received 21 mm valves; 62 patients, 23 mm valves; 60 patients, 25 mm valves; and 19 patients, 27 mm valves.

TABLE 5.2
Concomitant operative procedures performed at the time of heart valve replacement
with Hancock porcine xenograft valves

Valves replaced	Coronary artery bypass graft	Ascending aorta replacement	Mitral valve reconstruction	Aortic valve reconstruction
Aortic	25	6	7	–
Mitral	14	–	–	2
Multiple valves	2	–	–	–
Total	41 (12.6%)	6	7	2

Mitral valve replacement

In this group of 131 patients, there were 37 males and 94 females aged 25–75 (mean 54) years (*Table 5.1*). The predominant lesions were mitral stenosis in 79 and mitral regurgitation in 52 patients. There were two patients in functional class II, 80 patients in class III and 49 patients in class IV (NYHA). *Table 5.2* lists the concomitant surgical procedures performed at the time of mitral valve replacement. Aorta to coronary artery bypass grafts were performed in 14 patients and aortic commissurotomy in two patients. The distribution of valve sizes was as follows: 29 mm valves were inserted in 17 patients, 31 mm valves in 67 patients, 33 mm valves in 37 patients and 35 mm valves in 10 patients.

Multiple valve replacement

Forty patients underwent multiple valve replacement requiring two or more cardiac valves. Thirty-two patients underwent mitral and aortic valve replacement, six patients underwent mitral and tricuspid valve replacement and two patients had mitral, aortic and tricuspid valve replacement. There were 21 males and 19 females, aged 19–75 (mean 53) years (*Table 5.1*). In the group of 32 patients with mitral and aortic valve replacement there were 18 patients who had primarily left ventricular volume overload (predominant incompetence of both valves), six patients with primarily left ventricular pressure overload (predominant stenotic lesions of the two valves) and eight patients with mixed valvular lesions.

In the multiple valve replacement group 22 patients were in functional class III and 18 patients in class IV (NYHA).

OPERATIVE TECHNIQUE

The valve replacement operations were performed during extracorporeal circulation with a disposable bubble oxygenator and complete haemodilution. The heart–lung machine was primed with a solution consisting of 5 g/100 ml of albumin, 50 g of 50 per cent glucose and lactated Ringer's solution to simulate the normal serum constituents of glucose, albumin and electrolytes. The total priming volume for adult patients was approximately 2 ℓ. Intraoperative monitoring included systemic arterial pressure measured through a radial artery catheter, central venous pressure via a catheter in the internal jugular vein and urinary output through a catheter placed prior to the induction of anaesthesia. Anaesthesia for the majority of patients consisted of morphine, nitrous oxide and oxygen.

A median sternotomy was used for all valve replacements, including re-operations. The pericardium was suspended by sutures and cannulations made in the right atrium and in the ascending aorta after heparinization (3 mg/kg body weight). If the patients underwent single aortic valve replacement, only one venous drainage cannula was placed into the right atrium. Patients undergoing mitral valve replacement or double valve replacement had both venae cavae cannulated without caval tourniquets. The ascending aorta was cannulated with a size 20 or 22 French Bardic® cannula through a single purse-string suture of 3–0 Dacron. Heparin activity throughout the cardiopulmonary bypass was checked by activated clotting time and appropriate additional amounts of heparin were added. This test was also valuable in determining the protamine dosage following discontinuation of cardiopulmonary bypass. For patients who had neither aortic stenosis nor critical coronary artery lesions, and who were not anaemic a phlebotomy of 500–1000 ml of blood was performed between the induction of anaesthesia and the onset of heparinization. The blood was stored in the operating room and was auto-transfused following discontinuation of cardiopulmonary bypass and neutralization of heparin. In addition, the remaining oxygenator red cells were centrifuged and given back to the patient in the operating room or in the intensive care unit[10,45]. The cardiopulmonary bypass flow rates were approximately 1.5 ℓ/min/m² for adult patients, accompanied by systemic hypothermia of 28–30 °C. The perfusion pressure was maintained at approximately 75 mmHg.

Prophylactic antibiotic treatment was used in all patients. Antibiotics (1 g cephalosporin-Keflin) were given at the institution of anaesthesia just prior to the sternotomy. An additional 1 g dose was given in the heart–lung machine at the beginning of cardiopulmonary bypass and 1 g every six hours was continued intravenously for two days. Following this, oral cephalosporin (Keflex) was continued for the remainder of the prophylactic period of five days.

Myocardial protection in all cases of valve replacement was provided by hypothermic ischaemic arrest, accomplished by profound local topical hypothermia[9,19]. Lactated Ringer's solution at a temperature of 4–5 °C was topically irrigated over the heart throughout the period of ischaemic arrest and the excess fluid was removed from the pericardium by a wall suction device. For optimal cooling, the patient was placed approximately 30° head up and the table tilted slightly to the left so that the left ventricle became the dependent structure and received the maximum cooling during the entire operative procedure. The interior of the left ventricle was also frequently irrigated with the same cold solution.

For multiple valve replacement or combined valve replacement and coronary artery bypass grafting (CABG), cardioplegic solution was also added for myocardial protection; 1 ℓ of 5 per cent dextrose in 0.2 per cent sodium chloride with 30 mEq of potassium chloride and 5 ml of bicarbonate (pH 7.5 and osmolality 340 mmol) was used. The solution was administered in multiple doses through a 13 gauge plastic catheter placed in the most superior portion of the ascending aorta following cross-clamping of the aorta distal to the infusion point.

The mitral valve was approached through a left atrial incision posterior to the interatrial groove. Valve insertion has been carried out using two different suture techniques. Horizontal mattress sutures of 2-0 Ethibond or simple sutures were passed through the mitral annulus.

The aortic valve was exposed through a low oblique aortotomy extending into the non-coronary sinus. Horizontal mattress sutures or simple sutures were used to attach the valve passing from above downward in order to evert the aortic annulus. In cases of calcific aortic stenosis, careful debridement of all annular calcium was done to secure the seating of the valve on a flexible, supple annulus. When aortic and mitral replacement was performed the mitral valve was inserted first followed by the aortic valve. The valve was handled as little as possible during all the steps of the operation to minimize any possibility of trauma to the valve cusps.

Following the placement of the valve sutures, hypothermia was reversed and the patient warmed to 37 °C. At the conclusion of the valve replacement and closure of the appropriate cardiac chamber, the aortic cross-clamp was removed after ensuring that the patient was placed in the Trendelenburg position with the ascending aorta the highest structure with regard to the innominate artery. An air vent needle was used in the ascending aorta, the left ventricular apex, and in the uppermost portion of the left atrium between the aorta and the superior vena cava. The patients were defibrillated with electrical counter-shock into sinus rhythm as soon as possible after the removal of the aortic cross-clamp. Experimental work by Hottenrott and associates[24] has shown that the hypertrophied left ventricle is at risk with prolonged ventricular fibrillation. After resumption of sinus rhythm, a variable period of time from 10-30 min was used for resuscitation of the heart and weaning the patients off the cardiopulmonary bypass.

In patients undergoing concomitant myocardial revascularization by saphenous vein bypass grafts, the following technique was used. After the institution of local hypothermia the distal ends of the vein grafts were anastomosed to the coronary arteries. Following this, the valve replacement was carried out and the aortic or atrial incision closed. The heart was electrically defibrillated and during resuscitation, the proximal ends of the saphenous vein grafts were anastomosed to the ascending aorta, using continuous, monofilament sutures.

In most instances, a catheter was placed in the left atrium through the right superior pulmonary vein. This left atrial catheter was then used to wean patients off cardiopulmonary bypass by ensuring the appropriate degree of left ventricular filling. Once the heart-lung bypass was discontinued the heparin was neutralized and the perfusion cannulae removed. A pacing wire was placed on the anterior aspect of the right ventricle in all patients and a right atrial placing wire was used in those patients who had a hypertrophied and/or non-compliant ventricle for possible post-operative atrial pacing. Chest drainage tubes were placed in the precordial space. In more than 90 per cent of our patients neither pleural space was violated and, therefore, no intrapleural drainage tubes were required.

Optimal post-operative care was directed toward maintaining maximal cardiac output in each patient. This was accomplished by balancing filling pressures, heart rate and myocardial contractility appropriately. The use of right and left atrial pressure monitors, atrial and ventricular pacing wires, appropriate cardio-vascular medications such as dopamine or nitroprusside were used to improve contractility or reduce systemic afterload respectively.

The policy for anticoagulant treatment in this series of patients with porcine xenograft valve replacement was as follows. Patients with aortic valve replace-ment and in sinus rhythm were not anticoagulated. In the unusual situation of patients with aortic valve replacement and chronic atrial fibrillation, long-term anticoagulation was given. All patients with mitral valve replacement were anti-coagulated for approximately 4–6 weeks post-operatively, and the prothrombin time was maintained at twice the normal level. Following this period of time a decision was made with respect to either discontinuation or permanent use of prothrombin depressants. In patients with sinus rhythm the anticoagulants were withdrawn. The anticoagulants were also gradually discontinued in young patients with atrial fibrillation but with a small left atrium and good evidence of adequate cardiac output. In patients with a large left atrium, suboptimal cardiac output and chronic atrial fibrillation anticoagulation was continued indefinitely[12].

CLINICAL RESULTS AND FOLLOW-UP OF PATIENTS WITH GLUTARALDEHYDE-TREATED PORCINE XENOGRAFTS—PETER BENT BRIGHAM HOSPITAL EXPERIENCE (1972–1977)

All patients in this clinical series were evaluated by either personal examination, telephone conversation or letters, or through information obtained following patients' examination by their personal physician. The evaluation was performed at a minimum interval of six months following operation (July 1977). The evaluation consisted of physical examination, history of thromboembolism, anti-coagulation medication intake and assessment of functional status. Patient survival and rate of thromboembolism were expressed in actuarial form using the methods of Cutter and Ederer[14].

Aortic valve replacement

The operative mortality in this group was 6.5 per cent (ten out of 152 patients). The ten early deaths resulted from acute myocardial infarction in two patients, post-operative low cardiac output following cardiopulmonary bypass in five patients and technical errors in three patients. Five of the ten operative deaths occurred in patients undergoing concomitant coronary artery bypass grafts or replacement of the ascending aorta. The average age of patients who died at operation was 64 years.

There were 13 late deaths, an incidence of 8.5 per cent. Three patients died of post-operative infective endocarditis (2 per cent), four patients died of congestive cardiac failure, four died due to ischaemic heart disease and myo-cardial infarction and two patients, near 80 years old, died of stroke (*Table 5.3*). The mean age of this group was 67 years. The follow-up period for patients with aortic porcine xenograft valve replacement has been 6–66 (mean 24) months. The actuarial survival rate at 60 months post-operatively was 69 per

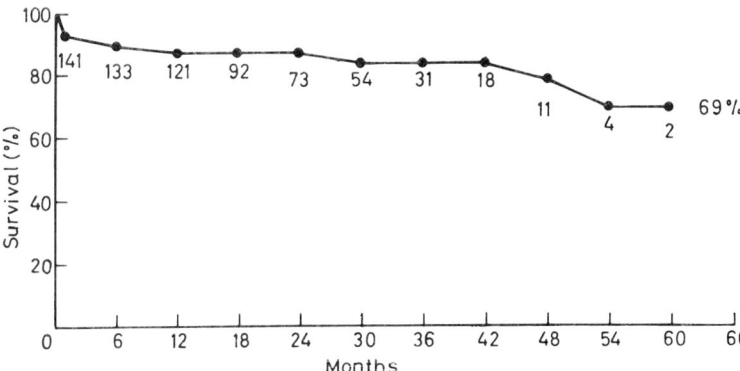

1972 - 1977
152 Cases

Figure 5.3 Actuarial curve for survival rate of patients following aortic valve replacement
with Hancock porcine xenografts (operative mortality included)

cent (*Figure 5.3*). Functional evaluation indicated that 98 patients were, at the
latest examination, in functional class I, 25 in class II, two patients in class III
and none in class IV (NYHA).

The embolic complications in the 152 patients are presented in *Table 5.4*.
There was one embolus in the late post-operative period (0.65 per cent). This
embolus occurred in a 72 year old man who had been in chronic atrial fibrillation pre-operatively and who could not be cardioverted following the operation.
He had not been on anticoagulation and sustained a femoral embolus six months
post-operatively. Femoral embolectomy restored normal blood flow. Four

TABLE 5.3
Causes of late death in patients having heart valve replacement
with Hancock porcine xenografts

Cause of death	Number of patients
Congestive heart failure	9
Cerebrovascular accident	5
Myocardial infarction	4
Infective endocarditis	3
Chronic renal failure	2
Carcinoma	2
Left atrial thrombosis	1
Myeloid metaplasia	1
Gastrointestinal haemorrhage	1
Arrhythmia	1
Chronic pulmonary disease	1
Lupus erythematosus	1
Total	31

TABLE 5.4

Incidence of embolic complications in 323 patients having heart valve replacement
with Hancock porcine xenografts

| Valves replaced | Number of patients | Emboli | | Episodes/100 patient years |
		Number	Per cent	
Aortic	152	1	0.65	0.4
Mitral	131	11	8.4	3.8
Multiple valves	40	2	5.0	1.8

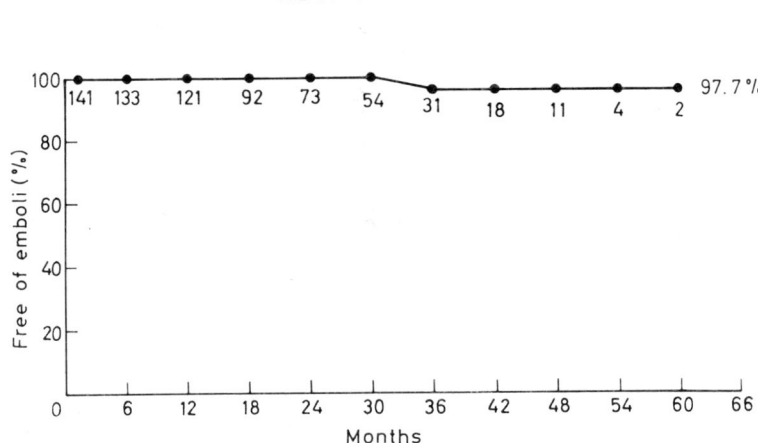

1972 - 1977
152 Cases

Figure 5.4 Actuarial curve for patients free from emboli following aortic valve replacement
with Hancock porcine xenografts

patients are on long-term anticoagulation because of chronic atrial fibrillation.
All the other patients (125) are off anticoagulation and have not had embolic
episodes. The percentage of patients free from emboli is actuarially computed in
Figure 5.4 (97.7 per cent at 60 months post-operatively). There were 0.4 emboli
per 100 patient years in the aortic valve replacement group.

Mitral valve replacement

There were six operative deaths in 131 patients undergoing mitral valve replacement, an operative mortality of 4.6 per cent. Three patients, who were in class
IV NYHA pre-operatively, died in the early post-operative period due to severe
low cardiac output. One patient died of bleeding from a tear in the posterior
wall of the left atrium, one other patient bled intractably from a perforation of
the posterior wall of the left ventricle produced by a strut of the valve, and one

patient suffered irreparable damage to the circumflex branch of the left coronary artery during the operation. Three of the six patients who died had associated coronary artery bypass grafts. The mean age of the deceased was 66 years.

There were 12 late deaths, an incidence of 10 per cent (*Table 5.3*). Four non-cardiac deaths were due to cancer in two patients, lupus erythematosus in one, and chronic renal failure in one patient. Two patients died of cerebral vascular accidents, probably embolic in origin, one died of chronic pulmonary disease which was well established prior to operation, one patient died of arrhythmia and four patients died of congestive heart failure and chronic low cardiac output. All cardiac deaths (8 patients) occurred in cases with severe pre-operative mitral regurgitation and markedly depressed left ventricular function. The actuarial survival curve for patients with mitral valve replacement is shown in *Figure 5.5*. The projected survival rate at 66 months is 86.8 per cent.

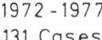

1972 - 1977
131 Cases

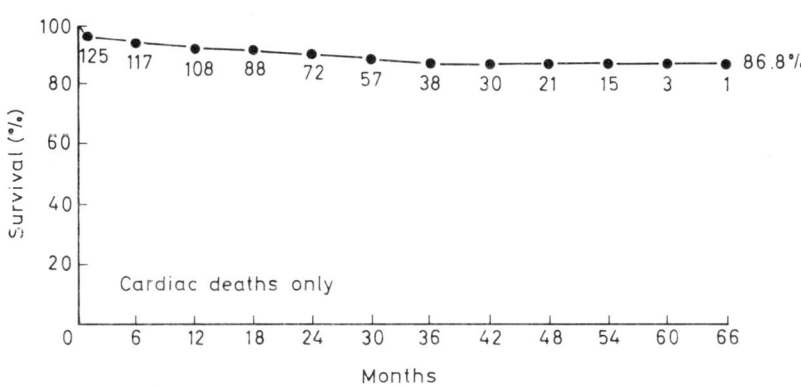

Figure 5.5 Actuarial curve for survival rate of patients following mitral valve replacement with Hancock porcine xenografts (operative mortality included)

There were nine non-fatal and two fatal thromboembolic complications in the 131 patients with mitral valve replacement, an incidence of 8.4 per cent (3.8 episodes/100 patient years). The actuarial curve for this complication showed that 72.9 per cent of patients are expected to be free from thromboemboli at 66 months post-operatively (*Figure 5.6*). As shown in *Table 5.4* there were 3.8 embolic episodes/100 patient years.

Post-operative functional classification showed that 76 patients were, at the latest assessment, in class I, 25 patients in class II, five in class III and one was in class IV (NYHA).

The patients were also analysed for post-operative emboli in relation to their post-operative cardiac rhythm. Forty patients were in sinus rhythm and 73 in atrial fibrillation following the operation. Ten emboli occurred in the group of 73 patients in atrial fibrillation, while only one embolus was noted in the group of 40 patients in sinus rhythm. Forty-two patients or 38 per cent of the entire patient group are taking therapeutic warfarin sodium indefinitely. Thirty-six of

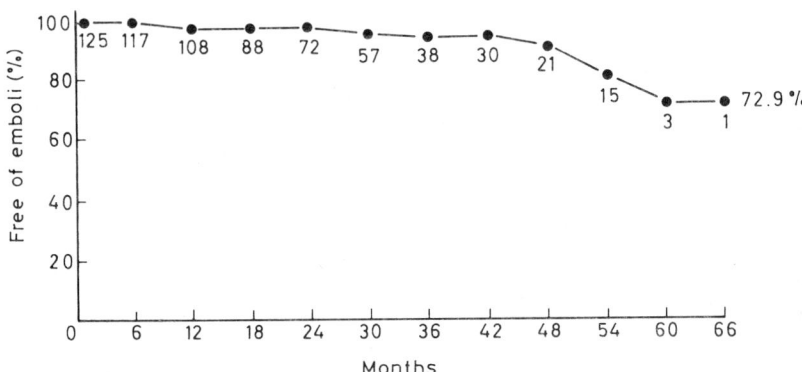

Figure 5.6   Actuarial curve for patients free from emboli following mitral valve replacement with Hancock porcine xenografts

these 42 patients are in atrial fibrillation. Previous work[5] has demonstrated that the incidence of thromboemboli in patients who are in sinus rhythm is significantly lower than in those patients who are in atrial fibrillation following mitral valve replacement with the Hancock porcine xenograft. If a patient remains in atrial fibrillation following mitral valve replacement with a Hancock porcine valve, the incidence of emboli is higher than in patients in sinus rhythm and not significantly different from patients with prosthetic valves. This would suggest, therefore, that embolization in patients with atrial fibrillation occurs as a result of the primary, underlying cardiac disease and not necessarily because of the type of valve substitute employed.

Multiple valve replacement

In the group of 40 patients who were subjected to multiple valve replacement there was one operative death in a patient who underwent mitral and tricuspid valve replacement, an incidence of 2.5 per cent (*Table 5.5*). This patient was class IV (NYHA) with end-stage mitral and tricuspid regurgitation and died in the early post-operative period due to low cardiac output syndrome. *Table 5.5* summarizes the early and late deaths in the three categories of multiple valve replacements.

Six patients died in the late post-operative period, four following aortic and mitral valve replacement and two patients after mitral and tricuspid valve replacement. One patient with mitral and aortic replacement died of a thrombosed mitral valve one month post-operatively. This patient was in atrial fibrillation and fully anticoagulated at the time of the incident. He developed a massive hinged thrombus originating at the valve suture line. By flopping over into the mitral valve the thrombus prevented the egress of blood from the left atrium. Three patients died of non-cardiac causes; one from renal failure, one from leukaemia, and one from gastrointestinal haemorrhage. A fifth patient, with

TABLE 5.5
Early and late mortality in 40 patients having multiple heart valve replacement
with Hancock porcine xenografts

Valves replaced	Number of patients	Operative mortality	Late mortality
Mitral and aortic	32	–	4
Mitral and tricuspid	6	1	2
Mitral, aortic and tricuspid	2	–	–
Total (per cent)	40	1 (2.5)	6 (15)

mitral and tricuspid replacement, died of a cerebral haemorrhage and a sixth patient, also with mitral and tricuspid valves, died of a generalized and progressive cardiomyopathy. The actuarial survival curve, which does not include deaths due to non-caridac causes, for this entire group is shown in *Figure 5.7.* The projected survival rate at 66 months with a mean follow-up of 33 months was 89.8 per cent. Functional classification showed that at the latest evaluation 24 patients were in class I, six. in class II, one in class III and one in class IV (N YHA).

The incidence of embolization in this patient group is shown in *Table 5.4.* There have been two embolic episodes, an incidence of 5 per cent. One additional patient was re-operated upon because of thrombotic stenosis of the aortic valve. Ten patients are on chronic long-term anticoagulation because of the persistence of atrial fibrillation. The percentage of patients free from emboli, on an actuarial basis, is shown in *Figure 5.8* (84.6 per cent). There were 1.8 embolic episodes/ 100 patient years of follow-up.

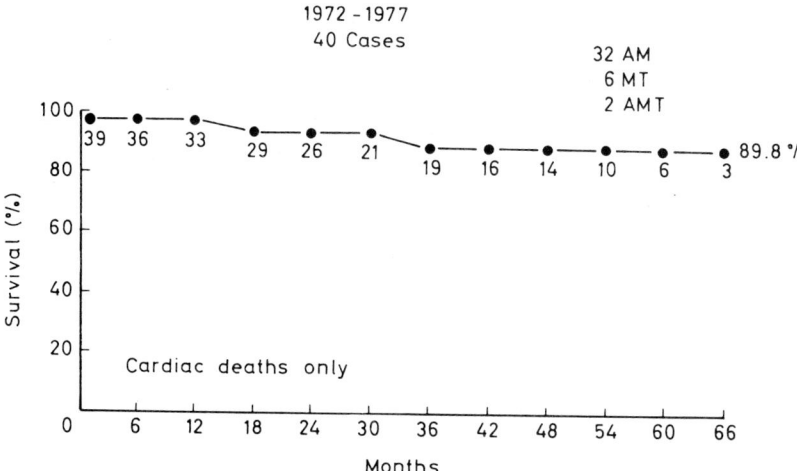

Figure 5.7 Actuarial curve for survival rate of patients following multiple valve replacement with Hancock porcine xenografts. (Deaths due to non-cardiac causes were not included in this calculation.) A = aortic; M = mitral; T = tricuspid

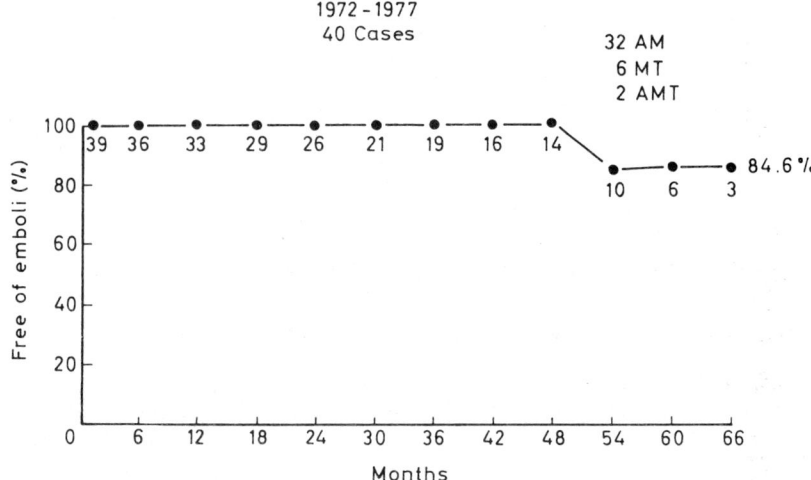

Figure 5.8 Actuarial curve for patients free from emboli following multiple valve replacement with Hancock porcine xenografts. A = aortic; M = mitral; T = tricuspid

Infective endocarditis

In the entire series of 323 patients, there have been seven cases of proven bacterial endocarditis, an incidence of 2.2 per cent. There have been no cases of immediate post-operative endocarditis. The seven cases occurred from 6–66 months post-operatively. Three patients with aortic valve endocarditis died because of severe aortic incompetence and congestive heart failure. In one patient, who had both aortic and mitral valve replacement, the aortic valve developed an infection in two of the cusps and was replaced with another Hancock valve without incident at 66 months post-operatively. In the mitral replacement group, there were three patients who developed endocarditis. All three valves were sterilized with intensive antibiotic therapy without re-operation.

PATHOLOGY OF THE HANCOCK PORCINE XENOGRAFT VALVE– PETER BENT BRIGHAM HOSPITAL

All valves from patients who died in the immediate post-operative period or from those who died late post-operatively were recovered either at the post-mortem examination or during re-operation and were examined by the cardiac pathologist at the Peter Bent Brigham Hospital, Dr. Michael Fishbein. This pathological experience, combined with that of the West Roxbury Veterans Hospital was reported recently[18].

All valves recovered in the immediate post-operative period were normal except for one valve infected with a fungus.

Those valves which were recovered from patients who died late following the operation have shown a variety of pathological findings as indicated in *Table 5.6.*

The major pathological alterations have been calcification, endocarditic changes, torn leaflet in one patient (primary tissue failure) and thrombotic stenosis (*Figure 5.9*). The incidence of primary tissue failure has been extremely low involving only one valve in our series of 363 tissue valves inserted (*Table 5.6*). The two patients in whom calcification occurred were both treated with chronic renal dialysis and were subjected to shifts in serum calcium and other electrolytes. Because of these problems and the potential bacteraemia associated with repeated haemodialyses we advise and employ prosthetic valves in such patients. Thrombotic stenosis occurred in two patients. This fibrosis of organized thrombus in the cuspal sinuses occurred in an 80 year old man treated with oestrogens for carcinoma of the prostate and in a 40 year old man at six months following double valve replacement. This second patient suffered from intermittent atrial fibrillation and was not on anticoagulant treatment.

TABLE 5.6
Pathologic findings in 11 Hancock porcine xenograft valves removed from nine patients

Patient number	Valve	Time of examination following insertion (months)	Pathologic diagnosis
1	Aortic	66	Infection
2	Aortic	31	Infection
3	Mitral	31	Torn cusp
4	Aortic	13	Normal
5	Aortic	11	Thrombotic stenosis
6	Aortic	6	Calcification*
	Mitral	6	Thrombosis
7	Mitral	5	Thrombosis fibrosis*
8	Aortic	4	Normal
	Mitral	4	Normal
9	Aortic	4	Thrombotic stenosis

*Patients number 6 and 7 had been treated with chronic haemodialysis

Spray and Roberts[42] have published the results on the structural changes of the Hancock porcine xenograft from the National Institutes of Health. Of 51 valves, four were removed surgically and 47 were obtained at post-mortem examinations. Their study showed that the porcine xenografts were not biologically inert in the human circulation, although clinical dysfunction has been extremely uncommon. The histologic changes documented were thrombus in the cuspal sinus or outflow in 26 out of 26 valves examined which were obtained early post-operatively. In valves removed late after their insertion there was thrombus formation in the outflow area in 14 and in the inflow area in nine out of 18 valves examined. Inflammatory cells, including plasma cells and macrophages were found on the leaflets of 19 out of 26 valves removed early and 12 out of 18 valves removed late post-operatively. Foreign body type of giant cells were seen in 12 and focal invasion of the leaflets by host and giant cells in eight out of 18 valves removed late after insertion. Three atrioventricular valves examined microscopically, late after the operation showed complete disruption of the cusp tissue.

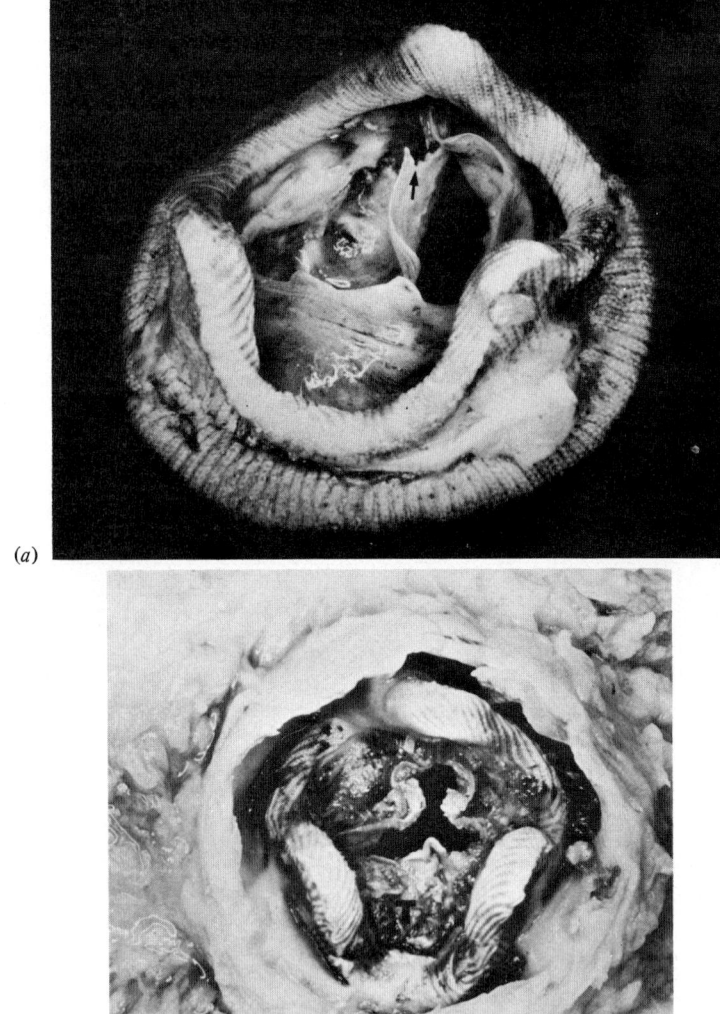

Figure 5.9 Hancock porcine xenograft valves recovered following implantation. (*a*) Primary valve dysfunction in a xenograft removed from the mitral position 31 months after its insertion. The arrow points towards a torn leaflet near to the commissure. (*b*) Thrombotic stenosis of a xenograft inserted in the aortic position. T indicates cuspal thrombus

CLINICAL EXPERIENCE WITH THE HANCOCK PORCINE XENOGRAFT REPORTED FROM OTHER SURGICAL CENTRES

Since the first clinical usage of the Hancock porcine xenograft in May 1970[46], there has been an increasing number of surgical groups utilizing this valve for aortic, mitral and tricuspid replacement, so that by 1977, more than 35 000

Hancock valves have been implanted. At the outset, six institutions, in addition to the Peter Bent Brigham Hospital, began using the valve and, therefore, have the longest cumulative experience. These insitutions were: Stanford University[37,38], Henry Ford Hospital[15], University of Padua[8], the National Institutes of Health[33], University of Kansas[21] and the Cardiology Associates of Oklahoma City[46]. The follow-up time was approximately four years, and in some instances the observation period extended beyond seven years.

The experience from five centres with the Hancock porcine xenograft in the aortic position is shown in *Table 5.7*. Approximately 20 per cent of the operations performed had concomitant coronary artery bypass grafting or ascending aorta replacement. *Table 5.7* summarizes the number of patients, length of follow-up actuarial survival rate, incidence of thromboemboli and the number of primary dysfunctional valves. In the aortic position the actuarial survival rate was comparable to results reported with prosthetic valves but the incidence of emboli was markedly reduced, although the great majority of patients did not receive long-term anticoagulant treatment. The incidence of valve dysfunction was also extremely low, less than one per cent at a follow-up of 4–6 years.

TABLE 5.7
Clinical experience with the Hancock porcine xenograft in the aortic position.
Data from reported series

| Authors (year of publication) | Number of patients | Follow-up period (years) | | Actuarial survival rate (%) | Emboli | Number of valve dysfunction |
		Maximum	Mean			
Oyer et al.[37] (1977)	251	5.0	1.2	90	99% free	3
Pipkin, Buch and Fogarty[38] (1976)	75	4.0	1.5	65	2.4 episodes/ 100 patient years	1
Cevese et al.[8] (1977)	102	6.0	3.0	92	0	2
Jones et al.[26] (1978)	129	2.5	1.0	92*	1.6 episodes/ 100 patient years	1
Davila, Magilligan and Lewis[15] (1977)	59	6.0	4.0	92*	96% free	1

*Hospital mortality excluded

Table 5.8 summarizes essential data from five published reports concerning the actuarial survival rate, embolic incidence and number of dysfunctional valves in patients who underwent mitral valve replacement. Most patients in these series were placed on anticoagulants in the immediate post-operative period (except for the National Institutes of Health group) and then the anticoagulants were gradually discontinued in patients who were in sinus rhythm, or even in patients

TABLE 5.8

Clinical experience with the Hancock porcine xenograft in the mitral position.
Data from reported series

Authors (year of publication)	Number of patients	Follow-up period (years)		Actuarial survival rate (%)	Emboli	Number of valve dysfunction
		Maximum	Mean			
Oyer et al.[37] (1977)	338	5.5	1.8	78	92% free	3
Hannah and Reis[21] (1976)	104	5.0	2.5	6% early deaths 12% late deaths	93% free	3
McIntosh et al.[33] (1975)	111	5.0	2.6	77	1.9% incidence	1
Cevese et al.[8] (1977)	335	6.0	3.0	77	1.9% incidence	3
Davila, Magilligan and Lewis[15] (1977)	124	6.0	4.0	93*	87% free	0

* Hospital mortality excluded

with atrial fibrillation but who had small left atria. The incidence of thrombo-emboli was higher than in the aortic position but this undoubtedly represents the results of the underlying chronic atrial fibrillation.

The dysfunctional valves which have been recovered fall into three categories, as indicated in our own pathological review; primary valve dysfunction from tissue fatigue which was exceedingly unusual, thrombotic stenosis, particularly in low cardiac output situations, and those valves recovered from patients who had some other mechanical or metabolic problems such as chronic renal failure and haemodialysis which may predispose to calcification.

HAEMODYNAMIC CHARACTERISTICS OF THE GLUTARALDEHYDE-PRESERVED PORCINE XENOGRAFT VALVE

The foregoing material would support conclusions that the glutaraldehyde preserved porcine xenograft in both the aortic and mitral positions is a relatively durable and considerably less thrombogenic valve, when compared with pros-thetic valves. Since there is a frame upon which the porcine aortic xenograft is mounted in addition to the tissue thickness of the valve itself, there are less effective orifice areas and higher transvalvular pressure gradients in porcine valves of small sizes. This section details objective haemodynamic studies in patients, discusses some of the latest results of the *in vitro* testing of the valve, and focuses on new modifications of the Hancock porcine valve which have been made in order to reduce the haemodynamic problems related to the smaller sized valves.

Table 5.9 summarizes essential haemodynamic data from patients catheterized following heart valve replacement with Hancock xenografts. In the mitral position, Lurie, Miller and Maxwell[32], Johnson *et al.*[25], McIntosh *et al.*[33], and Hannah and Reis[21] have shown that the Hancock valve is haemodynamically a very satisfactory mitral valve substitute, comparable to similar sized prosthetic devices. Mean transvalvular pressure gradients range from 3.6-7.9 mmHg, while calculated valve areas measure from 1.84-2.3 cm^2.

TABLE 5.9

Mean transvalvular gradients and valve surface areas in patients having mitral or aortic Hancock porcine xenograft valve replacement. Data from reported series

Authors (year of publication)	Number of patients	Transvalvular gradient (mmHg)		Calculated valve area (cm^2)	
		Mean	Range	Mean	Range
MITRAL REPLACEMENT					
Lurie, Miller and Maxwell[32] (1977)	14	7.9	1-13	1.84	0.7-3.2
Johnson *et al.*[25] (1975)	14	6.5	4-14	2.15	0.9-3.5
McIntosh *et al.*[33] (1975)	37	4.0	0-15	2.0	0.7-3.2
Hannah and Reis[21] (1976)	31	3.6	0-9	2.3	2.1-3.1
AORTIC REPLACEMENT					
Lurie, Miller and Maxwell[32] (1977)	12	19	3-52	1.33	0.75-2.5
Hannah and Reis[21] (1976)	10	16	0-35	–	–
Jones *et al.*[26] (1978)	23	21	17-28	–	0.99-1.42
Cohn, Sanders and Collins[12] (1976)	7	16	5-32	1.4	0.90-2.9

In the aortic position there has been documentation of significant transvalvular pressure gradients and reduced valve areas in the small sized conventional Hancock xenografts. In *Table 5.9* the mean left ventricular–aortic gradients range from 16-21 mmHg and the mean calculated valve areas average 1.4 cm^2. Hancock xenografts with 19, 21 and 23 mm annulus diameter were found to have calculated valve areas in the range of 1.0 cm^2 which is considered to be in the operable range for moderate aortic stenosis. In our own experience, prior to recent developments in the fabrication of the Hancock xenograft, patients with a 19 or 21 mm aortic annulus diameter received Björk–Shiley prosthetic aortic valves. The Björk–Shiley valve has the best hydraulic performance when compared with prosthetic valves of any size on the market today[40]. Other surgeons have taken a different approach believing that, because of the low thrombogenicity of the porcine xenograft, certain technical manoeuvres were warranted for the insertion of a porcine xenograft even in small aortic annuli, particularly in younger patients with endocarditis or congenital aortic stenosis with hypoplasia of the aortic annulus. Hatcher[23], Lamberti[29], Konno *et al.*[28] and

Kinsley[27] have advocated various surgical techniques for enlargement of the aortic annulus by annuloplastic procedures. These include either cutting into the anterior leaflet of the mitral valve, incising into the right ventricular outflow tract or using a prosthetic gusset onto the base of the aortic annulus in order to enlarge the aortic outflow tract to allow the insertion of a larger porcine aortic valve. In certain selected cases, annular expansion may be preferable to the insertion of small sized aortic prostheses which require long-term anticoagulation.

The nature of the obstruction in the small sized porcine valves is the muscular base of the right coronary cusp which assumes greater importance as the annulus diameter becomes smaller. *Figure 5.10* shows that during systole there is partial obstruction to the lumen of the valve produced by this cusp which cannot open because of the muscular bar at its base. The adjacent valve in *Figure 5.10*, the so-called Modified Orifice (MO) Hancock Valve Model No. 250, shows that during systole there is complete opening of the valve orifice for maximal egress of blood. This was accomplished by removing the obstructive right coronary muscular cusp and substituting it with a non-coronary cusp from another animal. Thus, the Modified Orifice Hancock Valve contains one left coronary and one non-coronary cusp in continuity and one non-coronary cusp from another porcine aortic valve.

In vitro studies were carried out and the transvalvular pressure gradient (delta P) was measured in the Hancock model No. 242, the Hancock MO No.250 and the Björk–Shiley aortic valve prosthesis. The size of these valves ranged from 19–25 mm annulus diameter. The valves were mounted at the base of a model aorta and were subjected to sinusoidally varied pulsatile flow. The mean systolic pressure gradients were measured at various mean systolic ejection flow rates over a simulated range of heart rates from resting values to maximal exercise. The results indicated that the Hancock Modified Orifice No. 250 represents a clear hydraulic improvement over the standard model throughout the size range tested and has advantages over comparable sizes of Björk–Shiley prostheses. These studies have demonstrated that the mean systolic pressure gradient (mmHg) at various mean systolic ejection flows (ml/s) across the 19 mm annulus diameter valves was better with the Hancock Modified Orifice valve than with either the Björk–Shiley prosthesis or the standard model Hancock valve[20]. The difference in gradients between the Björk–Shiley prosthesis and the Hancock MO valve was less apparent in valves with 23 and 25 mm annulus diameter. John Wright at the University of Liverpool has made careful measurements of the flow dynamics across tissue and prosthetic valves and his important contributions to hydraulic testing of valves are described in Chapter 2. A number of small size valves of these modified orifice Hancock porcine xenografts have been used at our Institution since October 1976. In 15 patients there was no evidence of post-operative obstruction to left ventricular ejection. One patient, a 67 year old female, who underwent aortic valve replacement with a 21 mm annulus diameter MO Hancock xenograft, was re-catheterized and there was no pressure gradient between the left ventricle and the aorta at normal cardiac output. Levine, Buckley and Austen[31] have measured intraoperative gradients in 12 patients having aortic valve replacement with the MO Hancock xenograft. There were six patients with 21 mm and six patients with 23 mm annulus diameter valves. The mean transvalvular gradients were 0–15 (mean 6) mmHg with the 21 mm size and 0 in all six patients with 23 mm valves.

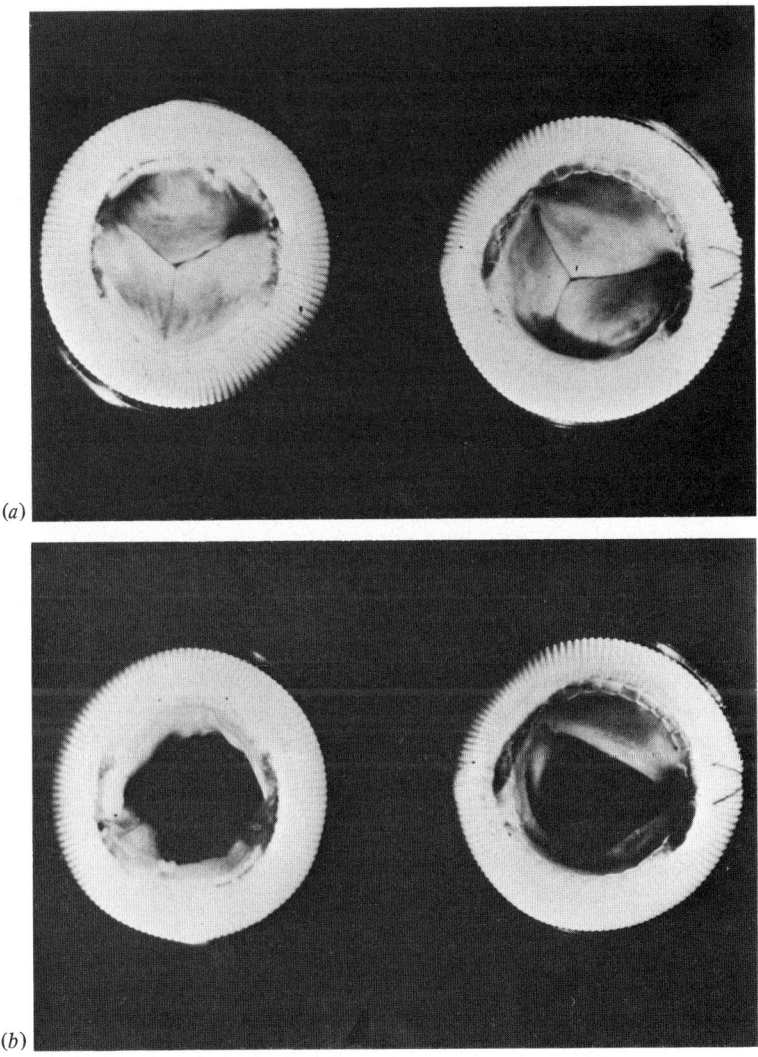

Figure 5.10 Inflow aspect of standard model and Modified Orifice model of Hancock xenograft valves: (*a*) diastole; (*b*) systole. On the right of the figures is the standard model of the Hancock valve and on the left the Modified Orifice model. Note the complete opening of the Modified Orifice model as compared with the standard one in which the muscle bar at the base of the right coronary cusp restricts the excursion of this cusp and limits the valvular opening

CONCLUSIONS AND SUMMARY

The glutaraldehyde treated porcine xenograft valve is an effective and relatively non-thrombogenic device for replacement of diseased human cardiac valves. We have reviewed our six years' experience at the Peter Bent Brigham Hospital, and the experience of others, with these valves in the aortic, mitral and tricuspid positions. The durability of these valves at six to seven years' follow-up seems to be quite adequate with less than 1 per cent of the valves undergoing primary valvular dysfunction. Extremely careful handling is a necessity to prevent any operative injury to the valve cusps which may result in tissue valve failure at a later date. Shrink temperature and tensile elongation curves of xenografts recovered as late as four years post-operatively would indicate that the durability of the valve was maintained up to this length of time. The pathological changes in valves recovered from patients who had not had valvular dysfunction were minimal. Thrombotic stenosis of the valve has occurred in a few patients and valve calcification was observed, in our experience, in some patients who were treated with chronic artificial haemodialysis.

The glutaraldehyde porcine xenografts are clearly less thrombogenic than valvular prostheses. In the aortic position, the porcine xenograft is virtually non-thrombogenic in the absence of long-term anticoagulation. In the mitral position, patients with xenografts, and in sinus rhythm, had a very low incidence of systemic emboli. On the other hand, there was relatively little difference in the thromboembolic rate between patients with xenografts and in atrial fibrillation and patients with mitral prosthetic valves. Therefore, long-term anticoagulation should be maintained in patients with xenografts and atrial fibrillation.

The haemodynamic characteristics of the glutaraldehyde stabilized porcine xenografts of larger sizes are satisfactory and equal those of prosthetic valves. The haemodynamic performance of the very small size porcine xenografts in both the mitral and aortic areas has been a problem but the recent modification in the fabrication of the smaller valves has made an improvement in the haemodynamic function of the valves, particularly in the aortic region. Whether or not this may compromise the durability of the xenograft because of the new fabrication techniques is unclear.

The porcine glutaraldehyde xenograft valve is a relatively non-thrombogenic and relatively durable biological valve which has achieved a prominent place in the armamentarium of surgeons performing heart valve replacement.

REFERENCES

[1] Binet, J. P., Duran, C. G., Carpentier, A. and Langlois, J. 'Heterologous aortic valve transplantation', *Lancet*, **2**, 1275 (1965)

[2] Binet, J. P., Planché, C. and Weiss, M. 'Heterograft replacement of the aortic valve', In *Biological Tissue in Heart Valve Replacement*. Ed. by M. I. Ionescu, D. N. Ross and G. H. Wooler, pp. 409–444. London; Butterworths (1972)

[3] Blank, R. H., Pupello, D. F., Bessone, S. N., Harrison, E. E. and Sbar, S. 'Method of managing the small aortic annulus during valve replacement', *Annals of thoracic Surgery*, **22**, 356 (1976)

[4] Brewer, R. J., Deck, J. D., Capati, F. and Nolan, S. P. 'The dynamic aortic root', *Journal of thoracic and cardiovascular Surgery*, **72**, 413 (1976)

[5] Buch, W. S., Kosek, J. C. and Angell, W. W. 'Deterioration of formalin-treated aortic heterografts', *Journal of thoracic and cardiovascular Surgery*, **69**, 673 (1970)

[6] Carpentier, A., Blondeau, P. and Marcel, P. 'Remplacement des valves mitrales et tricuspides par des heterogrefes', *Annales de Chirurgie thoracique et cardiovasculaire*, **7**, 33 (1968)

[7] Carpentier, A., Deloche, A., Relland, J., Fabiani, J. N., Forman, J., Camillieu, J. P., Soyer, R. and Dubost, C. 'Six-year follow-up of glutaraldehyde preserved heterografts', *Journal of thoracic and cardiovascular Surgery*, **68**, 771 (1974)

[8] Cevese, P. G., Gallucci, V., Morea, M., Volta, S. D., Fasoli, G. and Casarotto, D. 'Heart valve replacement with the Hancock bioprosthesis. Analysis of long-term results', *Circulation*, **56** (*Suppl. II*), 111 (1977)

[9] Cohn, L. H. and Collins, J. J. Jr. 'Local cardiac hypothermia for myocardial protection', *Annals of thoracic Surgery*, 17, 135 (1974)

[10] Cohn, L. H., Anderson, W., Fosberg, A. and Collins, J. J. Jr. 'Effects of phlebotomy, haemodilution and autologous transfusion on blood utilization in open-heart surgery', *Chest*, 68, 283 (1975)

[11] Cohn, L. H., Lamberti, J. J., Castaneda, A. R. and Collins, J. J. Jr. 'Cardiac valve replacement with the stabilized glutaraldehyde porcine aortic valve: indications, operative results and follow-up', *Chest*, 68, 162 (1975)

[12] Cohn, L. H., Sanders, J. J. and Collins, J. J. Jr. 'Actuarial comparison of Hancock porcine and prosthetic disc valves for isolated mitral valve replacement', *Circulation*, 54 (*Suppl. III*), 60 (1976)

[13] Cohn, L. H., Sanders, J. J. and Collins, J. J. Jr. 'Aortic valve replacement with the porcine xenograft', *Annals of thoracic Surgery*, 22, 221 (1976)

[14] Cutter, S. J. and Ederer, T. 'Maximum utilization of the life-table method in analysing survival', *Journal of chronic Diseases*, 8, 699 (1958)

[15] Davila, J. C., Magilligan, D. J. and Lewis, J. W. 'Is the Hancock valve the best cardiac valve substitute today?' *Annals of thoracic Surgery* (*in print*).

[16] Duran, C. G. and Gunning, A. J. 'Heterologous aortic valve transplantation in the dog', *Lancet*, 2, 114 (1965)

[17] Edwards Laboratories, Personal communications (1977)

[18] Fishbein, M. C., Gissen, S. A., Collins, J. J. Jr., Barsamian, E. M. and Cohn, L. H. 'Pathologic findings after cardiac valve replacement with glutaraldehyde-fixed porcine valves', *American Journal of Cardiology*, 40, 331 (1977)

[19] Griepp, R. B., Stinson, E. B. and Shumway, N. E. 'Profound local hypothermia for myocardial protection during open-heart surgery', *Journal of thoracic and cardiovascular Surgery*, 66, 731 (1973)

[20] Hancock Laboratories, Personal communications (1977)

[21] Hannah, H. and Reis, R. L. 'Current status, porcine heterograft prostheses: a five-year appraisal', *Circulation*, 54 (*Suppl. III*), 27 (1976)

[22] Harken, D. E., Soroff, H. S., Taylor, W. J., Lefemine, A. A., Gupta, S. K. and Lunzer, S. 'Partial and complete prostheses in aortic insufficiency', *Journal of thoracic and cardiovascular Surgery*, 40, 744 (1960)

[23] Hatcher, C. R. 'Aortic valve replacement: The problem of the small aortic annulus', *Annals of thoracic Surgery*, 22, 400 (1976)

[24] Hottenrott, C. E., Towers, B., Kurkji, H. T., Maloney, J. V. and Buckberg, G. 'The hazard of ventricular fibrillation in hypertrophied ventricles during cardiopulmonary bypass', *Journal of thoracic and cardiovascular Surgery*, 66, 742 (1973)

[25] Johnson, A. D., Daily, P. O., Peterson, K. L., LeWinter, M., DiDona, G. J., Blair, G. and Niwayama, G. 'Functional evaluation of the porcine heterograft in the mitral position', *Circulation*, 52 (*Suppl. I*), 40 (1975)

[26] Jones, E. L., Craver, J. M., Morris, D. C., King, S. B., Douglas, J. S. Jr., Franch, R. H., Hatcher, C. R. Jr. and Morgan, E. A. 'Haemodynamic and clinical evaluation of the Hancock xenograft bioprosthesis for aortic valve replacement', *Journal of thoracic and cardiovascular Surgery*, 75, 300 (1978)

[27] Kinsley, R. H. 'The narrow aortic annulus', *American heart Journal*, 93, 759 (1977)

[28] Konno, S., Imai, Y., Iida, Y., Nakajima, M. and Tatsuno, K. 'A new method for prosthetic valve replacement in congenital aortic stenosis with hypoplasia of the aortic valve ring', *Journal of thoracic and cardiovascular Surgery*, 70, 909 (1975)

[29] Lamberti, J. J. 'Patch aortoplasty for insertion of the porcine xenograft', *Journal of thoracic and cardiovascular Surgery*, 72, 86 (1976)

[30] Laskowski, L. F., Marr, J. J. and Spernoga, J. F. 'Fastidious mycobacteria grown from porcine prosthetic heart valve cultures', *New England Journal of Medicine*, 297, 101 (1977)

[31] Levine, F. H., Buckley, M. J. and Austen, W. G. 'Hemodynamic evaluation of Hancock modified orifice aortic position bioprostheses', *Circulation*, 58, (*Suppl. I*), 33 (1978)

[32] Lurie, A. J., Miller, R. R. and Maxwell, K. S. 'Haemodynamic assessment of the glutaraldehyde-preserved porcine heterograft in the aortic and mitral positions', *Circulation*, 56 (*Suppl. II*), 104 (1977)

[33] McIntosh, C. L., Michaelis, L. L., Marion, A. G., Itscoitz, S. B., Redwood, D. R. and Epstein, S. E. 'Atrioventricular valve replacement with the Hancock xenograft', *Surgery*, 78, 768 (1975)

[34] Murray, G. 'Homologous aortic valve segment transplants as surgical treatment for aortic and mitral insufficiency', *Angiology*, 7, 446 (1956)

[35] O'Brien, M. F. and Clarebrough, J. K. 'Heterograft aortic valve transplantation for human valve disease', *Australian medical Journal*, 2, 228 (1966)

[36] O'Brien, M. F. 'Heterologous replacement of the aortic valve'. In *Biological Tissue in Heart Valve Replacement*. Ed. by M. I. Ionescu, D. N. Ross and G. H. Wooler, pp. 445–466. London; Butterworths (1972)

[37] Oyer, P. E., Stinson, E. B., Griepp, R. B. and Shumway, N. E. 'Valve replacement with the Starr–Edwards and Hancock prostheses', *Annals of Surgery*, 186, 301 (1977)

[38] Pipkin, R. O., Buch, W. S. and Fogarty, T. J. 'Evaluation of aortic valve replacement with a porcine xenograft without long-term anticoagulation', *Journal of thoracic and cardiovascular Surgery*, 71, 179 (1976)

[39] Reis, R. L., Hancock, W. D., Yarbrough, J. W., Glancy, D. L. and Morrow, A. G. 'The flexible stent', *Journal of thoracic and cardiovascular Surgery*, 62, 683 (1971)

[40] Roschke, E. J. and Harrison, E. C. 'Size comparisons of commercial prosthetic valves', *Medical Instruments*, 7, 277 (1973)

[41] Shiley Laboratories. Personal communication (1977)

[42] Spray, T. L. and Roberts, W. C. 'Structural changes in porcine xenografts used as substitute cardiac valves. Gross and histologic observations of 51 glutaraldehyde-preserved Hancock valves in 41 patients', *American Journal of Cardiology*, 40, 319 (1977)

[43] Starr, A., Edwards, M. L., McCord, C. W. and Griswold, H. E. 'Aortic replacement. Clinical experience with a semi-rigid ball valve prosthesis', *Circulation*, 27, 779 (1963)

[44] Thomson, F. J. and Barratt-Boyes, B. G. 'The glutaraldehyde-treated heterograft', *Journal of thoracic and cardiovascular Surgery*, 74, 317 (1977)

[45] Tucker, W. Y. and Cohn, L. H. 'Intraoperative use of the Haemonetics Cell Saver in open-heart surgery', *Proceedings of the Haemonetics Research Seminar*, 7, 25 (1976)

[46] Zuhdi, N. 'The porcine aortic valve bioprosthesis', *Annals of thoracic Surgery*, 21, 573 (1976)

6

The Ionescu-Shiley Pericardial Xenograft Heart Valve

Marian I. Ionescu
and Anand P. Tandon

Le temps use l'erreur et polit la vérité.

G. de Lévis
Maximes et préceptes (1808)

INTRODUCTION

Although heart valve replacement with prosthetic devices has generally proved to be a safe and beneficial operation, the quality of the long-term results continues to remain sub-optimal, primarily because of thromboembolic episodes and the complications associated with anticoagulant treatment[30,37]. With the aim of creating a valve which could be safely used without the administration of prothrombin depressants and which, in addition, would incorporate optimal hydraulic characteristics and long-term durability, work began in 1970 for the construction and testing of the glutaraldehyde stabilized pericardial xenograft[3,38]. In March, 1971 a systematic clinical evaluation of this valve was instituted. Based on the gratifying results obtained over the initial period of five years[40], the Ionescu-Shiley pericardial xenograft* was released for general use in 1976.

Over a period of 7.5 years, 411 patients were operated upon at our institution for heart valve replacement and received a total of 458 pericardial xenografts.

Between March 1971 and April 1976 the valves were constructed in our own hospital laboratory in a limited number, and used for single valve replacement only. Since May 1976, when the pericardial xenograft became available from Shiley Laboratories, it has been used in all our patients for both single and multiple valve replacements.

This chapter describes the clinical and laboratory experience with this valve substitute and analyses the results obtained.

CLINICAL MATERIAL

Since March 1971, glutaraldehyde stabilized pericardial xenografts were used for heart valve replacement in 411 patients. There were 369 patients with single valve replacement (216 aortic, 150 mitral and 3 tricuspid) and 42 patients with multiple replacements (31 mitral and aortic, 6 mitral and tricuspid and 5 mitral, aortic and tricuspid). As the group of patients with multiple valve insertions is a small one and the follow-up is shorter, only essential data from this group, related to patients' condition and valve function, will be presented and discussed.

TABLE 6.1
Age distribution of 369 patients subjected to single heart valve replacement
with pericardial xenografts

Valve replaced	Age groups in years						Total	Mean age
	11–20	*21–30*	*31–40*	*41–50*	*51–60*	*61–70*		
Aortic	2	14	36	56	71	37	216	49.5
Mitral	3	7	30	61	37	12	150	44.9
Tricuspid		1	2				3	31.7
Total	5	22	68	117	108	49	369	47.5

*Shiley Laboratories Inc., Irvine, California, U.S.A.

TABLE 6.2
Sex distribution of 369 patients with single heart valve replacement

Valve replaced	Male		Female	
	Number	*Percentage*	*Number*	*Percentage*
Aortic	158	73	58	27
Mitral	55	37	95	63
Tricuspid	1	33	2	67
Total	214	58	155	42

The age and sex of the 369 patients with single valve replacement are shown in *Tables 6.1* and *6.2*. The mean ages were 49.5 for the aortic, 44.9 for the mitral and 31.7 for the tricuspid valve replacement group. For the entire group of patients with single valve replacement the age ranged from 14–70 years and the mean was 47.5 years. There were 214 males and 155 females. The type and aetiology of the valve lesions of these patients are shown in *Tables 6.3* and *6.4*. In the aortic group 13 patients had previous cardiac operations (three open valvotomy, one pericardiectomy and nine aortic valve replacement) while in the mitral group there were 48 patients with previous cardiac surgery (43 had

TABLE 6.3
Clinical lesions in 369 patients with single heart valve replacement

Valve lesion	*Aortic*	*Mitral*	*Tricuspid*	*Total*
Predominant stenosis	75	56		131
Regurgitation	61	31	2	94
Mixed disease	71	59	1	131
Malfunction of previous valve substitute	9	4		13
Total	216	150	3	369

TABLE 6.4
Aetiology of valve lesion in 369 patients with single heart valve replacement

Lesion	*Aortic*	*Mitral*	*Tricuspid*
1. Rheumatic	94	137	2
2. Congenital	39	3	
3. Indeterminate	49	2	
4. Ruptured chordae tendinae		3	
5. Endocarditis	7	1	
6. Syphilis	4		
7. Marfan's disease	9		
8. Rheumatoid arthritis	5		
9. Malfunction of previous valve substitutes	9	4	
10. Traumatic			1
Total	216	150	3

TABLE 6.5
Associated valve lesions in 369 patints with single heart valve replacement

Associated lesions	Aortic	Mitral	Tricuspid	Total
Aortic stenosis		12		12
Aortic incompetence		5		5
Aortic valve disease		13		13
Mitral stenosis	14			14
Mitral incompetence	19			19
Mixed mitral valve disease	9		1	10
Tricuspid incompetence	1	29		30
Total	43	59	1	103

TABLE 6.6
Additional surgical procedures performed in 369 patients at the time of
valve replacement with pericardial xenografts

Surgical procedure	Aortic	Mitral	Tricuspid	Total
Aorta coronary SVBG	27	9		36
Removal LA thrombus		15		15
Closure PDA, VSD, ASD	5	1		6
Resection LV muscle	51	1		52
Ascending aorta replacement	12			12
Tricuspid annuloplasty	1	13		14
Mitral commissurotomy	11			11
Mitral annuloplasty	14		1	15
Mitral patch repair	2			2
Mitral decalcification	25			25
Permanent pacemaker insertion	8	4		12
Resection arterial aneurysm	2			2
Plication atrial septum		1		1
Decalcification LA wall		2		2
Total	158 (113)	46 (32)	1 (1)	205 (146)

SVBG = saphenous vein bypass graft; LA = left atrium; PDA = patent ductus arteriosus;
VSD = ventricular septal defect; LV = left ventricle
Figures in parentheses denote the number of patients with additional surgical procedures

TABLE 6.7
Number of patients having multiple heart valve
replacement with pericardial xenografts

Valves replaced	Number of patients
Mitral and aortic	31
Mitral and tricuspid	6
Mitral, aortic and tricuspid	5
Total	42

closed mitral valvotomy, one mitral annuloplasty and four mitral valve replacement). From the total of 369 patients 103 had associated valve lesions as detailed in *Table 6.5*. These valve lesions varied from trivial to severe. Pre-operatively 55 per cent of patients in the aortic and 88 per cent in the mitral group were in class III and IV of the New York Heart Association (NYHA) classification. At the time of valve replacement 205 additional cardiovascular surgical procedures were performed in 146 patients as shown in *Table 6.6*. The majority of these procedures were aorto–coronary saphenous vein bypass grafts and conservative operations on other heart valves. The number and distribution of patients subjected to multiple valve replacement are shown in *Table 6.7*.

DESCRIPTION OF THE PERICARDIAL XENOGRAFT

The pericardial xenograft[83] consists of bovine pericardium mounted onto a Dacron* covered support stent (*Figure 6.1*). The support stent is made of pure titanium which is biocompatible and has a high fatigue resistance. The frame is covered with a thin layer of Dacron* cloth to facilitate tissue ingrowth and encapsulation without increasing the bulk of the valve. The sewing rim contains porous Dacron* fabric covered with a thin layer of Dacron cloth. The configuration of the sewing rim is the same for all valve sizes and is made in such a way as to permit insertion of the valve in both aortic and atrioventricular positions, either sub- or supra-annular. The geometry of the valve and sewing rim are specifically designed to offer the optimum orifice diameter/implantation (annulus) diameter ratio which is essential in small size valves.

The pericardium is obtained from calves 6–18 months old, raised specifically for human food purposes and inspected and certified by the USDA† as being fit for human consumption. From the time of collection, sterile procedures are observed during the whole process of valve manufacture. Pericardial tissue portions of perfectly uniform thickness are selected, accurately measured for each valve size and mechanically cleaned and trimmed. Following this the pericardial strips are placed in sterile Hanks solution for a period of 3–6 h to remove

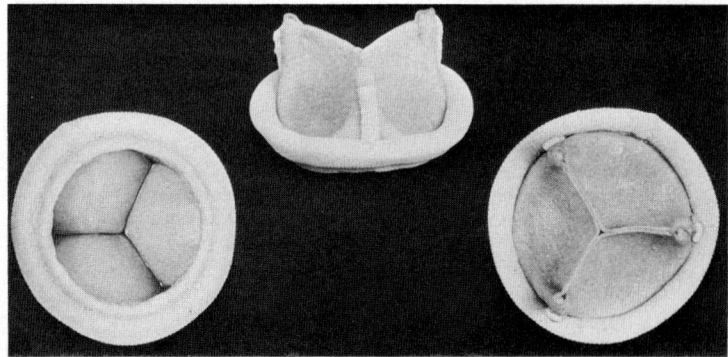

Figure 6.1 The glutaraldehyde-stabilized pericardial xenograft

*Dupont TM
†United States Drug and Food Administration

soluble proteins and other soluble components. The tissue strips are then rinsed with fresh sterile Hanks solution followed by a sterile physiological saline rinse. The cleaned pericardial strips are then stored in 0.5 per cent Purified Glutaraldehyde* buffered to pH 7.4 with 0.067 M phosphate, at 4 °C for a minimum of two weeks. The native structure of the pericardial tissue is permanently stabilized by the formation of inter- and intramolecular covalent bonds between the amino groups of lysine and hydroxylysine residues (present in collagen, elastin, glycoproteins and proteoglycans) and various forms of glutaraldehyde. The total tissue antigenicity is significantly reduced by this chemical immobilization and stabilization process with Purified Glutaraldehyde.

The tissue cross-link density, evaluated by tissue temperature shrinkage techniques, is optimum when 0.5 per cent Purified Glutaraldehyde is used as the chemical stabilizing agent[86]. The details of tissue stabilization with glutaraldehyde and the chemical reactions involved are outlined in Chapter 10.

During the entire process of valve fabrication, aseptic procedures are observed and all accessory materials (Dacron covered frames, sutures, etc.) and instruments are pre-sterilized. The construction and inspection of the valves take place in specially designed and controlled clean-air rooms. The valves are manufactured individually and rigorously inspected before release.

For construction of the valve, the stabilized pericardium is attached onto the outer aspect of the Dacron cloth covered titanium stent, thus maintaining intact the central opening of the valve which is the inside diameter of the fabric covered support stent. Due to this technique and to the thinness of the pericardium, the orifice diameter/implantation (annulus) diameter ratio of the pericardial xenograft is superior to all other commercially available tissue valves, and particularly advantageous in small aortic sizes (*Table 6.8*). After fabrication is completed, the valve is placed in a chemically compatible container surrounded with batting to prevent damage to the cusps. The container is filled with 4 per cent formaldehyde solution, buffered to pH 5.4 with 0.2 M acetate. After two days at room temperature, the solution is checked for both bacterial and fungal contaminants using standard Millipore filtrations as well as microbiological and mycological assay techniques. The container is then refilled with fresh 4 per cent buffered formaldehyde solution, sealed and quarantined for at least two weeks pending

TABLE 6.8
Essential dimensions of pericardial xenografts

Valve	Annulus diameter (mm)	Orifice diameter (mm)	Orifice area (mm²)
15 ISU	15	11.4	102
17 ISU	17	13.4	141
19 ISU	19	15.4	186
21 ISU	21	17.4	238
23 ISU	23	19.4	296
25 ISU	25	21.4	360
27 ISU	27	23.4	430
29 ISU	29	25.4	507
31 ISU	31	27.4	590
33 ISU	33	29.4	679

*Shiley Laboratories Inc., Irvine, California, U.S.A.

the results of the sterility assay. Storage in formaldehyde follows the permanent and complete stabilization of tissue by glutaraldehyde induced cross-links. Formaldehyde lowers the residual antigenicity of the pericardial tissue*, maintains its optimal pliability and, being a safer and more stable sterilizing agent[85], provides an additional margin of safety for long-term storage of the valves.

Between March 1971 and April 1976 all the pericardial xenografts were manufactured in our own hospital laboratory. The principle of the technique of valve construction was essentially the same as the one used at present by Shiley Laboratories. However, the 'home-made' valves did not benefit from the accuracy of a standardized procedure. The thickness and pliability of the valve cusps were not measured and independent quality control was non-existent. Moreover, during the initial five years of the experience the pericardial tissue was treated, prior to glutaraldehyde fixation, with sodium metaperiodate and ethylene glycol as initially advocated by Carpentier and Dubost[15]. The glutaraldehyde used in our laboratory was a simple dilution of commercially available non-purified glutaraldehyde with an unknown and unstable proportion of monomers and polymers.

TABLE 6.9
Yearly distribution of patients with pericardial xenograft valve replacement according to the time of operation

Year of operation	Valve replacement				
	Aortic	Mitral	Tricuspid	Multiple	Total
1971†	9	8			17
1972	27	16	3		46
1973	30	10			40
1974	35	15			50
1975	34	13			47
1976	29	27		1	57
1977	26	28		22	76
1978†	26	33		19	78
Total	216	150	3	42	411

†Less than 12 months

Since 1976 the pericardial xenografts are being manufactured by Shiley Laboratories using standardized techniques and highly accurate methods for the measurement of pericardial thickness and flexibility in order to obtain uniform movement of all three cusps of the particular valve. Using elaborate chemical methods a solution of 'purified glutaraldehyde' was obtained with the optimum proportion of monomeric and polymeric forms and an ideal cross-link density achieved by controlling the concentration and pH of the solution as well as the temperature and time of exposure.

Between 1971 and 1976, 220 'home-made' xenografts were inserted in 220 patients. Since 1976, 238 Ionescu–Shiley pericardial xenografts have been implanted in 191 patients for single, as well as for multiple, valve replacement.

*Slanczka, D. J., Bajpai, P. K. University of Dayton, Dept. of Biology and Wright State Univ., Dept. of Physiology, School of Med., Dayton, Ohio. *Clinical Research*, **26**, 124A (1978).

For the entire series 53.5 per cent of patients received 'home-made' valves and 46.5 per cent Shiley valves. *Table 6.9* outlines the number of patients operated upon yearly since 1971 and shows the increase in pericardial xenograft usage from 1976 onwards.

OPERATIVE TECHNIQUES

There are a variety of established techniques for aortic, mitral and tricuspid valve replacement. Any of the standard methods are applicable to the surgical implantation of pericardial xenografts. Due to the relatively low profile of the valve and the configuration of the sewing rim, the pericardial xenografts can be placed in either sub- or supra-annular positions for mitral and tricuspid replacement.

In our series, all valve replacements were performed through a median sternotomy and with the aid of conventional cardiopulmonary bypass. During the first six years of our experience, continuous, selective coronary perfusion was employed for aortic valve replacement and the heart was allowed to contract. For mitral valve replacement, intermittent hypoxia with topical hypothermia was the routine procedure. Since January 1977 moderate total body hypothermia (29-32 °C) with cold cardioplegia and topical hypothermia were used for all patients receiving mitral, aortic or multiple valve replacements.

The size of the xenografts used in 369 patients with single valve replacement and the type of suturing for implantation are shown in *Table 6.10*.

TABLE 6.10

Details of pericardial xenograft size and type of suturing to the heart valve annuli in 369 patients with single valve replacement

Valve replaced	Implantation diameter of xenograft (mm)						Type of sutures used		
	19	21	23	25	27	29	Interrupted	Continuous	Mixed*
Aortic	13	59	79	56	9		201	1	14
Mitral				11	108	31	15	108	27
Tricuspid					2	1			3
Total	13	59	79	67	119	32	216	109	44

*Denotes placement of interrupted sutures on one-third or less of the circumference of the valve and one continuous suture for the remaining two-thirds of the circumference

RESULTS

The definition of terms used in this chapter is as reported in previous publications[1,38]. Standard statistical formulae were used for the calculation and the analysis of results.

Early mortality

From the series of 369 patients with single valve replacement, 22 patients (5.9 per cent) died during the early postoperative period. There were 12 deaths (5.5 per cent) in the aortic and ten (6.7 per cent) in the mitral valve replacement group. The causes of early deaths are shown in *Table 6.11*. The majority of early deaths were due to cardiac causes and none of the patients died from a valve related complication. There were four deaths (9.5 per cent) in the group of 42 patients with multiple valve replacement. Two patients died from myocardial failure and one each from myocardial infarction and renal failure.

TABLE 6.11
Causes of early deaths in patients having single heart valve replacement
with pericardial xenografts

Cause of death	Aortic	Mitral
Cardiac		
Myocardial failure	4	4
Ventricular dysrhythmia	3	
Myocardial infarction	2	2
Non-cardiac		
Septicaemia		1
Mediastinitis	1	
Gastrointestinal haemorrhage	1	1
Cerebral infarction	1	1
Bronchopneumonia		1
Total (per cent)	12 (5.5)	10 (6.7)

Follow-up

All hospital survivors have been examined personally by the senior author and by one cardiologist at monthly intervals for the first three post-operative months, followed by six-monthly examinations for the entire duration of follow-up. This schedule was observed invariably for every patient irrespective of the patients

TABLE 6.12
Duration of follow-up for patients having heart valve replacement
with pericardial xenograft

Valves replaced	Number of patients	Hospital survivors	Total follow-up (months)	Mean follow-up (months)
Aortic	216	204	7388	37.8
Mitral	150	140	3948	35.8
Tricuspid	3	3	212	70.6
Multiple	42	38	347	9.2
Total	411	385	11 895	30.8

being seen by their own physicians. In addition to physical examination, chest radiographs and electrocardiograms were obtained in all patients at yearly intervals, or more often if indicated. Other laboratory investigations, including haemodynamic and angiographic studies were performed in a series of patients.

The 385 hospital survivors have been observed over a period of 6–90 months, for a total of 11 895 months (mean 30.8). In the aortic group 204 patients were observed for 7388 months (mean 37.8); in the mitral group 140 patients were followed for 3948 months (mean 35.8); the three patients with tricuspid valve replacement were followed for 212 months (mean 70.6); and the 38 patients with multiple valve replacement were observed for 347 months (mean 9.2). As shown in *Tables 6.9* and *6.12* the patients with multiple valve replacement have had a short follow-up period.

Late deaths

The late mortality for the entire pericardial xenograft series was 5.6 per cent. In the single valve replacement series 23 patients (6.2 per cent) died during the follow-up period of 7.5 years. There have been 15 deaths (6.9 per cent) in the aortic group and eight deaths (5.3 per cent) in the mitral. None of the patients with tricuspid or multiple valve replacement died during the follow-up period. The causes of late deaths are outlined in *Table 6.13*.

In nine patients (six aortic and three mitral) the death was valve related and was the consequence of endocarditis in seven patients (four aortic and three mitral) and of mechanical problems in two aortic patients (one valve cusp tear and one perivalvular leak).

TABLE 6.13
Causes of late deaths in patients having single heart valve replacement
with pericardial xenografts

Cause of death	Aortic	Mitral
Valve related		
Infective endocarditis	4	3
Cusp tear, haemolysis, re-op., haemorrhage*	1	
Perivalvular leak, mitral disease, re-op., brain damage†	1	
Cardiac causes		
Myocardial failure	1	3
Ventricular dysrhythmia	1	
Myocardial infarction	2	
Non-related causes		
Malignancy	1	1
Mesenteric vein thrombosis	1	
Dissection descending aorta	1	
Chronic cor-pulmonale	1	
Cerebral infarction	1	
Perforation of the colon		1
Total (per cent)	15 (6.9)	8 (5.3)

*The patient had had three previous open heart procedures
†The patient had had two previous open heart procedures

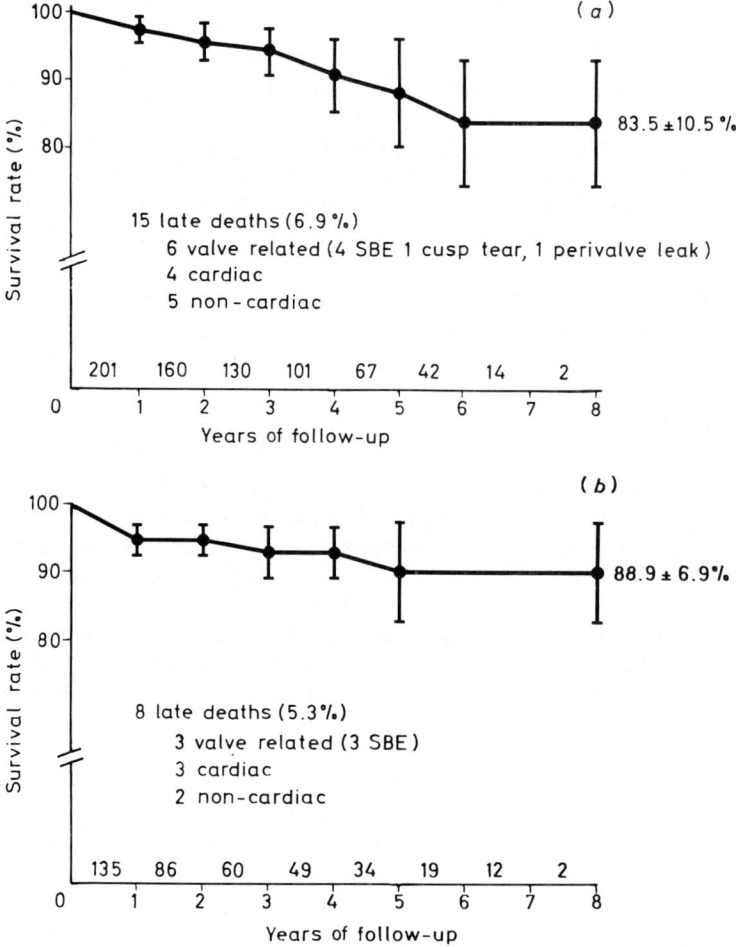

Figure 6.2 Actuarial representation of expected survival rate for patients having heart valve replacement with pericardial xenografts. The figures above the horizontal axes show the number of patients at the beginning of each year of the observation period. (*a*) Patients with aortic and (*b*) patients with mitral valve replacement

The actuarial analysis of survival rate for both aortic and mitral groups is shown in *Figure 6.2*. The expected survival rate for patients with aortic valve replacement is 87.0 ± 7.8 per cent at five years and 83.5 ± 10.5 per cent at eight years of follow-up. For patients with mitral replacement the expected survival is 88.9 ± 6.9 per cent both at five and eight years following valve insertion.

Valve thrombosis

Thrombosis of the pericardial xenografts has not been encountered in the entire series of 411 patients.

Embolic complications

Routine long-term treatment with prothrombin depressants or with anti-platelet drugs has not been used in this series. Between March 1971 and May 1976 none of the patients having pericardial xenografts, whether in the aortic, mitral or tricuspid position, received anticoagulants at any time. Since June 1976 all patients with either mitral replacement (76 patients) or with multiple valve replacement (42 patients) were treated for 4–6 weeks following valve insertion with warfarin sodium. The prothrombin time of these patients was maintained around, or slightly below the double of normal. Since June 1976 there have not been any embolic episodes in patients with mitral replacement and only one episode in a patient with multiple valve replacement.

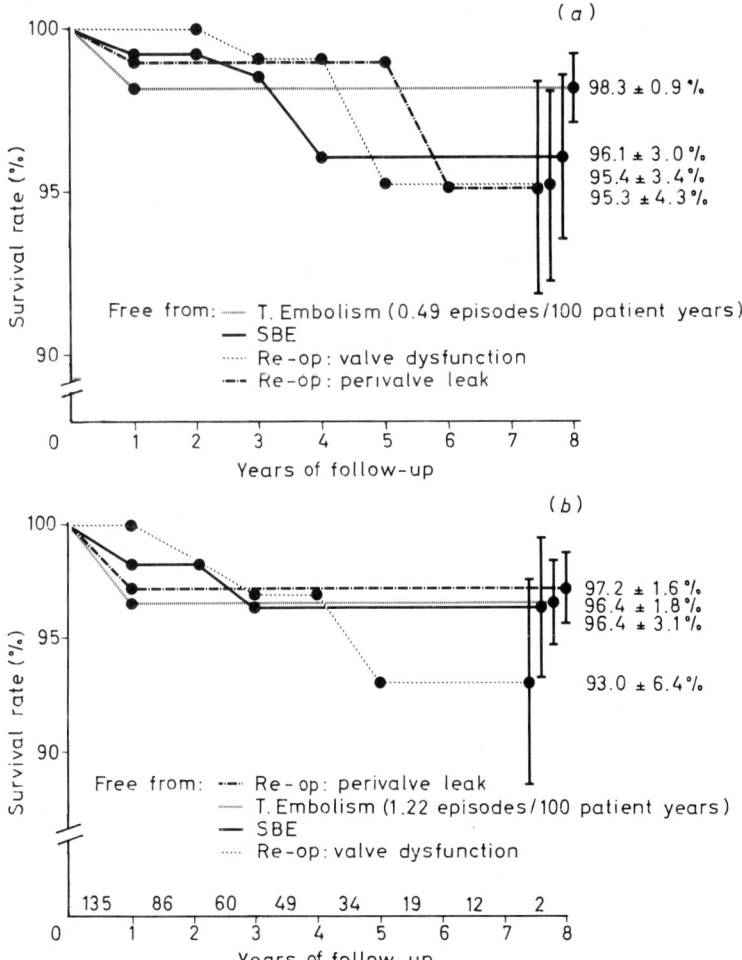

Figure 6.3 Actuarial analysis of results following heart valve replacement with pericardial xenografts. (*a*) Patients with aortic and (*b*) patients with mitral valve replacement. The data are expressed as per cent for individual event free curves. The figures above the horizontal axes denote the number of patients entering each year of follow-up

In the entire series there were eight instances of systemic embolization (1.9 per cent or 0.81 episodes/100 patient years). All embolic episodes occurred within six weeks following valve replacement, were mild and left no sequelae.

In the aortic replacement group there were three embolic episodes (0.49 episodes/100 patient years). Two patients developed transient visual field defects at four and 16 days postoperatively, following electrical cardioversion for atrial fibrillation. One of these patients had mitral commissurotomy at the time of aortic valve replacement. The third had transient facial paralysis 15 days postoperatively.

Four patients in the mitral replacement group had mild and transient pareses at 3, 17, 30 and 42 days following valve insertion. All four patients had grossly enlarged left atria and were in atrial fibrillation. The incidence of embolization for the mitral group was 1.22 episodes/100 patient years.

Among the 42 patients with multiple valve replacement there has been one slight paresis which occurred two days following the operation.

The actuarial representation of the event-free curves for embolism is shown in *Figure 6.3*. For patients having aortic valve replacement 98.3 ± 0.9 per cent are expected to be free from embolization at one and eight years of follow-up. For patients with mitral replacement 96.4 ± 1.8 per cent are expected to be free from embolism at one and eight years following valve insertion.

Endocarditis

Fungal endocarditis has not been encountered in this entire series. Bacterial endocarditis occurred in five patients (1.2 per cent) early post-operatively (within three months of valve insertion)[27] and in seven patients (1.7 per cent) late during the follow-up. Of the 12 patients with infected valves (six aortic and six mitral) five are alive. Four of them had re-operation and replacement of the infected valve with another pericardial xenograft and one had antibiotic treatment only. Seven patients died, five following re-operation, one shortly after admission to hospital in a moribund condition and the last one died suddenly two years after successful eradication of the infection with antibiotics. At post-mortem examination the aortic pericardial xenograft of this last patient was intact but the heart was considerably enlarged and the left ventricle grossly hypertrophied as it was described at the time of operation. The actuarial representation of the event-free curves for infective endocarditis are depicted in *Figure 6.3*. The curve for patients with aortic replacement shows that 96.1 ± 3.0 per cent are expected to be free from infection at four and eight years of follow-up. The curve for patients with mitral replacement shows that 96.4 ± 3.1 per cent are expected to be free from infection at three and eight years post-operatively.

Re-operation

In this series, 21 patients (5.1 per cent) underwent re-operation, nine of them because of endocarditis or its sequelae, as already described. Of the 12 remaining patients six had aortic and six mitral valve replacement.

In the aortic group three patients had closure of perivalvular leak at 4, 7 and 65 months post-operatively respectively. Two patients are alive and well. The third patient, who was re-operated upon at 65 months following valve insertion, developed, in addition to the perivalvular leak, progressively severe mitral valve disease. Closure of the leak and mitral valve replacement were performed. At re-operation, which was the third open heart procedure (previous aortic Starr valve) he sustained air embolism and died shortly after from neurological damage. Three other patients with aortic valve replacement were operated upon because of valve dysfunction as described in the next paragraph. Two of these three patients are alive and well.

In the mitral group three patients had closure of perivalvular leak at two, three and four months following valve insertion. Two patients are alive and well. The third one developed faecal peritonitis due to perforation of the colon and died. Three other patients in the mitral group were re-operated upon because of valve dysfunction as described in the next paragraph.

The actuarial representation of the event free curves of re-operation for perivalvular leak is shown in *Figure 6.3*. The percentage of patients expected to be free from re-operation for perivalvular leak at eight years of follow-up is 95.3 ± 4.3 for the aortic group and 97.2 ± 1.6 for the mitral replacement group.

Valve dysfunction

Seven patients (1.7 per cent) in the whole series (four aortic and three mitral) developed mechanical dysfunction of the pericardial xenograft valve.

One patient with aortic replacement developed an early diastolic murmur at 26 months post-operatively. Although the regurgitation was haemodynamically insignificant, re-operation became necessary six months later because of chronic intravascular haemolysis. At re-operation, which was the fourth median sterno-tomy (three previous aortic valve replacements) irreparable laceration of the right ventricle occurred. One cusp of the aortic pericardial valve was found to have a vertical tear, about 4 mm long, near to a commissure. The valve tissue was otherwise unchanged. A second patient with aortic replacement was re-operated upon when he became symptomatic at 57 months following valve insertion. A tear along the base of one cusp was found, the valve removed and replaced with another pericardial xenograft and the patient is now asymptomatic. The third aortic patient developed progressive symptoms of aortic restenosis and was operated upon at 57 months after valve replacement. Light, diffuse calcification of all three cusps of the xenograft was found and the valve was successfully re-placed. The last patient in the aortic group died from a cerebral tumour 60 months following valve insertion. At post-mortem examination an indentation, 1 mm deep was found at the free margin of a cusp near to the commissure. From the cardiac view point the patient was completely asymptomatic prior to his death.

There were three cases of xenograft dysfunction in the mitral series. Two patients developed clinical signs of progressive mitral regurgitation and within a few weeks of the appearance of the murmur both required re-operation, which was performed at 13 and 31 months following valve insertion. In these two xenografts the mechanical lesion was similar, one cusp became disinserted from the support stent along the suture line. The commissural areas were intact. The third patient developed, over a period of 18 months, clinical signs of mitral re-stenosis. At re-operation, 60 months following valve insertion, the pericardial xenograft was found lightly and diffusely calcified and a small section of one cusp was disinserted from the stent at the suture line. All three patients had the defective valves removed and successfully replaced with pericardial xenografts. The actuarial event free curves of re-operation for valve dysfunction are shown in *Figure 6.3*. All seven valve dysfunctions occurred in the 220 patients operated upon during the first five years of our experience and all were 'home-made' xenografts treated with sodium metaperiodate and ethylene glycol prior to glutaraldehyde fixation. Mechanical valve dysfunction has not been observed in any of the 238 Ionescu–Shiley pericardial xenografts inserted in 191 patients since May 1976.

Heart valve murmurs

A total of 16 patients (3.9 per cent) in the entire series have cardiac murmurs. In the aortic replacement group 15 patients (6.9 per cent) developed early diastolic murmur. In 13 of them the murmur appeared in the early post-operative period, whereas in two patients the murmur was noted, 31 and 36 months following valve insertion. In seven of these patients perivalvular leaks were detected at the time of valve replacement and attempts were made to obliterate them. Aortic root angiography has been performed in 12 patients with early diastolic murmur and in all 12 the presence of perivalvular leak was clearly demonstrated. All 15 patients continue to remain in class I NYHA, with no clinical deterioration or statistically significant changes in cardiothoracic ratio or electrocardiogram over a period of observation of 9–64 months (mean 34) following the appearance of the murmur.

In the mitral replacement group one patient (0.7 per cent) developed an apical systolic murmur 49 months following valve insertion. He has been followed-up for 30 months since the appearance of the murmur and continues to be asymptomatic and working full-time.

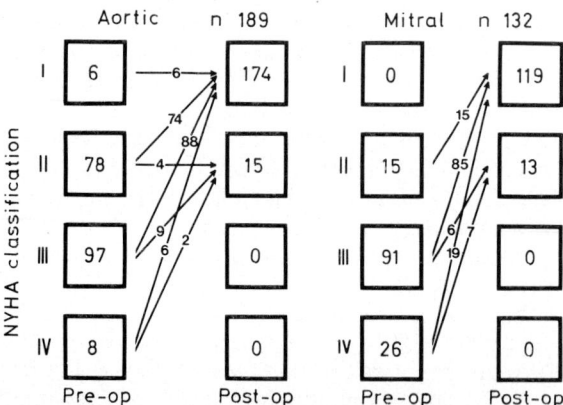

Figure 6.4 Diagrammatic presentation of the pre- and latest post-operative NYHA functional classification of 189 long-term survivors with aortic and 132 with mitral pericardial xenograft valve replacement

Clinical condition

A comparison between the pre- and the most recent post-operative evaluation according to the NYHA classification was made and the results are shown in *Figure 6.4*. Following valve replacement 92.1 per cent of the aortic and 90.2 per cent of the mitral long-term survivors are in class I. Those patients who are in class II (7.9 per cent from the aortic and 9.8 per cent from the mitral group) have either associated chronic bronchitis or have developed ischaemic heart disease since the valve replacement operation.

Tricuspid valve and multiple valve replacement

There were neither early nor late deaths and no complications among the three patients with tricuspid xenograft valve replacement during a period of follow-up of over six years (mean 70.6 months). All the patients are in class I NYHA.

In the group of 42 patients with multiple valve replacement there were four early deaths, none of them being valve related. There have not been any late deaths during the period of observation of 6–18 months (mean 9.2). As mentioned previously, the only complication that occurred in this group of patients was one systemic embolus which left a slight degree of arm paresis. This episode occurred early post-operatively. Clinically all operative survivors were greatly benefited by valve replacement.

Electrocardiographic and radiological changes

As shown in *Figure 6.5*, there was a statistically significant reduction in the mean left ventricular voltage in patients following aortic valve replacement. This was not so in the mitral replacement group, with the exception of patients who had predominant mitral regurgitation pre-operatively, in whom the decrease in voltage was significant.

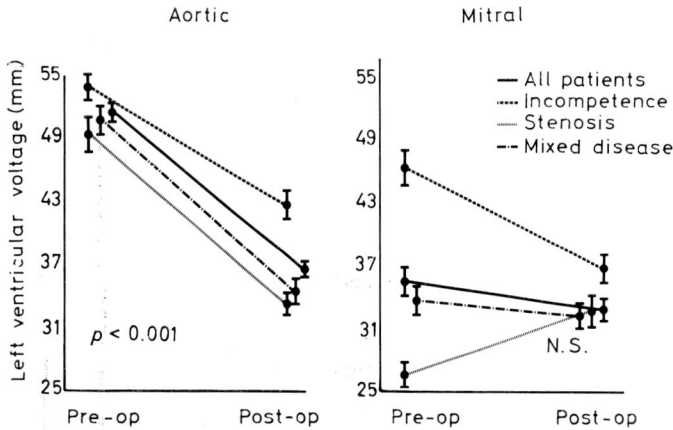

Figure 6.5 Graphic presentation of the pre- and latest post-operative left ventricular voltage in long-term survivors with aortic and mitral pericardial xenograft valve replacement

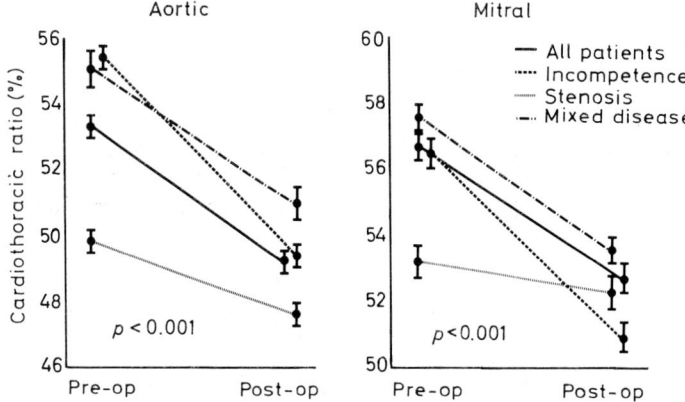

Figure 6.6 Graphic presentation of the pre- and latest post-operative cardiothoracic ratio in long-term survivors with aortic and with mitral pericardial xenograft valve replacement

There was also a statistically significant reduction in cardiothoracic ratio in all patients following either aortic or mitral valve replacement (*Figure 6.6*). Radiologically, there was no evidence of calcification of the pericardial xenograft during the period of observation, with the exception of the two patients already described.

Intravascular haemolysis

There was no clinical evidence of chronic intravascular haemolysis in this series with the exception of one patient with aortic valve replacement, already described, who developed a cusp tear. Laboratory investigations were performed for the detection of chronic intravascular haemolysis in 24 patients having single valve replacement with pericardial xenografts (12 with aortic and 12 with mitral replacement) at a mean interval of nine months after valve insertion. The investigations performed included haemoglobin level, haematocrit, reticulocyte count, total red blood cell count, fragment red cell count, serum bilirubin, SGOT level, serum lactic acid dehydrogenase level, haemopexin and haptoglobin estimation, and they were found to be within physiological range in all 24 patients.

Pathology of the pericardial xenograft

The pericardial xenografts recovered at re-operation or at autopsy (24 h to 65 months post-operatively) were examined. All valves, with the exception of the two calcified xenografts, were essentially unchanged when compared with unimplanted specimens. The sewing rim and exposed Dacron surfaces were covered with a thin, glistening layer of fibrous tissue in continuity with the endocardium.

Six of the eight xenograft valves recovered from patients with endocarditis had the substance of the cusps unaffected by the disease process. When vegetations attached to the sewing rim were removed the pericardial tissue appeared macroscopically essentially unchanged. Microscopic examination of valves removed at various periods of time after implantation showed that the histologic components of the pericardium had undergone little, if any, change when compared with unimplanted specimens. They have maintained their structure and organization despite the passage of time. There was practically no difference in the microscopic appearance between valves removed 2–3 weeks post-operatively and those which were implanted for up to 65 months. There was an insignificant (0.03–0.05 mm) layer of fibrin deposited in a regular fashion over the inflow aspect of the cusps (the non-cardiac, rough surface of the original calf pericardium). The thickness of this fibrin layer did not seem to have increased with the passage of time, as its thickness and general appearance were the same in all valves whether they were implanted for two weeks or for 65 months. There was no evidence of immune or inflammatory reaction in or around the valve cusps (*Figure 6.7*).

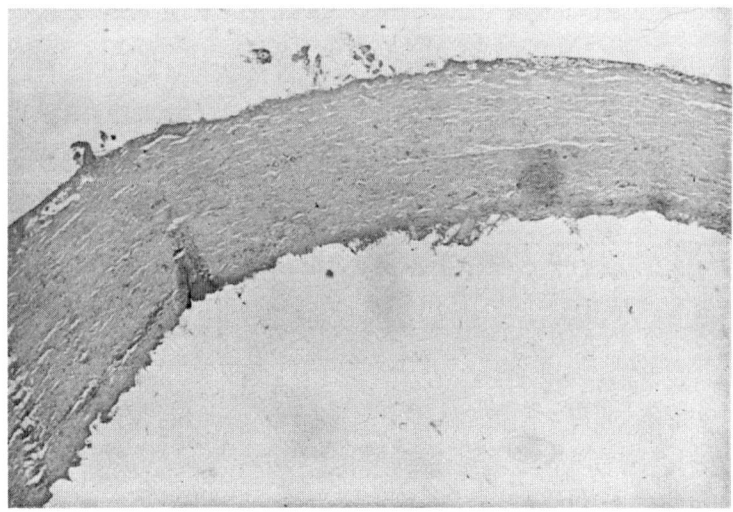

Figure 6.7 Microscopy section through a cusp of the pericardial xenograft removed from the aortic position 65 months following its insertion. The histological components of the pericardium are essentially unchanged when compared with unimplanted specimens. Haematoxylin and eosin × 30, reduced by 40% in printing

Two valves, one removed from the aortic position at 57 months and one from the mitral area at 60 months post-operatively, were lightly, but diffusely calcified. All three cusps were slightly thickened and uniformly impregnated with calcium which on microscopic examination was found to be deposited throughout the thickness of the pericardium. The collagen fibres were dissociated by the deposits.

It should be mentioned that amongst the xenografts examined all those obtained late post-operatively were 'home-made' valves implanted during the first five years of our experience.

Haemodynamic investigations

Haemodynamic studies were performed in 68 patients with single valve replacement. The number of patients investigated and the time of the studies are detailed in *Table 6.14*. The criteria for selection were the informed consent of the patient and either a duration of at least two years since valve replacement in patients for long-term study, or complete pre-operative investigations for patients to be subjected to sequential haemodynamic studies.

TABLE 6.14
Number of patients and time of haemodynamic and angiographic investigations

A. Long-term study

	Pre-operative	Post-operative		
	Number of patients	*Number of patients*	*Time of investigation* (months)	
			Mean	*Range*
Aortic	25	36	41.2	22–59
Mitral	21	29	40.2	24–59
Tricuspid	2	3	47.7	24–66

B. Sequential studies

	Pre-operative *Number of patients*	*Number of patients*	*Mean time* (months)	*Number of patients*	*Mean time* (months)
Aortic	13	13	9.9	13	42.2
Mitral	6	6	11.0	6	43.0

Thirty-six patients with aortic valve replacement underwent long-term study at a mean duration of 41.2 (range 22–59) months following valve insertion. Of these, 13 patients had three sequential haemodynamic investigations. In addition to the pre-operative catheterization, they underwent two post-operative cardiac studies at mean durations of 9.9 and 42.2 months following valve replacement. Twenty-nine patients with mitral valve replacement underwent long-term haemo-dynamic evaluation at 40.2 (range 24–59) months post-operatively. Of these, six patients had three sequential investigations, one pre-operatively and two at 11.0 and 43.0 months following valve replacement. The three patients with tricuspid valve replacement were investigated at a mean duration of 47.7 (range 24–66) months post-operatively.

The sizes of the valves of those patients subjected to haemodynamic studies are shown in *Table 6.15*.

All patients were hospitalized 24 h prior to the haemodynamic study. On admission, a detailed clinical history, estimation of functional capability, physical examination, haematological assessment, a chest radiograph, a 12 lead electro-cardiogram and a phonocardiogram were obtained in all patients. Electrocardio-grams and chest radiographs were analysed for rhythm, left ventricular voltage and cardiothoracic ratio.

All the patients underwent right and left heart catheterization in the post-absorptive state without any prior sedation. In addition, all patients with aortic

TABLE 6.15
Size of annulus diameter of the pericardial xenografts of patients subjected to
haemodynamic studies

Valve replaced	Annulus diameter (mm)						Total
	19	21	23	25	27	29	
Aortic	5	9	13	8	1		36
Mitral				2	15	12	29
Tricuspid					2	1	3

valve replacement had trans-septal catheterization. Pulmonary and systemic
pressures were transduced by strain gauge manometers with the zero level set
5 cm below the sternal angle, integrated electronically and recorded on a multi-
channel ultraviolet light recorder (SEM 3012)*. Cardiac output was measured by
the direct Fick method. Haemodynamic data were obtained during a 4-min
period of rest and between the fourth and sixth minutes of a 6-min period of
supine leg exercise on a bicycle ergometer. The same level of exercise was employed in all three studies of the sequential investigation. The ejection systolic
gradients across the aortic pericardial xenografts were measured by planimetric
integration of simultaneously recorded phasic left ventricular and aortic root
tracings. Similarly, the mean diastolic gradient across the mitral pericardial xenograft was measured by planimetric integration of simultaneously recorded phasic
left ventricular and pulmonary wedge tracings. Pulmonary and systemic vascular
resistance was calculated using the standard formula. The xenograft surface area
was calculated according to the hydraulic formula of Gorlin and Gorlin[29].
Ventricular and/or aortic root angiograms were performed in all the patients at
the completion of the study.

Aortic valve replacement

Long-term study The results are outlined in *Tables 6.16* and *6.17* and in
Figures 6.8, 6.9 and *6.10.*
   In the aortic replacement group there was a significant increase in cardiac output and reduction in mean pulmonary wedge and left ventricular end-diastolic
pressures both at rest and during exercise at the post-operative study as compared
with the pre-operative values. The mean cardiac index was 2.7 at rest and
4.6 ℓ/min/m^2 during exercise at the post-operative study, and the cardiac output
response to exercise was normal. Both the mean pulmonary wedge and left
ventricular end-diastolic pressures were normal at rest but were abnormally
elevated during exercise at the post-operative study. The mean peak systolic
gradient values during the post-operative study were 6.4 ± 1.0 mmHg at rest and
9.6 ± 1.6 mmHg on exercise. The corresponding figures for calculated xenograft
surface areas were 1.6 ± 0.07 cm^2 and 2.0 ± 0.1 cm^2.
   An analysis of the post-operative results as related to the xenograft size is

*Sheilds and Epstein Monitoring, Middlesex, UK

TABLE 6.16

Pre- and post-operative haemodynamic data (mean values ± SEM and statistical significance)
of 36 patients having aortic valve replacement with pericardial xenografts.
Investigations performed 22–59 (mean 41.2) months post-operatively

	Cardiac index (ℓ/min/m^2)		PWP (mmHg)		LVEDP (mmHg)		PSG (mmHg)		XSA (cm^2)	
	R	E	R	E	R	E	R	E	R	E
Pre-operative	2.4 ±0.2	4.2 ±0.3	13.7 ±1.7	31.4 ±5.2	19.1 ±2.8	32.7 ±5.8	83.3 ±10.0			
Post-operative (mean 41.2 months)	2.7 ±0.1	4.6 ±0.2	9.4 ±0.5	20.3 ±1.1	9.9 ±0.7	18.3 ±1.6	6.4 ±1.0	9.6 ±1.6	1.6 ±0.07	2.0 ±0.1
p value	< 0.05	< 0.05	< 0.05	< 0.01	< 0.01	<0.01	< 0.001			

SEM = standard error of the mean; PWP = pulmonary wedge pressure; LVEDP = left ventricular end-diastolic pressure; PSG = peak systolic gradient; XSA = calculated xenograft surface area; R = rest; E = exercise

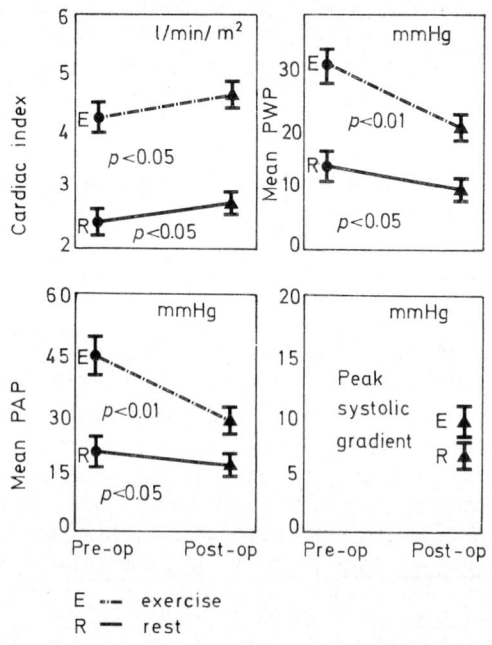

Figure 6.8 Graphic presentation of pre- and post-operative haemodynamic data from 36 patients with aortic pericardial xenograft valve replacement. The post-operative investigations were performed at a mean of 41.2 months (range 22–59) following valve insertion. The data are expressed as mean values, at rest and on exericse. Pre-op = pre-operative; Post-op = post-operative; p = statistical significance

TABLE 6.17

Post-operative haemodynamic data in 36 patients with aortic valve replacement as related to the pericardial xenograft size. Investigations performed 22–59 (mean 41.2) months post-operatively

Xenograft size (annulus diameter in mm)	In vitro surface area (cm²)	Number of patients	Cardiac index (ℓ/min/m²)		AVF (ml/s)		PWP (mmHg)		LVEDP (mmHg)		PSG (mmHg)		ESG (mmHg)		XSA (cm²)	
			R	E	R	E	R	E	R	E	R	E	R	E	R	E
19	1.86	5	2.8	4.3	192 ±33.9	249 ±24.0	10.6 ±1.8	24.5 ±4.1	11.3 ±1.8	25 ±4.9	8.3 ±2.7	12.3 ±2.7	14.3 ±3.2	22.6 ±6.4	1.1 ±0.07	1.3 ±0.07
21	2.38	9	2.6	4.4	194 ±11.9	282 ±16.5	9.6 ±1.4	19.3 ±2.9	10.6 ±2.0	20.3 ±3.2	7.9 ±1.6	13.3 ±2.3	12.9 ±1.2	20.3 ±6.2	1.4 ±0.1	1.8 ±0.03
23	2.96	13	2.9	4.8	204 ±13.8	324 ±13.2	8.9 ±0.5	19.8 ±0.4	9.2 ±0.5	18.1 ±1.9	3.2 ±1.6	10.0 ±2.6	10.8 ±1.6	17.3 ±1.6	1.6 ±0.1	2.1 ±0.1
25	3.60	8	2.6	4.3	260 ±19.3	367 ±22.2	9.5 ±1.1	18.1 ±1.6	9.2 ±0.6	13.0 ±1.9	3.3 ±1.1	5.7 ±2.5	7.5 ±1.2	13.0 ±1.9	1.8 ±0.08	2.1 ±0.1
27	4.30	1*	2.3	4.5	196	302	12	19	10	15	0	1.0	5	6	2.1	2.4
All patients		36	2.7	4.6	225 ±11	322 ±13.7	9.4 ±0.5	20.3 ±1.1	9.9 ±0.7	18.3 ±1.6	6.4 ±1.0	9.6 ±1.6	10.9 ±0.9	16.9 ±1.6	1.6 ±0.07	2.0 ±0.1

*Had additional mitral annuloplasty at the time of aortic valve replacement

Data expressed as mean values ± standard error of the mean.

AVF = aortic valve flow; PWP = mean pulmonary wedge pressure; LVEDP = left ventricular end-diastolic pressure; PSG = peak systolic gradient; ESG = ejection systolic gradient; XSA = calculated xenograft surface area; R = rest; E = exercise

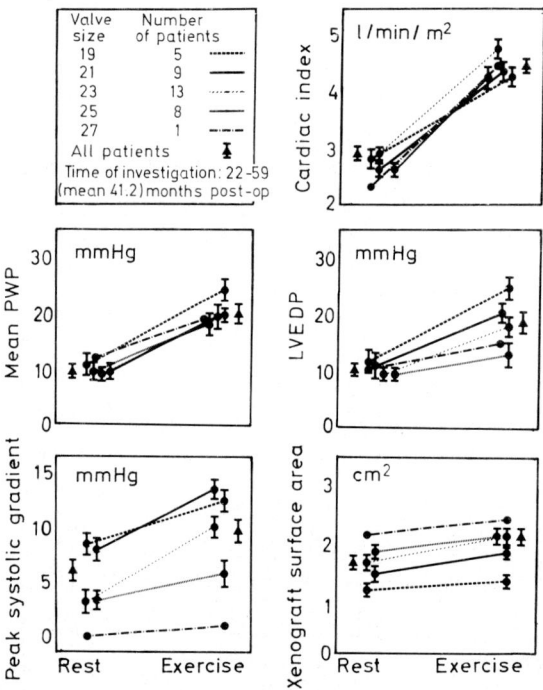

Figure 6.9 Graphic presentation of post-operative haemodynamic data at rest and on exercise, from 36 patients with aortic pericardial xenograft valve replacement, according to the size (annulus diameter in mm) of the xenograft inserted. PWP = pulmonary wedge pressure, LVEDP = left ventricular end diastolic pressure. (Mean values ± SEM)

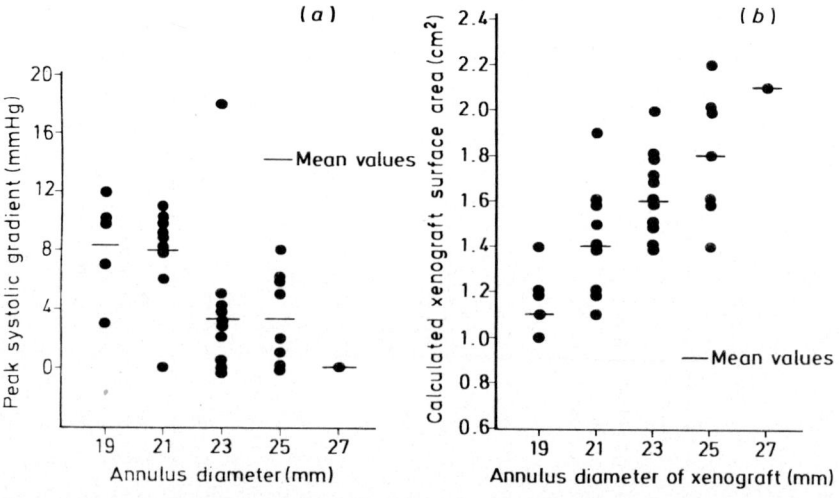

Figure 6.10 Graphic presentation of correlation between the annulus diameter of pericardial xenografts in the aortic position and both (*a*) the peak systolic gradient and (*b*) the calculated surface area

depicted in *Table 6.17* and in *Figures 6.9* and *6.10*. A normal increase in cardiac output and its response to oxygen uptake during exercise was found in all patients. The calculated flow across the pericardial xenograft ranged from 192 to 260 ml/s at rest and 249 to 367 ml/s during exercise. The aortic valve flow was directly related to the annulus diameter of the pericardial xenograft ($r = 0.861$ at rest and $r = 0.998$ on exercise). Although the mean pulmonary wedge and left ventricular end-diastolic pressures were normal at rest, an abnormal increase was found in all patients on exercise. The highest increments in both left ventricular end-diastolic and mean pulmonary wedge pressures were encountered in patients with smaller sizes of pericardial xenografts although there was only an insignificant obstruction to forward flow in these patients. However, the number of patients was too small for meaningful statistical analysis.

The peak systolic gradient ranged from 0–18 mmHg at rest and from 1–22 mmHg during exercise. The mean peak systolic gradient was 8.3 mmHg at rest and 12.3 mmHg during exercise in patients with the smallest xenograft (19 mm) studied and it decreased with corresponding increase in valve size, so that with the 27 mm xenograft it was 0 at rest and 1 mmHg during exercise (*Figure 6.10a*). The correlation was confirmed by statistical analysis ($r = 0.982$ at rest and 0.887 on exercise).

The calculated xenograft surface area varied from 1.0–2.1 cm² at rest and 1.2–2.6 cm² during exercise. As expected the calculated areas were lowest with the smallest xenografts studied and increased with a corresponding increase in the valve size (*Figure 6.10b*). A statistically significant correlation was found between the xenograft size and the calculated surface areas ($r = 0.996$ at rest and $r = 0.951$ on exercise).

All pericardial xenografts were competent at angiography.

Sequential haemodynamic study   The results of the sequential haemodynamic investigations are detailed in *Figures 6.11* and *6.12*.

The cardiac output increased significantly both at rest and during exercise between the pre-operative and the first post-operative study. The mean cardiac index was 2.4 ± 0.2 at rest and 4.6 ± 0.3 ℓ/min/m² during exercise at the pre-operative investigation while the corresponding figures at the first post-operative study were 2.7 ± 0.2 and 4.7 ± 0.2 ℓ/min/m². The mean stroke index increased from 29 ± 3.0 to 31 ± 2.2 ml/m² at rest and from 24 ± 3.7 to 41 ± 3.0 ml/m² during exercise between the pre-operative and the first post-operative studies. The cardiac output response to exercise was normal at the first post-operative study.

The peak systolic gradient was 49 ± 17.7 mmHg at rest at the pre-operative investigation and decreased significantly to 6 ± 1.6 mmHg at the first post-operative study. Exercise systolic gradients were only available in five patients with aortic incompetence at the pre-operative investigation and the mean level was 17 ± 2.1 mmHg. This decreased to 11 ± 1.9 mmHg at the first post-operative study. The calculated surface areas were 1.6 ± 0.1 cm² at rest and 2.0 ± 0.1 cm² during exercise at the first post-operative study.

Between the first and second post-operative investigations there were no significant changes in any of the parameters studied. The mean peak systolic gradient was 6 ± 1.2 mmHg at rest and 9 ± 1.7 mmHg during exercise at the second post-operative study while the corresponding calculated surface areas were 1.6 ± 0.1 and 2.1 ± 0.1 cm².

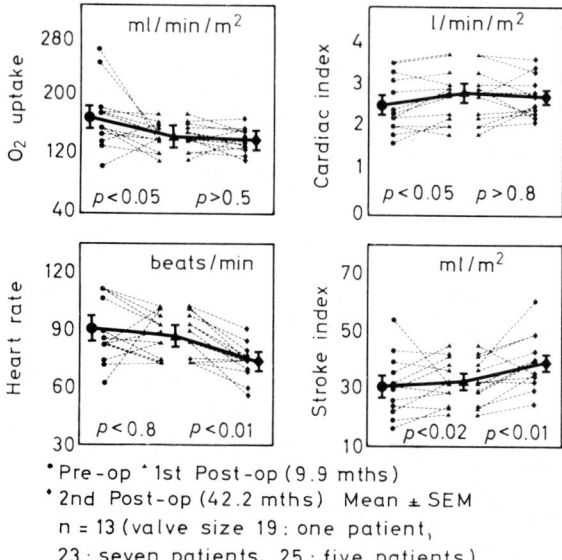

(a)

*Pre-op *1st Post-op (9.9 mths)
*2nd Post-op (42.2 mths) Mean ± SEM
n = 13 (valve size 19: one patient,
23 : seven patients, 25 : five patients)

(b)

*Pre-op *1st Post-op (9.9 mths)
*2nd Post-op (42.2 mths) Mean ± SEM
n = 13 (valve size 19: one patient,
23: seven patients, 25: five patients)

Figure 6.11 Sequential haemodynamic data at rest from 13 patients with aortic pericardial xenograft valve replacement. PAP = pulmonary artery pressure; PWP = pulmonary wedge pressure; LVEDP = left ventricular end diastolic pressure; Pre-op = pre-operative; Post-op = post-operative

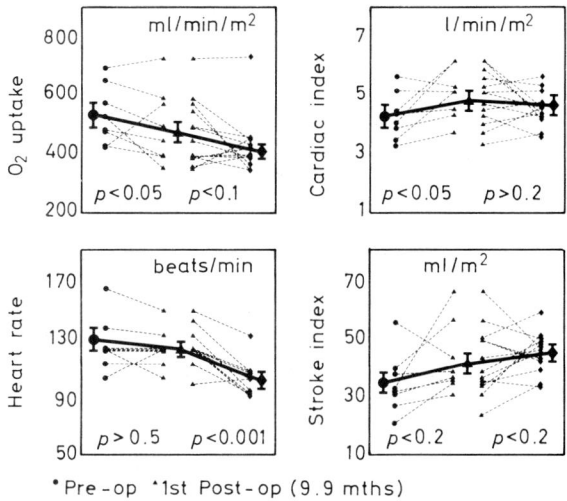

(a)

• Pre-op • 1st Post-op (9.9 mths)
• 2nd Post-op (42.2 mths) Mean + SEM
n = 13 (valve size 19: one patient,
23: seven patients, 25: five patients)

(b)

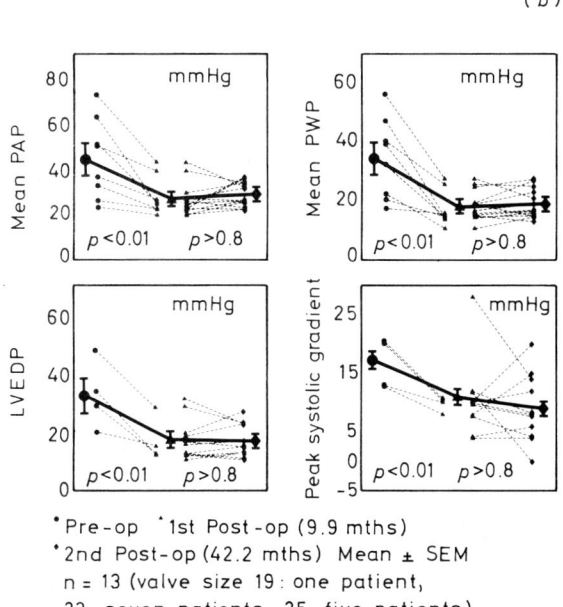

• Pre-op • 1st Post-op (9.9 mths)
• 2nd Post-op (42.2 mths) Mean ± SEM
n = 13 (valve size 19: one patient,
23: seven patients, 25: five patients)

Figure 6.12 Sequential haemodynamic data on exercise from 13 patients with aortic pericardial xenograft valve replacement. Abbreviations as in *Figure 6.11*

Mitral valve replacement

Long-term study   The results are given in *Table 6.18* and in *Figures 6.13* and *6.14.*

The long-term study undertaken in 29 patients with mitral valve replacement showed a significant increase in cardiac index and reduction in mean pulmonary wedge and pulmonary artery pressures and in the pulmonary vascular resistance.

The cardiac index was 2.6 ± 0.2 $\ell/min/m^2$ at rest and 4.1 ± 0.2 $\ell/min/m^2$ on exercise at the post-operative study. Both the oxygen consumption and the cardiac output response to exercise were, however, abnormal at the post-operative investigation.

The mean pulmonary wedge pressure at rest decreased from a pre-operative level of 23.0 ± 1.9 mmHg to a near normal level of 13.8 ± 0.8 mmHg at the post-operative study. The corresponding values during exercise were 40.4 ± 2.7 and 29.4 ± 1.5 mmHg. The mean pulmonary artery pressures at the post-operative study were 22.8 ± 1.0 and 42.0 ± 1.9 mmHg at rest and on exercise respectively. Thus, both the mean pulmonary wedge and pulmonary artery pressures were abnormally elevated during exercise at the post-operative study. A decrease in pulmonary pressures and pulmonary vascular resistance was also noted in ten patients with severe pre-operative pulmonary hypertension. Thus, in this series, the severity of pre-existing pulmonary hypertension did not seem to influence the post-operative haemodynamic improvement. The mean diastolic gradient was

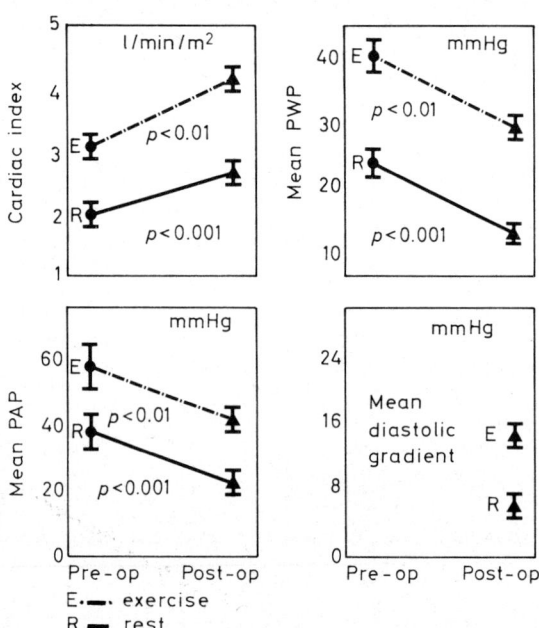

Figure 6.13 Graphic presentation of pre- and post-operative haemodynamic data from 29 patients with mitral pericardial xenograft valve replacement. The post-operative investigations were performed at a mean of 40.2 months (range 24–59) following valve insertion. The data are expressed as mean values at rest and on exercise. Pre-op = pre-operative; post-op = post-operative; p = statistical significance

TABLE 6.18

Pre- and post-operative haemodynamic data (mean values ± SEM and statistical significance) of 29 patients having mitral valve replacement with pericardial xenografts. Investigations performed 24–59 (mean 40.2) months post-operatively

	O_2 uptake (ml/min/m²)		Cardiac index (ℓ/min/m²)		PWP (mmHg)		PAP (mmHg)		PVR (dyn s cm⁻⁵ m²)		MDG (mmHg)		XSA (cm²)	
	R	E	R	E	R	E	R	E	R	E	R	E	R	E
Pre-operative	123.7 ±6.0	314.6 ±40.4	1.9 ±0.1	3.0 ±0.3	23.0 ±1.9	40.4 ±2.7	38.7 ±4.1	57.1 ±4.9	535.6 ±113.3	656.8 ±241.1				
Post-operative	136.3 ±4.0	406.5 ±14.4	2.6 ±0.2	4.1 ±0.2	13.8 ±0.8	29.4 ±1.5	22.8 ±1.0	42.0 ±1.9	285.0 ±20.7	260.3 ±26.3	6.4 ±0.5	15.3 ±0.9	2.0 ±0.1	2.3 ±0.1
p value	< 0.05	< 0.05	< 0.001	< 0.01	< 0.001	< 0.01	< 0.001	< 0.01	< 0.01	< 0.05				

SEM = standard error of the mean; PWP = mean pulmonary wedge pressure; PAP = mean pulmonary artery pressure; PVR = pulmonary vascular resistance; MDG = mean diastolic gradient; XSA = calculated xenograft surface area; R = rest; E = exercise

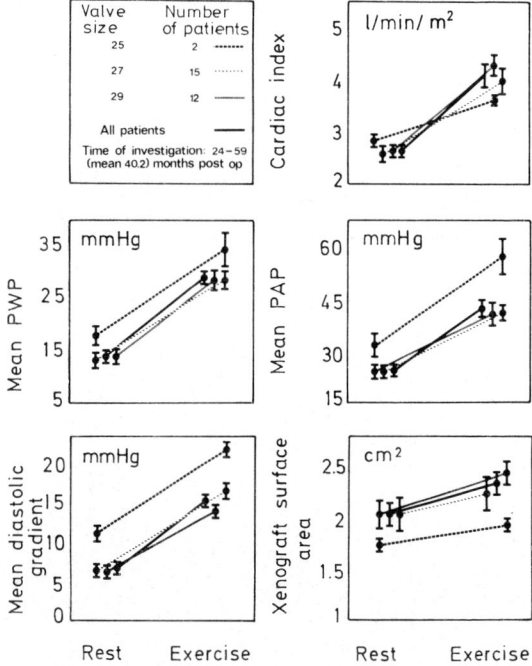

Figure 6.14 Graphic presentation of post-operative haemodynamic data, at rest and on exercise, from 29 patients with mitral pericardial xenograft valve replacement according to the size (annulus diameter in mm) of the xenograft inserted. PWP = pulmonary wedge pressure, PAP = pulmonary artery pressure. (Mean values ± SEM)

6.4 ± 0.5 mmHg at rest and 15.3 ± 0.9 mmHg during exercise at the post-operative study. The corresponding values for calculated xenograft surface areas were 2.0 ± 0.1 and 2.3 ± 0.1 cm^2.

The mean post-operative haemodynamic data as related to xenograft size are depicted in *Figure 6.14*. The three sizes of pericardial xenografts investigated were 25 mm in two patients, 27 mm in 15 patients and 29 mm in 12 patients. No difference was noted in the haemodynamic data both at rest and during exercise between patients with 27 mm and 29 mm pericardial xenografts.

All the pericardial xenografts investigated were competent at angiography.

Sequential haemodynamic study   The results of these investigations are illustrated in *Figures 6.15* and *6.16*.

Between the pre-operative and the first post-operative study both the cardiac output and stroke index increased significantly at rest. During exercise a statistically significant increase was noted only in stroke index. There was no change in the oxygen uptake either at rest or during exercise. The cardiac output response to exercise was impaired. A significant reduction both at rest and on exercise, was noted in the mean pulmonary artery and pulmonary wedge pressures and

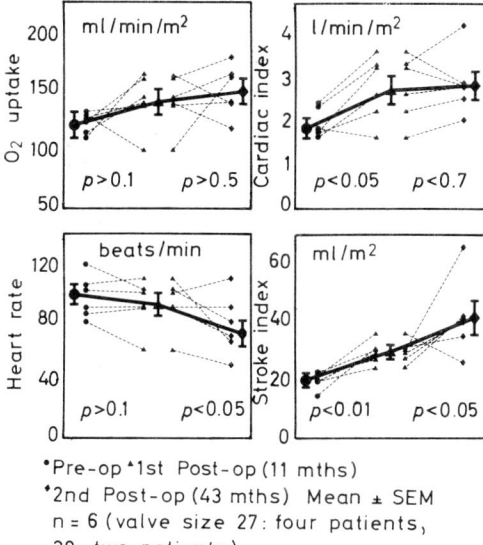

• Pre-op ▲ 1st Post-op (11 mths)
✦ 2nd Post-op (43 mths) Mean ± SEM
n = 6 (valve size 27: four patients,
29: two patients)

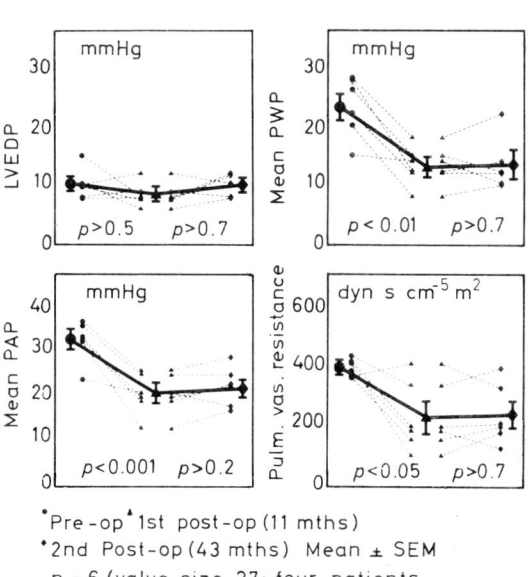

• Pre-op ▲ 1st post-op (11 mths)
✦ 2nd Post-op (43 mths) Mean ± SEM
n = 6 (valve size 27: four patients,
29: two patients)

Figure 6.15 Sequential haemodynamic data at rest from 6 patients with mitral pericardial xenograft valve replacement. LVEDP = left ventricular end diastolic pressure; PWP = pulmonary wedge pressure; PAP = pulmonary artery pressure; pre-op = pre-operative; post-op = post-operative

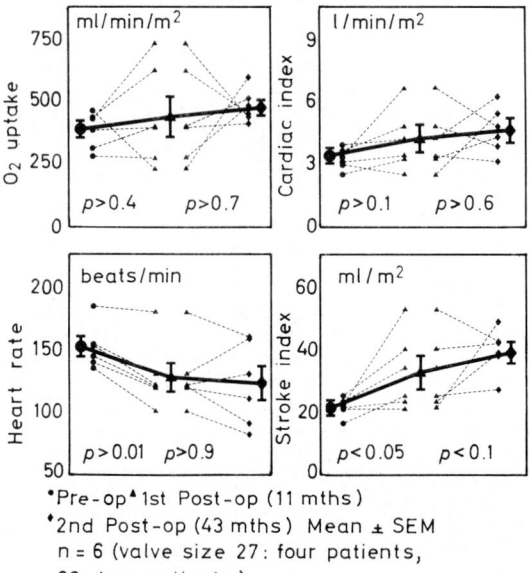

(a)

•Pre-op▲1st Post-op (11 mths)
•2nd Post-op (43 mths) Mean ± SEM
n = 6 (valve size 27: four patients,
    29: two patients)

(b)

•Pre-op▲1st Post-op (11 mths)
•2nd Post-op (43 mths) Mean ± SEM
n = 6 (valve size 27: four patients,
    29: two patients)

Figure 6.16 Sequential haemodynamic data on exercise from six patients with mitral pericardial xenograft valve replacement. Abbreviations as in *Figure 6.15*

pulmonary vascular resistance between the pre-operative and the first post-operative study. However, the pulmonary pressures increased abnormally during exercise at the first post-operative investigation.

There were no significant changes in the haemodynamic data between the first and the second post-operative studies.

Tricuspid valve replacement

The post-operative haemodynamic studies, performed in three patients with isolated tricuspid valve replacement showed a significant reduction in right sided pressures with marginal increase in cardiac index. The diastolic gradient across the tricuspid xenografts ranged from 2–4 mmHg. All the pericardial xenografts were competent.

Hydrodynamic studies

In vitro studies have been performed in order to assess the functional characteristics of the pericardial xenograft. Continuous flow measurements in a static rig were made with at least two valves of each size of the pericardial xenografts. Although there are limitations in the interpretation of figures derived from continuous flow measurements, the direct comparison between gradients obtained

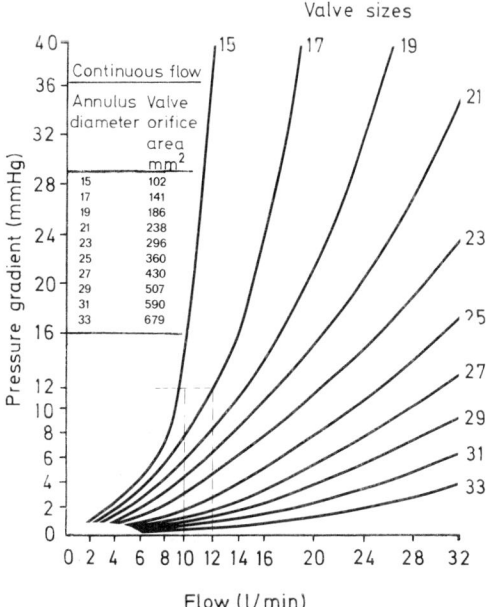

Figure 6.17 Pressure gradients across pericardial xenografts as measured in a continuous flow rig. The curves represent mean values obtained from measurements made with at least two valves of each size

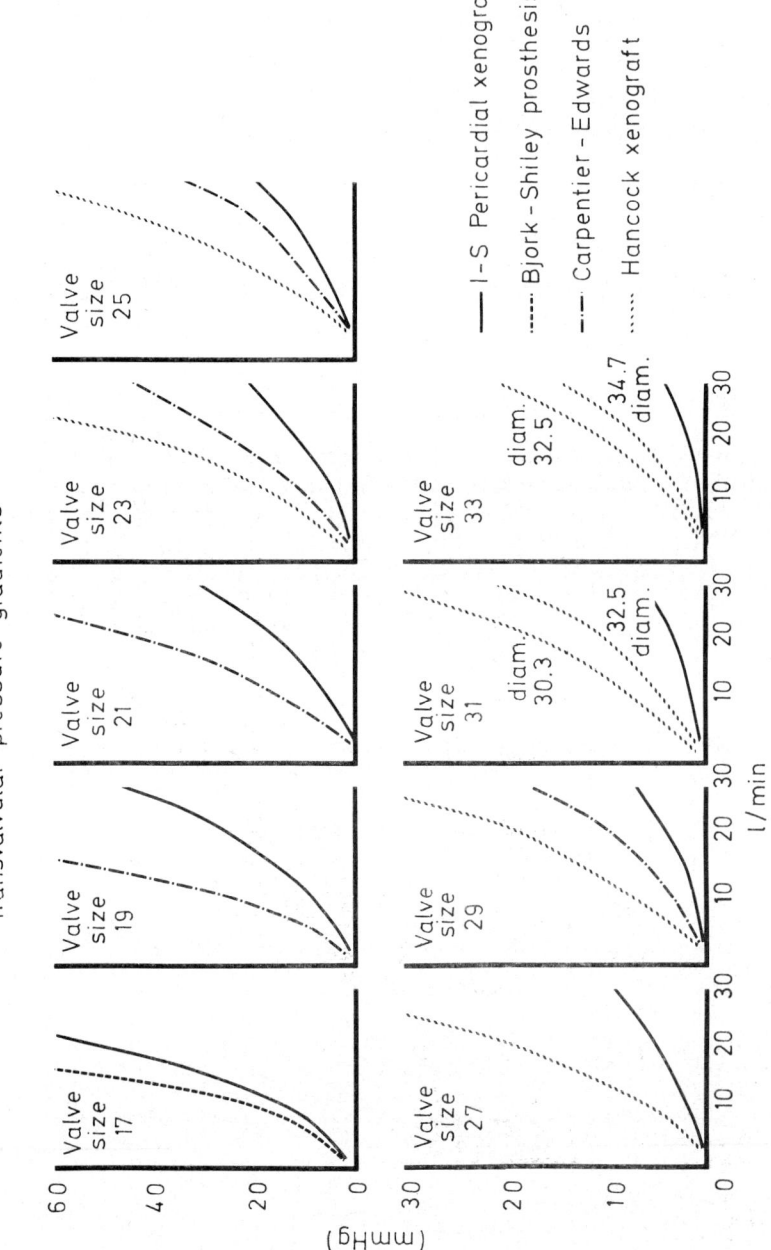

Figure 6.18 Pressure gradients measured in a continuous flow rig across four types of heart valve substitute

by the same method with different types of valves remains valid. At a flow rate of 10 ℓ/min the gradient across the 15 mm pericardial xenograft, the smallest available, is only 12 mmHg. The transvalvular gradient decreases progressively as the diameter of the valve increases (*Figure 6.17*). A direct comparison between transvalvular gradients of various valves measured in a static rig is depicted in *Figure 6.18*. The 15 mm pericardial xenograft is not shown as there is no other available heart valve substitute of this small size for comparison. When compared with other tissue valves (the Hancock and the Carpentier-Edwards bioprostheses) it becomes evident that the pericardial xenograft produces significantly lower gradients.

As the opening characteristics of a valve, especially a tissue valve, are as significant for its function, as the closure mechanism, a series of studies in a pulsatile flow rig have been performed. The transvalvular gradients of the valves studied have been found to be 19 and 22 per cent higher in the pulsatile system than in the continuous flow rig as already known from other studies[87].

The total surface area at the peak of diastole and the opening characteristics of three tissue valves have been investigated and compared under conditions of simulated pulsatile flow. The valves studied were the Hancock porcine valve, the Carpentier-Edwards porcine bioprosthesis and the Ionescu-Shiley pericardial xenograft. All were mitral substitutes of 29 mm implantation (annulus) diameter. *Figure 6.19* shows different and progressive stages of the opening phase of these three valves at increasing diastolic flow rates. It is evident that the two porcine valves have not only considerably smaller orifice areas than that of the pericardial xenograft but that they open their cusps sequentially and with an irregular, rigid,

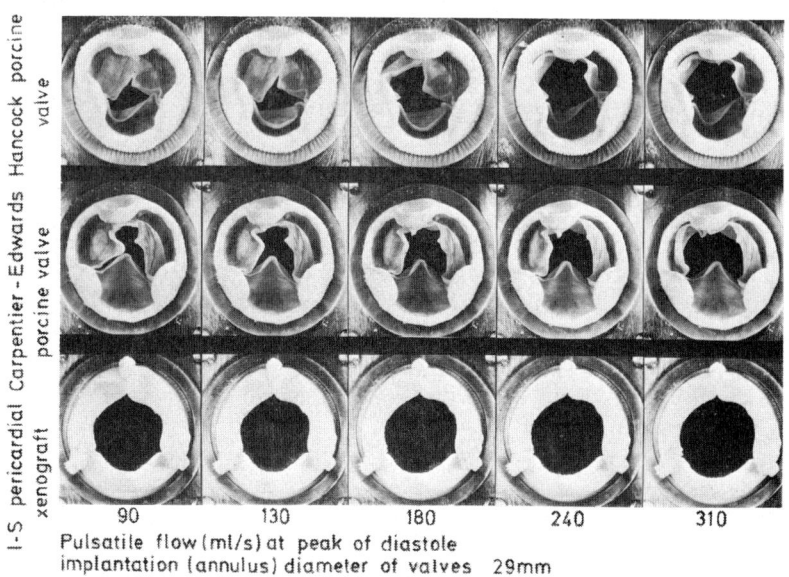

Figure 6.19 Comparison of the opening characteristics and surface area available to flow in three types of tissue valve substitutes. The test was performed under conditions of simulated pulsatile flow and with the valves mounted in the mitral position. All valves had the same implantation (annulus) diameter (29 mm). The photographs were taken at the peak of diastole. The flow rate was progressively increased from 90-310 ml/s

hinge-like movement. In the Carpentier-Edwards valve under test, the right coronary cusp, which is supported by the septal muscles, failed to open even at very high flow rates. In contrast, the cusp opening of the pericardial xenograft is regular, almost simultaneous for all three cusps and follows a smooth unfolding pattern. The orifice area of the pericardial xenograft is considerably larger than that of the porcine valves examined for each diastolic filling pressure and flow rate. The pericardial xenograft is almost fully open at a diastolic flow of 90 ml/s. *Figure 6.20* shows a pericardial xenograft of 23 mm implantation (annulus) diameter tested under similar conditions to the three valves shown in *Figure 6.19*. The 23 mm and smaller valves have the supporting prongs splayed outward in order to increase the secondary orifice area. This produces a proportionally greater opening of the smaller valves when compared with pericardial xenografts 25 mm implantation diameter and larger.

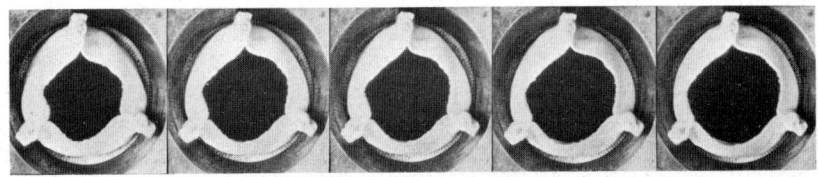

Figure 6.20 The opening characteristics and surface area of a pericardial xenograft with 23 mm annulus diameter. The photographs were made and the test conducted under identical conditions to those described in *Figure 6.19*. Due to the outward splayed prongs of valves 23 mm diameter and smaller the surface area available to flow is proportionately greater than in valves with 25 mm diameter and larger. This is evident when this figure is compared with *Figure 6.19*.

A series of pericardial xenografts (three valves for each size available—15–33 mm annulus diameter) have been tested for durability in a specially designed high speed fatigue machine. The tests were conducted at 20 °C and the fluid was tap water renewed every 14 days. The machine was set to cycle 760 times/min in order to avoid excessive vibration, and the flow rate was 15 ℓ/min. The pressures on either side of the valves (inflow and outflow) were maintained at 180 mmHg. A stroboscope was used to adjust the cycling and to inspect the valves. In addition, the valves under test were closely inspected every 14 days. So far the pericardial xenografts have been exposed to this accelerated fatigue challenge for an equivalent period of 26.5 years without any visible deleterious effect.

More detailed and specialized information on the hydrodynamics of different tissue valves is given in Chapter 2.

DISCUSSION

The three main goals for which the pericardial xenograft was created, namely, freedom from thromboembolic complications without long-term anticoagulant treatment, near normal haemodynamic characteristics and long-term maintenance of structural and functional integrity have been attained[39,40,78,80,81]. Detailed analysis of the results obtained from 411 patients with heart valve replacement over a period of 7.5 years has demonstrated not only that the glutaraldehyde stabilized pericardial xenograft compares favourably with other tissue and prosthetic valves in clinical use, but that with respect to haemo-dynamic performance and relative freedom from thromboembolism, the peri-cardial xenograft is superior[39,40,79,81,82]. Furthermore, the long-term clinical follow-up and various *in vivo* and *in vitro* laboratory investigations have brought to light previously unknown, beneficial characteristics of the pericardial xeno-graft heart valve.

The early mortality rate of 6.3 per cent for the entire series of 411 patients is similar to results reported with other types of valve replacement[9,13,47,50,51,64]. It is generally agreed that the hospital mortality is not directly related to the type of valve substitute used[70]. In this series none of the early deaths could be ascribed to the pericardial xenograft *per se*.

The most important determinants of the quality of a heart valve substitute are the long-term record of patients' survival and the paucity of valve related complications. As the experience with this original tissue valve during the initial stages was a 'journey into the unknown' and as we realized that the late morbid-ity and mortality depend, to some extent, on careful and close observation of the patients, we organized a rigorous programme of complete follow-up of all patients receiving pericardial xenografts irrespective of their geographical loca-tion. All 385 hospital survivors were followed-up personally by the authors. The period of observation totals 11 895 months (6–90 months). Of the total number of 362 long-term survivors 104 patients have completed four years of follow-up.

There were 23 late deaths (5.6 per cent) in the entire series and nine (2.2 per cent) were valve related. The causes of death of these nine patients were infec-tion in seven (1.7 per cent), a periaortic valve leak complicated by mitral disease in one patient and a cusp tear of an aortic xenograft in one patient.

The actuarial expected survival rate at eight years follow-up is 83.5 ± 10.5 per cent for patients with aortic and 88.9 ± 6.9 per cent for patients with mitral valve replacement. These compare very favourably with published reports con-cerned with the use of prostheses[9,13,24,42,50,51], and tissue valves[2,14,64,75].

Although the long-term survival of patients with valve replacement depends on many other factors[20,41,70,71], the complications directly related to the valve substitute are reported to contribute significantly to the overall late mortality of patients with other types of valve replacement[6,10,41,50,70,74]. However, in the present series the incidence of deaths from mechanical dysfunction of the valve was 0.24 per cent or 0.1 episodes/100 patient years.

Relative freedom from thromboembolism in the absence of long-term anti-coagulation is one of the major advantages of tissue valves. Long-term anticoagu-lant treatment has never been used in any of the patients in this series. Between March 1971 and May 1976 anticoagulants were not used at all, not even in the early post-operative period.

Valve thrombosis, which has been described with both prostheses[5,9,24,26,50] and porcine valves[17,25,33,44] has not been encountered in this series.

The incidence of embolization for the whole series was 0.81 episodes/100 patient years. There were no deaths attributable to embolic phenomena. All emboli occurred within six weeks following valve replacement, were mild and left no sequelae. The number of episodes/100 patient years was 0.49 for patients with aortic replacement, 1.22 for patients with mitral, none for the tricuspid patients and 3.4 for the multiple replacement group. These figures compare very favourably with those reported from patients with prosthetic valves and long-

TABLE 6.19

Incidence of embolism in patients having mitral valve replacement with Hancock porcine bioprosthesis.
Data from published reports

Institution and authors	Years of valve replacement	Number of patients in series	Embolic episodes/ 100 patient years	Anticoagulant regimen
Peter Bent Brigham Cohn, L.H. and Collin, J.J.[17]	1972–1977	131	3.8	4-6 weeks post-operatively Long-term in patients with AF or large LA
University of Kansas Hannah, H. and Reis, R.L.[32]	1970–1975	104	4.8*	Only if LA thrombus present
Stanford University Oyer, P.E. et al.[62]	1971–1975	338	4.1	60 per cent of patients for 3 months post-operatively 17 per cent of patients long-term anticoagulation
Henry Ford Hospital Davila, J.C. and Magilligan, D.H.[22]	1971–1975	288†	4.7	23 per cent of patients no anticoagulants 23 per cent short-term anticoagulants 54 per cent long-term anticoagulants

*Embolic rate estimated from data available and average time of follow-up
†Includes patients with single mitral, as well as multiple replacements including the mitral valve
AF = atrial fibrillation, LA = left atrium

term anticoagulation[5,26,30,41,47,60,78]. Furthermore the embolic rate in the present series was lower than that encountered in patients with porcine valves in either aortic or mitral positions, whether or not the patients received anticoagulant treatment[14,17,18,22,32,33,62,64,75]. *Table 6.19* shows the incidence of embolism in patients having mitral valve replacement with Hancock porcine bioprostheses[17,22,32,62] and these figures are certainly higher than the incidence of embolization in the present series. However, the number of patients in the various published reports is too small for any valid statistical comparison. Indeed from the entire spectrum of published data with tissue valves there is neither clinical nor statistical evidence to support or refute the contention that patients with tissue valves require prothrombin depressants at any time following valve replacement. Neither is there any scientific data available to prove that treatment with prothrombin depressants protects patients with tissue valves in the mitral position from the risk of thromboembolism. However, because all emboli in our series occurred during the first six post-operative weeks, we started, since June 1976, to administer warfarin sodium to all patients receiving mitral (76 patients) or multiple valve (42 patients) replacement. The anticoagulant treatment was continued for 4-6 weeks following the operation. Based on our experience with a very low incidence of embolic complications prior to June 1976, the prothrombin level was deliberately maintained at or slightly below, the double of the control value. Since June 1976 there have not been any embolic episodes in patients with mitral replacement and only one early episode in the multiple replacement group.

An anlysis of embolism, which occurred in this series of patients during the five years preceding the operation, showed an incidence of 2.5 episodes/100 patient years (1.3 for aortic and 5.1 for mitral valve disease). This is definitely a higher incidence than that observed post-operatively. The embolic rate in the present series of patients with mitral valve replacement is similar to the incidence reported following mitral valvuloplasty[23,56].

The advantage of a very low embolic rate and the absence of valve thrombosis without long-term treatment with prothrombin depressants becomes even more significant when considering both the psychological anxieties and the haemorrhagic risks associated with long-term anticoagulant therapy[35,41,43,50].

Although at present there is not sufficient scientific evidence concerning either the precise aetiology of thromboembolism or the intimate mechanism of thrombus formation in patients with mitral valve surgery, two facts emerged from the clinical experience. One is the extremely high risk of thromboembolism in patients with prosthetic replacement of the mitral valve without correct anticoagulation and the second one is the very low propensity for thromboembolism of tissue valves. The experience with the pericardial xenograft in the mitral position has shown complete absence of valve thrombosis, a reduced risk of embolism when compared with porcine valves and the absence of embolic phenomena beyond the first six post-operative weeks. Whether the administration of prothrombin depressants to some of our mitral patients during the early post-operative period has in real terms reduced the embolic risk remains circumstantial.

The occurrence of valve thrombosis and the slightly higher embolic rate encountered with porcine valves may be partly explained by the configuration of these valves. The pig aortic valve, one must assume, has the ideal shape for its function. Following its removal from the pig's aortic root, its slight, but certain stiffening by glutaraldehyde fixation and its mounting on a bulky irregular structure, which is the cloth-covered support frame, this valve becomes, from a hydraulic view point, a sub-optimal structure. *Figure 6.19* shows the irregular pattern of cusp movement and the crevices formed at the base of the artificially created sinuses of Valsalva. Furthermore when compared with the pericardial xenograft, all porcine valves at present available have a large surface of Dacron cloth exposed to the blood. Indeed from the total surface area of the outflow aspect of the porcine valves, half is exposed Dacron cloth as compared with only 8 per cent in the pericardial xenograft.

In addition to our own observations[80], there is ample evidence concerning the sequential, rather delayed, and often incomplete opening of at least one of the cusps of the Hancock and other porcine valves in a low pressure system as occurs in the atrioventricular position[28,36,84,87]. The shape and the opening characteristics of the frame mounted porcine valves might explain, at least in part, the presence of microscopic thrombus formation on the cusps[27,73], the partial or complete thrombotic obstruction of some of these valves[17,25,39,44], and the marginally higher rate of embolization[14,17,18,22,32,33,62,64,75], when compared with the pericardial xenograft. There appears also to be an increased tendency in several centres to use long-term anticoagulation in patients with porcine mitral valves.

The pericardial xenograft is a more regular, streamlined structure with very little Dacron fabric exposed to the blood and with practically no recesses or crevices. It opens fully even at low flow rates and the three cusps of each valve have an identical shape and their thickness and pliability are accurately matched. Due to the very low gradient across the valve, the pericardial xenograft closes with a slight amount of regurgitation which averages 5.9 per cent of the stroke volume (1.6 per cent for a 15 mm valve and 11 per cent for a 31 mm valve). These geometrical and hydraulic characteristics may have a bearing on the reduced thrombogenicity of the pericardial xenograft.

The incidence of bacterial endocarditis was 1.2 per cent early following valve replacement (within three months) and 1.7 per cent late during the follow-up period (up to four years post-operatively). The early occurrence is considered to be related to contamination during the surgical procedure or to obvious infections in non-cardiac areas which may be present in the early post-operative period. The cases of endocarditis of late occurrence are commonly attributed to un-treated infective processes, but in general, infective endocarditis does not seem to be related to a particular type of valve substitute. Its incidence in this series is similar to that in other published reports[41,42,48,50,53,74]. Fungal endocarditis has not been enountered in this series.

The incidence of perivalvular leaks that required re-operation was small and not different from other published reports. There were three patients in each aortic and mitral groups and in all patients the cause was found to be the poor quality of the heart valve annulus. The patients from the aortic group had previous prosthetic valve replacement while those from the mitral group had obvious connective tissue abnormalities.

The incidence of early diastolic murmurs (6.9 per cent) in patients with aortic valve replacement is relatively high but similar to that reported with both prosthetic[6,47,60] and tissue valve replacement[2,18,19,64]. In all patients with diastolic murmur the local anatomic circumstances were conducive to the occurrence of perivalvular leaks (heavy calcification of the aortic annulus, or operations following previous aortic valve replacement). During the early part of the experience with the pericardial xenograft the size and shape of the sewing rim were altered. The early uncushioned rims might have contributed to the appearance of perivalvular leaks.

In general the occurrence of perivalvular leaks is more related to the quality of the heart valve annulus to which the valve substitute is attached and to the surgical technique than to the valve itself. Since we learned from haemodynamic investigations that the pericardial xenograft produces insignificant gradients even with small sizes, we no longer endeavour to insert the largest possible valve in the aortic position.

Aortic root angiography[11] established the diagnosis of perivalvular leak in the majority of patients with early diastolic murmur by demonstrating the regurgitation of contrast material taking place outside the metal support frame of the valve. All patients with aortic diastolic murmur continue to remain asymptomatic 9–64 months (mean 31) following the apperance of the murmur. Although the systolic stress for tissue valves is greater in the mitral area, there is only one patient in the present series with an apical systolic murmur, which occurred late post-operatively (49 months). This patient has been observed for more than 30 months since the appearance of the murmur and he continues to remain asymptomatic and without changes in cardiothoracic ratio or left ventricular voltage on the electrocardiogram.

Mechanical dysfunction of pericardial xenografts occurred in seven patients (1.7 per cent for the whole series or 0.7 episodes/100 patient years). This involved four aortic and three mitral valves. Only one patient died as a consequence of mechanical dysfunction (0.24 per cent or 0.1 death/100 patient years). This particular patient died of irreparable cardiac laceration during his fourth median sternotomy operation.

In one of these seven patients an indentation, about 1 mm deep, was found at necropsy, on the free margin of one of the aortic valve cusps. The patient had died of a cerebral tumour 60 months following valve replacement. From the cardiac view point he was asymptomatic prior to his death. In the other six patients, physical signs of valve dysfunction appeared 12–45 months post-operatively and re-operation took place 13–60 months following the original pericardial xenograft valve insertion. The interval between the appearance of murmurs or symptoms and the time of re-operation varied from 1–18 months. This emphasizes again the well-known fact that tissue valves do not fail suddenly and that there is always time to assess the situation and to perform elective re-operation.

The lesion, which was incidentally discovered at necropsy, was more of a cosmetic defect but was, nevertheless, considered in the group of mechanical faults. The other six valves had three types of lesions. Two xenografts from the mitral area had one of the cusps partly detached from the frame at the suture line, which in the 'home-made' valves followed the scalloped margin of the support frame. This lesion was most probably due to a combination of local trauma during construction of the valve with sutures placed close together through the pericardium and poor chemical treatment with sodium metaperiodate. Both these valves failed early (the murmurs appeared at 12 and 28 months and the valves were removed at 13 and 31 months post-operatively respectively). Two other valves, both from the aortic position, developed a tear of the pericardial tissue, one starting at the free margin of a cusp and the second one at the base of a cusp. The diastolic murmur was first heard at 26 and 40 months and re-operation performed at 32 and 57 months post-operatively respectively. The last two valves with mechanical dysfunction, one from the mitral and one from the aortic position became calcified. Murmurs of valve stenosis appeared at 42 and 45 months and the valves were replaced at 60 and 57 months respectively following their insertion.

Calcification of tissue valves is known to have occurred sporadically with different tissue preparations and in various cardiac locations and it is considered to be due, at least in part, to a metabolic propensity of some patients for calcification[17,25,68,73]. In this series it affected two valves out of a total of 458 xenografts implanted. Whether calcification in these two cases might have been related to the chemical treatment of the early valves with sodium metaperiodate remains speculative.

All seven cases of mechanical dysfunction occurred in xenografts from the early series of 220 'home-made' valves used during the first five years of the experience. As mentioned before, the accuracy of valve fabrication, in our early experience, was far from perfect and the chemical treatment of the pericardium[15] proved to be at least traumatic if not deleterious. Sodium metaperiodate, which was used in the pre-treatment of the tissue, is known to be a strong oxidizing agent and to exert a damaging action on the connective tissue. Also, the glutaraldehyde employed was a simple dilution of commercially available Cidex of doubtful concentration and with unknown chemical characteristics. In retrospect, it is surprising that only so few mechanical problems have arisen with the 'home-made' valves over a relatively long period of follow-up.

It is interesting to note that the signs of valve dysfunction in these six patients appeared relatively early after valve insertion, between 12 and 45 months, and not late in the follow-up period, which now extends beyond 90 months. It seems, therefore, that valve dysfunction in the present series was not a time-related phenomenon, dependent upon the ageing of the pericardium, but most probably a consequence of faulty valve construction and traumatic chemical treatment of the tissue. Both these factors have been eliminated.

Since May 1976, the pericardial xenografts are being manufactured by Shiley Laboratories, using highly accurate and standardized techniques. An optimum density of cross-links is achieved with the 'purified glutaraldehyde'. The superiority of the pericardial xenograft manufactured by Shiley Laboratories is documented by elaborate *in vitro* studies[86,87] and by the excellent clinical results and the absence of valve related complications experienced in more than 110 cardiac centres using the pericardial xenograft. In our own series, 191 patients received, since May 1976, 238 Shiley valves, and until the time of this writing there have not been any valve related complications in patients with either single or multiple valve replacements.

From the six patients with symptomatic mechanical dysfunction of the valve, three developed signs or symptoms of valve malfunction and had their valves removed within 31 months of the original operation. The follow-up with the Shiley valve has reached 30 months and the complete absence of valve related complications is very encouraging.

The improvement in the clinical condition of patients operated upon, as well as the changes in cardiothoracic ratio and electrocardiogram (left ventricular voltage in particular) are similar to those already reported with this type of valve replacement[38-40]. The 14 long-term survivors having tricuspid pericardial xenografts (isolated or combined with other replacements) have not developed any complications and three of these patients have been observed for more than six years.

As expected with a full orifice tissue valve there was no intravascular haemolysis as demonstrated by clinical and laboratory investigations.

Table 6.20 summarizes some of the essential clinical data related to our experience with the pericardial xenograft over a period of observation of 7.5 years. These data are expressed as episodes/100 patient years because as some of the complications are not necessarily time related and most probably not different from events encountered with other valve substitutes. Infective endocarditis and perivalvular leaks are in this group. The cases of embolization, as already discussed have all occurred within the first six post-operative weeks. For the valve dysfunction group, there is sufficient evidence available to believe that all episodes of mechanical dysfunction were related to the sub-optimal quality of the pericardial xenograft manufactured in our own hospital laboratory during the early part of the series. Although the incidence of valve dysfunction was low and only one death in the entire series was valve related it is expected that with valves manufactured by Shiley Laboratories the occurrence of such complications will be prevented or minimized.

TABLE 6.20
Incidence of complications in patients having heart valve replacement
with pericardial xenografts

			Episodes per 100 patient years			
Valves replaced	*Number of patients*	*Years of follow-up*	*Endocarditis*	*Perivalve leak**	*Embolism†*	*Valve dysfunction*
Aortic	216	615.7	0.65	0.48	0.48	0.65
Mitral	150	329.0	0.91	0.91	1.22	0.91
Tricuspid	3	17.7	–	–	–	–
Multiple	42	29.9	–	–	3.34	–
Total	411	991.3	0.70	0.60	0.80	0.70

*Patients re-operated upon for perivalvular leak
†All 8 embolic episodes occurred within 6 weeks post-operatively and were transient

The results of the haemodynamic investigations have demonstrated a significant circulatory improvement in all patients with either aortic or mitral valve replacement. The sequential catheter studies have established that the functional integrity of the pericardial xenograft was maintained intact over a period of 59 months following valve insertion.

In patients with aortic valve replacement, the cardiac output increased marginally, but significantly and its reponse to exercise was normal. The oxygen utilization also improved and on exercise it was normal. Similar findings have been previously reported[6,7,12,38,61,81,82].

The left ventricular end-diastolic and mean pulmonary wedge pressures decreased significantly both at rest and on exercise at the post-operative study. However, both these pressures rose abnormally during exercise. Similar observations of raised left ventricular end-diastolic pressure on exercise, following successful aortic valve replacement, have been previously published[7,12,54,61,67].

A probable explanation for this phenomenon could be the presence of a certain degree of irreversible left ventricular dysfunction. Furthermore, the abnormal elevation of the left ventricular end-diastolic and pulmonary wedge pressures during exercise in the present series appears to be related to the size of the xenograft implanted. To our knowledge such an observation has not been previously recorded.

Published data regarding systolic gradients with the most commonly used aortic valve substitutes are given in *Table 6.21*. The pericardial xenograft, when compared with these other valves offers the least resistance to forward flow. For each annulus diameter, the systolic gradient is lower both at rest and during exercise across pericardial xenografts when compared with Björk-Shiley, Lillehei-Kaster and Hancock porcine valves[7,46,72].

TABLE 6.21
Post-operative systolic gradients in patients with various aortic valve substitutes
according to annulus diameter

Authors	Valve substitute	Peak systolic gradient (mmHg)					
		19	21	23	25	27*	Mean
Björk et al.[7] (1971)	Björk–Shiley valve		21 (39)	17 (20)	7 (10)	11 (17)	12.5 (17.0)
Sigwart et al.[72] (1976)	Lillehei–Kaster valve		30†	32.7†	21.7† (48.5)	14.1†	27.1†
Jones et al.[46] (1978)	Hancock bioprosthesis	33 (43)	22 (51)	19 (33)	19 (31)	15 (21)	22.0 (32.0)
Ionescu and Tandon Present study (1978)	Ionescu–Shiley pericardial xenograft	8.3 (12.3)	7.9 (13.3)	3.2 (10.0)	3.3 (5.7)	0 (1)	6.4 (9.6)

*Annulus diameter (mm) of the valve substitute
†Mean ejection systolic gradient
The figures in parentheses are systolic gradients during exercise

It is now well recognized that the smaller sizes of Hancock porcine valve are associated with high transvalvular gradients and there is general agreement that for clinical use valves larger than 23 mm annulus diameter should be preferred for aortic replacement[19,32,45,46,55]. High gradients have also been reported with the small sizes of Lillehei-Kaster prostheses. Nicoloff[59] found a mean peak systolic gradient of 46 mmHg (range 28-70) in 10 patients with number 14 Lillehei-Kaster valve (21 mm annulus diameter). Sigwart et al.[72] propose that Lillehei-Kaster valves of at least 18 mm internal diameter (25 mm annulus diameter) should be used for aortic replacement in adults in order to minimize the prosthesis induced stenosis.

Because of the high gradients produced by the valves mentioned, several authors have advocated and used rather complicated surgical manoeuvres for enlarging the aortic annulus, in order to overcome the prosthesis induced stenosis associated with the use of the small prosthetic and porcine valves[8,46,49,57,58]. The present study has established that the gradients across the pericardial xenograft, even of small sizes, are insignificant and therefore such elaborate surgical procedures for aortic root enlargement are unnecessary when the pericardial xenograft is used.

In practical terms the most important haemodynamic determinant of a valve substitute is the effective surface area available to flow as measured *in vivo*. None of the patients investigated in the present series had a calculated surface area of less than 1 cm² (*Figure 6.10*). Surface areas below 1 cm² are common findings in patients with the smaller sizes of porcine valves in the aortic position[19,32,45,46,55].

Because of its superior haemodynamic characteristics, we consider the pericardial xenograft to be the valve substitute of choice for patients with small aortic annulus and for children.

The sequential haemodynamic studies performed at mean intervals of 9.9 and 42.2 months following aortic valve replacement demonstrated that the post-operative circulatory improvement obtained in these patients was maintained and the transvalvular gradients did not change with the passage of time[81].

In the mitral replacement group the results of the long-term, as well as the sequential haemodynamic studies showed a post-operative increase in cardiac output and oxygen uptake both at rest and during exercise. However, the cardiac output response to exercise was impaired. The pulmonary artery and pulmonary wedge pressures approached normal values at rest but rose to abnormal levels with exercise. This seems to be a universal finding with all currently used mitral valve substitutes[4,10,24,31,34,44,52,63,65,69,72,76,79].

The post-operative reduction in the pulmonary pressures and in the pulmonary vascular resistance was not influenced by the severity of pre-operative pulmonary hypertension. This study confirmed the previously reported reversibility of pulmonary hypertension following mitral valve replacement[21,63,88].

The mean diastolic gradient across the mitral pericardial xenograft was 6.4 mmHg and this figure compares favourably with gradients obtained with currently used mitral valve substitutes as shown in *Table 6.22*. All available mitral valve replacements seem to be associated with obstruction to forward flow. The most significant single factor responsible for the obstruction to forward flow is the presence of the rigid rings of all currently used valves. These rigid structures do not expand during diastole and therefore encroach upon the normal functional mechanism of the mitral valve annulus[78].

Although the number of patients with sequential haemodynamic investigations was small the results obtained are of considerable importance. They established that maximum circulatory improvement was obtained by the end of the first year following valve insertion and that the functional integrity of the pericardial xenografts was maintained intact with the passage of time[80].

The shape of the pericardial xenograft was arrived at by repeated studies of different configurations in a pulse duplicator. During these experiments it was established that flexibility of the support frame would not improve the long-term function of the valve as the stress is distributed equally over the entire surface of the cusps and not only at the commissures, as it occurs to a certain extent with the porcine valves. Furthermore, the real deflection under physiological load of the prongs of the Hancock valve[66] was recently questioned[84] and in a clinical series there was no difference in long-term performance between Hancock valves with rigid and with flexible stents[16].

The hydrodynamic studies performed on the pericardial xenograft and on other tissue valves have established that the hydraulic characteristics of the

TABLE 6.22
Haemodynamic results following mitral valve replacement with various valve substitutes

Authors	Mitral valve substitute	Time of post-operative study (months)	Cardiac index (l/min/m²)		PWP (mmHg)		MDG (mmHg)	
			R	E	R	E	R	E
Pietras et al.[63] (1974)	Starr-Edwards valve Model 6300	16.3	3.2	4.8	13.2	30.0	11.6	24.5
Tandon et al.[78] (1978)	Björk-Shiley valve	22.7	2.2	4.3	16.4	34.2	6.2	17.6
Sigwart et al.[72] (1976)	Lillehei-Kaster valve	1-6*	3.0		16.0		9.0	
Luire et al.[52] (1976)	Hancock porcine xenograft	1-15*	2.5		15.0		8.0	
Ionescu and Tandon Present study (1978)	Ionescu-Shiley pericardial xenograft	40.3	2.6	4.1	13.8	29.4	6.4	15.3

*Mean period not available

PWP = mean pulmonary wedge pressure; MDG = mean diastolic gradient; R = rest; E = exercise

glutaraldehyde stabilized pericardial xenograft are superior to those exhibited by the frame mounted porcine valves. Similar conclusions have been reached by other authors[84,87]. The surface area of the pericardial xenograft, available to flow (corrected for regurgitation and fluid density) is significantly larger than that of the Hancock and Carpentier–Edwards porcine valves for each valve size in the series. This is simply explained by the anatomy of the valves. The porcine aortic valve, which has a thick aortic annulus is mounted inside the support frame reducing its inner diameter. In addition, the right coronary cusp of the pig's valve has a limited opening due to the muscle bar at its base. The amount of regurgitation associated with the pericardial xenograft is slightly higher than with other tissue valves, but well below the level of clinical significance. The slightly higher regurgitation, which is the direct consequence of very low gradients across the pericardial xenograft, should be considered beneficial. By the washout mechanism it could be responsible for the lower incidence of thromboembolism encountered in patients with pericardial valves. With both, continuous and simulated pulsatile flows, gradients across the pericardial xenograft are insignificant and considerably lower than with other tissue valves. Due to the pliability of its cusps and the shape of the valve, the pericardial xenograft displays the least sequential delay in its opening among the series of valves tested. The significance of equally distributed stress and strain on all three cusps of a valve has been previously emphasized[77]. Accelerated fatigue testing, still in progress, has shown so far that the pericardial xenograft is expected to maintain its mechanical and functional integrity up to 26.5 years. Whether data obtained in the rigid fatigue machine should be extrapolated to clinical situations remains, however, questionable.

SUMMARY AND CONCLUSIONS

The glutaraldehyde stabilized pericardial xenograft has been in clinical use for a period of 7.5 years. At our institution a total of 458 valves have been inserted in 411 patients. There were 369 patients with single valve replacement and 42 with multiple replacements. The 385 hospital survivors have been observed over a period of 6–90 months for a total of 11 895 months (mean 30.8). The expected survival rate for patients with aortic valve replacement is 83.5 ± 10.5 per cent at eight years of follow-up. The corresponding figure for patients with mitral valve replacement is 88.9 ± 6.9 per cent. The incidence of valve dysfunction was 1.7 per cent for the entire series (0.7 episodes/100 patient years). Only one patient died as a consequence of mechanical dysfunction of the valve (0.24 per cent or 0.1 deaths/100 patient years).

Microscopic examination of valves removed up to 65 months after implantation has shown good preservation of the histologic components of the pericardium and absence of immune or inflammatory reaction.

The great majority of patients obtained considerable clinical improvement following valve replacement. The incidence of endocarditis and perivalvular leaks was similar to that encountered following the use of other types of valve substitutes. Valve thrombosis has not been encountered in the entire series. Long-term anticoagulation has not been used in any of the patients with pericardial xenografts. Prothrombin depressants were given for a period of 4–6 weeks post-operatively only to the 42 patients with multiple valve replacement and to 76 patients from the group of 150 patients with single mitral valve replacement. The incidence of embolization for the whole series was 0.81 episodes/100 patient years. All emboli occurred within six weeks following valve insertion, were mild and left no sequelae. The incidence of embolization with the pericardial xenograft was lower than that reported with the use of porcine valves. In view of the very low embolic rate in this series, and the occurrence of emboli only in the early post-operative period, we consider the administration of prothrombin depressants beyond the first six post-operative weeks unwarranted. Patients with aortic pericardial xenografts should not require anticoagulant treatment at any time.

The results of haemodynamic investigations performed in 68 patients have demonstrated a significant circulatory improvement in all patients with either aortic, mitral or tricuspid valve replacement. The gradients across the aortic pericardial xenografts are negligible, even with valves of small diameter, and significantly lower than those reported with other valve substitutes currently available. In the mitral area the transvalvular gradients compare favourably with those obtained with other valve replacements. The effective surface areas available to flow are larger in all sizes of pericardial xenografts than in the corresponding porcine valves. The results obtained with the sequential haemodynamic investigations performed at two separate intervals post-operatively, are of considerable importance. They established that the circulatory improvement, obtained after valve replacement, as well as the functional integrity of the pericardial xenografts in both aortic and mitral positions, were maintained intact up to 59 months post-operatively.

The long-term durability of the glutaraldehyde stabilized pericardial xenograft has been established by the very good record of patients' survival, the sequential haemodynamic investigations and the microscopy studies performed.

Elaborate laboratory investigations have determined that the optimum stabilization of the pericardial tissue is obtained by exposure to 0.5 per cent 'purified glutaraldehyde' for a period of two weeks. After the formation of stable cross-links with glutaraldehyde, the pericardial valves are stored in 4 per cent formaldehyde. The storage in formaldehyde following glutaraldehyde stabilization, maintains the optimum pliability of pericardial tissue and ensures a higher degree of sterility of the valve. Recent studies have shown that this treatment with formaldehyde following glutaraldehyde stabilization results in lower tissue antigenicity than that obtained with glutaraldehyde alone, and this may prove to be of considerable importance for the long-term function of the pericardial xenograft.

Based on our experience over the past 7.5 years, we consider the pericardial xenograft to be the valve of choice for a multitude of clinical circumstances.

Acknowledgements

We should like to gratefully acknowledge the invaluable help given by Miss Anne Tunnicliffe in the preparation of this manuscript.

REFERENCES

[1] Anderson, R. P., Bonchek, L. I., Grunkemeier, G. L., Lambert, L. E. and Starr, A. 'The analysis and presentation of surgical results by actuarial methods', *Journal of surgical Research*, **16**, 224 (1974)

[2] Barratt-Boyes, B. G. Discussion of Karp *et al., Circulation,* 50, (Suppl. 2), 163 (1974)

[3] Bartek, I. T., Holden, M. P. and Ionescu, M. I. 'Frame-mounted tissue heart valves: Techniques of construction', *Thorax,* 29, 51 (1974)

[4] Björk, V. O., Book., K. and Holmgren, A. 'The Björk–Shiley mitral valve prosthesis', *Annals of thoracic Surgery,* 18, 379 (1974)

[5] Björk, V. O. and Henze, A. 'Prosthetic replacement of heart valves; Eight years experience with the Björk–Shiley tilting disc valve'. In *Tissue Heart Valves.* Ed. by M. I. Ionescu. London; Butterworths (1979)

[6] Björk, V. O., Henze, A. and Holmgren, A. 'Five years' experience with the Björk–Shiley tilting disc valve in isolated aortic valvular disease', *Journal of thoracic and cardiovascular Surgery,* 68, 393 (1974)

[7] Björk, V. O., Holmgren, A., Olin, C. and Ovenfors, C. 'Clinical and haemodynamic results of aortic valve replacement with the Björk–Shiley tilting disc valve prosthesis', *Scandinavian Journal of thoracic and cardiovascular Surgery,* 5, 177 (1971)

[8] Blank, R. H., Pupello, D. F., Bessone, L. N., Harrison, E. E. and Starr, S. 'Methods of managing the small aortic annulus during valve replacement', *Annals of thoracic Surgery,* 22, 356 (1976)

[9] Bonchek, L. I. and Starr, A. 'Ball-valve prostheses: Current appraisal of late results', *American Journal of Cardiology,* 35, 843 (1975)

[10] Book, K. 'Mitral valve replacement with Björk–Shiley tilting disc valve–A clinical and haemodynamic study in patients with isolated mitral valve lesions'. *Scandinavian Journal of thoracic and cardiovascular Surgery,* 12, (Suppl. 2) (1974)

[11] Brandt, P. W. T., Roche, A. H. G., Barratt-Boyes, B. G. and Lowe, J. B. 'Radiology of homograft aortic valves', *Thorax,* 24, 129 (1969)

[12] Bristow, J. D. and Kremkau, E. L. 'Haemodynamic changes after valve replacement with Starr–Edwards prostheses', *American Journal of Cardiology,* 35, 716 (1975)

[13] Brown, J. W., Myerowitz, P. D., Cann, M. S., Colvin, S. B., McIntosh, C. L. and Morrow, A. G. 'Clinical and haemodynamic comparisons of Kay–Shiley, Starr–Edwards No. 6520, and Hancock porcine xenograft mitral valves', *Surgery,* 76, 983 (1974)

[14] Buch, W. S., Pipkin, R. D., Hancock, W. D. and Fogarty, T. J. 'Mitral valve replacement with the Hancock–stabilized glutaraldehyde valve: Clinical and laboratory evaluation', *Presented at the twenty-third scientific meeting of the International Cardiovascular Society, Boston, Mass., June 19-20,* (1975)

[15] Carpentier, A. and Dubost, C. 'From xenograft to bioprosthesis: Evolution of concepts and techniques of valvular xenografts'. In *Biological Tissue in Heart Valve Replacement.* Ed. by M. I. Ionescu, D. N. Ross and G. H. Wooler, p. 515–541. London; Butterworths (1972)

[16] Cevese, P. G., Gallucci, V., Morea, M., Dalla Volta, S., Fasoli, G. and Casarotto, D. 'Heart valve replacement with the Hancock bioprosthesis: Analysis of long-term results', *Circulation,* 56 (Suppl. 2), 111 (1977)

[17] Cohn, L. H. and Collins, J. J. 'The glutaraldehyde stabilized porcine xenograft valve'. In *Tissue Heart Valves.* Ed. by M. I. Ionescu. London; Butterworths (1979)

[18] Cohn, L. H., Lamberti, J. J., Castaneda, A. R. and Collins, J. J. Jr. 'Cardiac valve replacement with the stabilized glutaraldehyde porcine aortic valve: Indications, operative results and follow-up', *Chest,* 68, 162 (1975)

[19] Cohn, L. H., Sanders, J. H. and Collins, J. J. 'Aortic valve replacement with the Hancock porcine xenograft', *Annals of thoracic Surgery,* 22, 221 (1976)

[20] Copeland, J. G., Griepp, R. B., Stinson, E. B. and Shumway, N. E. 'Long-term follow-up after isolated aortic valve replacement', *Journal of thoracic and cardiovascular Surgery,* 74, 875 (1977)

[21] Dalen, J. E., Matloff, J. M., Evans, G. L., Hoppin, F. G., Jr., Bhardwaj, P., Harken, D. E. and Dexter, L. 'Early reduction of pulmonary vascular resistance after mitral valve replacement', *New England Journal of Medicine,* 277, 387 (1972)

[22] Davila, J. C. and Magilligan, D. J., Jr. 'Experience with the Hancock porcine xenograft for mitral valve replacement'. In *Second Henry Ford Hospital International Symposium on Cardiac Surgery.* Ed. by J. C. Davila, p. 485. New York: Appleton-Century-Crofts (1977)

[23] Ellis, L. B., Singh, J. B., Morales, D. D. and Harken, D. E. 'Fifteen to twenty years' study of 1000 patients undergoing closed mitral valvuloplasty', *Circulation,* 48, 357 (1973)

[24] Fernandez, J., Morse, D., Spagna, P., Lemole, G., Gooch, A., Sang-Yang, S. and Maranhao, V. 'Results of mitral valve replacement with the Beall prosthesis in 209 patients', *Journal of thoracic and cardiovascular Surgery,* 71, 218 (1976)

[25] Fishbein, M. C., Gissen, S. A., Collin, J. J. Jr., Barsamian, E. M. and Cohn, L. H. 'Pathologic findings after cardiac valve replacement with glutaraldehyde-fixed porcine valves', *American Journal of Cardiology*, **40**, 331 (1977)

[26] Forman, R., Back, W. and Barnard, C. N. 'Results of valve replacement with the Lillehei-Kaster disc prosthesis', *American heart Journal*, **94**, 282 (1977)

[27] Freeman, R. 'Microbiological aspects of open heart surgery: Diagnosis and management'. In *Current Techniques in Extra Corporeal Circulation.* Ed. by M. I. Ionescu and G. H. Wooler, pp. 369–395. London; Butterworths (1976)

[28] Gabbay, S., McQueen, D., Yellin, E. L., Backer, R. M. and Frater, R. W. M. '*In vitro* hydrodynamic performance of mitral valve prostheses in high flow rates'. Read at the *48th Annual Meeting of the American Association for Thoracic Surgery, New Orleans, Louisiana, May 8-10*, (1978)

[29] Gorlin, R. and Gorlin, N. G. 'Hydraulic formula for the calculation of the area of the stenotic mitral valve, other cardiac valves and control circulatory shunts', *American heart Journal*, **41**, 1 (1951)

[30] Gott, V. L., Brawley, R. K. and Jones, M. 'Mitral valve prostheses: The problem of thromboembolism'. In *Second Henry Ford Hospital International Symposium on Cardiac Surgery.* Ed. by J. C. Davila, p. 395. New York; Appleton-Century-Crofts (1977)

[31] Haerten, K., Both, A., Loogen, F. and Bricks, W. 'Haemodynamics after mitral valve replacement with Starr–Edwards, Björk–Shiley and Lillehei–Kaster prostheses', (Abstr.) *Circulation*, **53, 54** *(Suppl. 2)* 181 (1976)

[32] Hannah, H., III and Reis, R. L. 'Current status of porcine heterograft prostheses: A five-year appraisal', (Abstr.) *Circulation*, **52** *(Suppl. 2)* 30 (1975)

[33] Horowitz, M. D. Discussion of Johnson *et al., Circulation*, **52**, *(Suppl. 1)*, 40 (1975)

[34] Hultgren, H., Hubis, H. and Shumway, N. E. 'Cardiac functions following mitral valve replacement', *American heart Journal*, **75**, 302 (1968)

[35] Hume, M., Sevitt, S. and Thomas, D. P. *Venous Thrombosis and Pulmonary Embolism.* p. 455. Cambridge, Mass.; Harvard University Press (1970)

[36] Imamura, E., Kay, M. P. and Davis, G. D. 'Radiographic assessment of leaflet motion on Gore-tex laminate trileaflet valves and Hancock xenograft in tricuspid position in dogs', *Circulation*, **56**, 1053 (1977)

[37] Ionescu, M. I. and Mary, D. A. S. 'Durability of mitral valve substitues', In *Second Henry Ford Hospital International Symposium on Cardiac Surgery.* Ed. by J. C. Davila, p. 388. New York; Appleton-Century-Crofts (1977)

[38] Ionescu, M. I., Mary, D. A. S. and Abid, A. 'Tissue heart valves: Appraisal of late results', In *Late Results of Valvular Replacements and Coronary Surgery.* Ed. by G. Stalpaert, R. Suy and F. Vermeulen, p. 56. Ghent; European Press (1976)

[39] Ionescu, M. I. and Tandon, A. P. 'Long-term clinical and haemodynamic evaluation of the Ionescu-Shiley pericardial xenograft heart valve', *Thoraxchirurgie, Vaskuläre Chirurgie*, **26**, 250 (1978)

[40] Ionescu, M. I., Tandon, A. P., Mary, D. A. S. and Abid, A. 'Heart valve replacement with the Ionescu–Shiley pericardial xenograft', *Journal of thoracic and cardiovascular Surgery*, **73**, 31 (1977)

[41] Isom, O. W., Spencer, F. C., Glassman, E., Teiko, W., Boyd, A. D., Cunningham, J. N. and Reed, G. E. 'Long-term results in 1375 patients undergoing valve replacement with the Starr–Edwards cloth-covered steel ball prosthesis', *Annals of Surgery*, **186**, 310 (1977)

[42] Isom, O. W., Williams, C. D., Falk, E. A., Glassman, E. and Spencer, F. C. 'Long-term evaluation of cloth-covered metallic ball prostheses', *Journal of thoracic and cardiovascular Surgery*, **64**, 254 (1972)

[43] Isom, O. W., Williams, C. D., Falk, E. A., Spencer, F. C. and Glassman, E. 'Evaluation of anticoagulant therapy in cloth-covered prosthetic valves', *Circulation*, **47** *(Suppl. 3)* 48 (1973)

[44] Johnson, A. D., Daily, P. O., Peterson, K. L., LeWinter, M., DiDonna, G. J., Blaire, G. and Niwayama, G. 'Functional evaluation of the porcine heterograft in the mitral position', *Circulation*, **52** *(Suppl. 1)*, 40 (1975)

[45] Jones, E. L. In discussion of paper by Blank *et al., Annals of thoracic Surgery*, **22**, 365 (1976)

[46] Jones, E. L., Craver, J. M., Morris, D. C., King, S. B. III, Douglas, J. S. Jr., Franck, R. H., Hatcher, C. R. Jr. and Morgan, E. A. 'Haemodynamic and clinical evaluation of the Hancock xenograft bioprosthesis for aortic valve replacement (with emphasis on management of the small aortic root)', *Journal of thoracic and cardiovascular Surgery*, **75**, 300 (1978)

[47] Karp, R. B., Kirklin, J. W., Kouchoukos, N. T. and Pacifico, A. D. 'Comparison of three devices to replace the aortic valve', *Circulation,* 50 *(Suppl. 2),* 163 (1974)

[48] Kloster, F. E. 'Diagnosis and management of complications of prosthetic heart valves', *American Journal of Cardiology,* 35, 872 (1975)

[49] Konno, S., Imai, Y., Iida, Y., Nakajima, M. and Tatsuno, K. 'A new method for prosthetic valve replacement in congenital aortic stenosis associated with hypoplasia of the aortic valve ring', *Journal of thoracic and cardiovascular Surgery,* 70, 909 (1975)

[50] Levine, F. H., Copeland, J. G. and Morrow, A. G. 'Prosthetic replacement of the mitral valve, continuing assessment of the 100 patients reported upon during 1961–1965', *Circulation,* 47, 518 (1973)

[51] Lillehei, C. W., Kaster, R. L., Coleman, M. and Block, J. H. 'Heart valve replacement with Lillehei–Kaster pivoting disk prosthesis', *New York State Journal of Medicine,* 74, 1426 (1974)

[52] Lurie, A. J., Miller, R. R., Maxwell, K., Grehl, T. M., Vismara, L. A., Hurley, E. J. and Mason, D. T. 'Haemodynamic assessment of the glutaraldehyde-preserved porcine heterograft in the aortic and mitral positions', *Circulation,* 56, *(Suppl. 2),* 104 (1977)

[53] Magilligan, D. J., Jr., Quinn, E. L. and Davila, J. C. 'Bacteraemia, endocarditis and the Hancock valve', *Annals of thoracic Surgery,* 24, 508 (1977)

[54] McHenry, M. M., Smeloff, E. A. and Davey, T. B. 'Haemodynamic results with full-flow orifice prosthetic valves', *Circulation,* 35, *(Suppl. 1),* 24 (1976)

[55] Morris, D. C., Wickliffe, C. W., King, S. W., III, Douglas, J. S. Jr. and Jones, E. L. 'Haemodynamic evaluation of the porcine xenograft aortic valve', (Abstr.) *American Journal of Cardiology,* 37, 157 (1976)

[56] Mullin, M. J., Engelman, R. M., Isom, O. W., Boyd, A., Glassman, E. and Spencer, F. C. 'Experience with open mitral commissurotomy in 100 consecutive patients', *Surgery,* 76, 974 (1974)

[57] Najafi, H., Ostermiller, W. E. and Hushang, J. 'Narrow aortic root complicating aortic valve replacement', *Archives of Surgery,* 99, 690 (1969)

[30] Nicks, R., Cartmill, T. and Bernstein, L. 'Hypoplasia of the aortic root', *Thorax,* 25, 339 (1970)

[59] Nicoloff, D. M. In discussion of paper by: Starek, P. J. K., McLaurin, L. P., Wilcox, B. R. and Murray, G. F. 'Clinical evaluation of the Lillehei-Kaster pivoting-disc valve', *Annals of thoracic Surgery,* 22, 362 (1976)

[60] Nitter-Hauge, S., Hall, K. V., Froysaker, T. and Efskind, L. 'Aortic valve replacement: One year results with Lillehei-Kaster and Björk-Shiley disc prostheses: A comparative clinical study', *American heart Journal,* 88, 23 (1974)

[61] Olin, C. 'Evaluation of the Kay–Shiley disc valve prosthesis in the aortic position', *Scandinavian Journal of thoracic and cardiovascular Surgery,* 7 *(Suppl. 1),* (1970)

[62] Oyer, P. E., Stinson, E. B., Griepp, R. B. and Shumway, N. E. 'Valve replacement with the Starr-Edwards and Hancock prostheses: Comparative analysis of late morbidity and mortality', *Annals of Surgery,* 186, 301 (1977)

[63] Pietras, R. J., Long, D. M. and Rosen, K. M. 'Late postoperative clinical and haemodynamic assessment of the early cloth-covered Starr–Edwards mitral valve prosthesis', *Journal of thoracic and cardiovascular Surgery,* 67, 450 (1974)

[64] Pipkin, R. D., Buch, W. S. and Fogarty, T. J. 'Evaluation of aortic valve replacement with a porcine xenograft without long-term anticoagulation', *Journal of thoracic and cardiovascular Surgery,* 71, 179 (1976)

[65] Reid, J. R., Stevens, T. W., Segwast, W., Fulweber, R. C. and Alexander, J. L. 'Haemodynamic evaluation of the Beall mitral valve prosthesis', *Circulation,* 45 *(Suppl. 1)* 1 (1972)

[66] Reis, R. L., Hancock, W. D., Yarbrough, J. W., Glancy, D. L. and Morrow, A. G. 'The flexible stent: A new concept in the fabrication of tissue heart valve prostheses', *Journal of thoracic and cardiovascular Surgery,* 62, 683 (1971)

[67] Rodriguez, L. 'Haemodynamic and angiographic findings in patients with isolated aortic valvular disease before and after insertion of a Starr–Edwards ball-valve prosthesis', *Scandinavian Journal of thoracic and cardiovascular Surgery,* 5 *(Suppl. 1)* (1970)

[68] Ross, D. N., Martelli, V. and Wain, W. H. 'Allograft and autograft valves used for aortic valve replacement'. In *Tissue Heart Valves.* Ed. by M. I. Ionescu. London; Butterworths (1979)

[69] Russell, T., II, Kremkau, E. L., Kloster, F. and Starr, A. 'Late haemodynamic function of cloth-covered Starr–Edwards valve prostheses', *Circulation,* 45, 46 *(Suppl. 1),* 8 (1972)

[70] Salomon, N. W., Stinson, E. B., Griepp, R. B. and Shumway, N. E. 'Mitral valve replace-

ment: Long-term evaluation of prosthesis-related mortality and morbidity', *Circulation*, **56** *(Suppl. 2)*, 94 (1977)

[71] Salomon, N. W., Stinson, E. B., Griepp, R. B. and Shumway, N. E. 'Patient-related risk factors as predicators of results following isolated mitral valve replacement', *Annals of thoracic Surgery*, **24**, 519 (1977)

[72] Sigwart, U., Schmidt, H., Gleichmann, U. and Borst, H. G. *'In vivo* evaluation of the Lillehei–Kaster heart valve prosthesis', *Annals of thoracic Surgery*, **22**, 213 (1976)

[73] Spray, T. L. and Roberts, W. C. Structural changes in porcine xenografts used as substitute cardiac valves. Gross and histologic observations in 51 glutaraldehyde-preserved valves in 41 patients', *American Journal of Cardiology*, **40**, 319 (1977)

[74] Starr, A., Bonchek, L. I., Anderson, R. P., Wood, J. A. and Chapman, R. D. 'Late complications of aortic valve replacement with cloth-covered composite seat prostheses', *Annals of thoracic Surgery*, **19**, 289 (1975)

[75] Stinson, E. B., Griepp, R. B. and Shumway, N. E. 'Clinical experience with a porcine aortic valve xenograft for mitral valve replacement', *Annals of thoracic Surgery*, **18**, 391 (1974)

[76] Strom, J., Becker, R. M., Frishman, W., Salazar, C., Oka, Y., Bassell, G., Lin, Y. T. and Frater, R. W. M. 'Haemodynamic evaluation of the Ionescu–Shiley bovine heterograft valve'. Read at the *27th Annual Scientific Session of the American College of Cardiology, Anaheim, California, March 6–9* (1978)

[77] Swales, P. D., Holden, M. P., Dowson, D. and Ionescu, M. I. 'Opening characteristics of the three-cusp tissue heart valves', *Thorax*, **28**, 286 (1973)

[78] Tandon, A. P., Sengupta, S. M., Lukacs, L. and Ionescu, M. I. 'Long-term clinical and haemodynamic evaluation of the Ionescu-Shiley pericardial xenograft, Bruanwald–Cutter and Björk–Shiley prostheses in the mitral position'. Read at the *48th Annual Meeting of the American Association for Thoracic Surgery, New Orleans, Louisiana, May 8–10* (1978)

[79] Tandon, A. P., Smith, D. R. and Ionescu, M. I. 'Haemodynamic evaluation of the Ionescu–Shiley pericardial xenograft in the mitral position', *American heart Journal*, **95**, 595 (1978)

[80] Tandon, A. P., Smith, D. R. and Ionescu, M. I. 'Long-term haemodynamic behaviour of the Ionescu–Shiley pericardial xenograft heart valve'. Read at the *27th Annual Scientific Session of the American College of Cardiology, Anaheim, California, March 6–9* (1978)

[81] Tandon, A. P., Smith, D. R., Mary. D. A. S. and Ionescu, M. I. 'Sequential haemodynamic studies in patients having aortic valve replacement with the Ionescu–Shiley pericardial xenograft', *Annals of thoracic Surgery*, **24**, 149 (1977)

[82] Tandon, A. P., Smith, D. R., Whitaker, W. and Ionescu, M. I. 'Long-term haemodynamic evaluation of the aortic xenograft', *British heart Journal*, **40**, 602 (1978)

[83] Technical information on the Ionescu-Shiley pericardial xenograft heart valve *Shiley Laboratories, Inc.,* Irvine, California (1977)

[84] Thomson, F. J. and Barratt-Boyes, B. G. 'The glutaraldehyde-treated heterograft valve. Some engineering observations', *Journal of thoracic and cardiovascular Surgery*, **74**, 317 (1977)

[85] Tyras, D. H., Kaiser, G. C., Barner, H. B., Laskowski, L. F. and Marr, J. J. 'Atypical myobacteria and the xenograft valve', *Journal of thoracic and cardiovascular Surgery*, **75**, 331 (1978)

[86] Woodroof, E. A. 'The use of glutaraldehyde and formaldehyde for processing tissue heart valves'. In *Tissue Heart Valves.* Ed. by M. I. Ionescu, London; Butterworths (1979)

[87] Wright, J. T. M. 'Hydrodynamic evaluation of tissue valves'. In *Tissue Heart Valves.* Ed. by M. I. Ionescu. London; Butterworths (1979)

[88] Zener, J. C., Hancock, E. W., Shumway, N. E. and Harrison, D. C. 'Regression of extreme pulmonary hypertension after mitral valve surgery', *American Journal of Cardiology*, **30**, 820 (1972)

7

The Dura Mater Allograft Valve

Euryclides de Jesus Zerbini
and Luiz B. Puig

Le temps couvre et découvre toutes choses.
Sprichwörter und Sprüchreden der Deutschen (1842)

INTRODUCTION

Our comments derive from the experience obtained with a series of 10 790 patients, operated upon under total cardiopulmonary bypass at the Hospital das Clinicas, Sao Paulo, Brazil during the period from July 1958 to June 1977. Among these patients, 3040 (28.17 per cent) were subjected to heart valve replacement. In this group, 1377 patients (45.30 per cent) received some type of prosthesis and 1663 (54.70 per cent) had valve replacement with biological tissue, comprising 50 aortic valve allografts, 20 aortic xenografts and 1593 dura mater allograft valves.

The replacement of cardiac valves with prosthesis or biological tissue has produced gratifying results in patients with heart valve disease. At present the perioperative mortality is low due to continuous improvements made in cardiopulmonary bypass technology and to the better understanding of the immediate post-operative pathophysiology and the prevention and treatment of various conditions in specialized intensive care areas.

The long-term clinical and haemodynamic results, as well as the length and quality of life of patients having valve replacement, are satisfactory. The life expectancy of patients with heart valve replacement appears to be similar to the expected longevity of the normal population of the same age and sex groups, if aortic valve replacement is performed prior to significant cardiac enlargement[8] and if mitral replacement is undertaken before the age of 50 years, or prior to the occurrence of significant enlargement of the heart[33].

Heart valve substitutes may cause various complications of differing degrees, either early post-operatively or late during the follow-up period. Thrombosis and embolization are among the most severe complications associated with valve replacement and their incidence is higher following the use of prosthetic valves[18,46,52,54]. Significant mortality and neurological sequelae are caused by thromboembolism. The more recently introduced low profile heart valve prostheses carry a lower risk of thromboembolism when associated with the use of long-term anticoagulant treatment[1,3,5,7,10,27]. However, life-long treatment with prothrombin depressants introduces the additional risk of bleeding, especially in elderly persons, in children and in those patients in whom, for socioeconomic or geographic reasons, the control of anticoagulation is difficult or impossible.

The reported incidence of thromboembolic complications following prosthetic valve replacement varies considerably from one centre to another. At our institution the use of the locally manufactured Starr ball valve prosthesis has generated an incidence of mild, severe or fatal thromboembolic episodes of 27.4 per cent during the early and late post-operative period. This incidence diminished to 13.7 per cent with the introduction of Teflon coating of the above mentioned prosthesis. The use of the low profile disc type prostheses was followed, in our experience, by a very high incidence of thromboembolism (33.8 per cent) and in many cases massive valve thrombosis was observed. This catastrophic complication, infrequently encountered with the ball valve prosthesis, has also been described following implantation of the Björk–Shiley tilting disc valve[4,6,15,23] and of the Lillehei–Kaster pivoting disc valve[13,31,47]. Patients with such a complication frequently die in acute cardiac failure if re-operation is not promptly performed.

The biological tissue valves are considered to be virtually non-thrombogenic and the clinical experience with such valve substitutes has demonstrated the veracity of this assumption. However, the durability of such valves is not indefinite and some of the tissue preparations develop cusp tissue degeneration which causes valve dysfunction. In contrast with prosthetic dysfunction, the tissue valve dysfunction is a slow and insidious process, evolving almost like the pathology of a diseased natural valve and, therefore, it allows time for adequate planning and preparation for re-operation under optimal clinical conditions[49].

Our experience with allogeneic aortic valves was rather limited. During 1966, a series of 50 patients received aortic valve allografts, preserved in a buffered formaldehyde solution. Although our own results discouraged us to continue the use of aortic allografts, it seems that with different valve graft preservations, satisfactory results could be obtained.

The use of tissue valves, especially allografts, when prepared or manufactured locally by the surgical team, poses problems concerned with the difficulty of obtaining and harvesting the tissue, its preservation, sterilization, storage and the valve fabrication. The use of xenogeneic material[12,24] simplifies the task to a certain extent, and we believe that the treatment of porcine aortic valves with our method of glycerol preservation could produce a satisfactory heart valve substitute. Valves made of tissues other than cardiac valves have been successfully employed for heart valve replacement[26,43].

The clinical use of dura mater allograft valves began at our institution in January 1971[35,36,37,39,40,55,58]. The initial satisfactory results obtained have encouraged our group to use this type of biological valve exclusively, and until June 1977 a series of 1593 consecutive patients received dura mater valves for heart valve replacement. Mitral valve replacement was performed in 726 patients (45.57 per cent), aortic replacement in 645 patients (40.49 per cent), tricuspid replacement in 37 patients (2.32 per cent), pulmonary valve replacement in six patients (0.38 per cent) and multiple replacement in 179 patients (11.24 per cent).

This chapter deals with the late evaluation of a series of 272 patients operated upon during the period from January 1971 to April 1973. The survivors have been followed-up for a period of time from 51–78 months.

This series of 272 patients comprises our early experience with the dura mater allograft and consequently provides the patients with the longest follow-up. In order to draw valid conclusions from the analysis of the results we decided to include only patients with at least 50 months of post-operative observation, as the long-term results and durability are the most important factors in the assessment of a tissue heart valve substitute. Inherently, there is a drawback in analysing this initial group of patients as they represent a higher risk group and because they did not benefit from our experience gained with the passage of time.

CLINICAL MATERIAL AND METHODS

In this series of 272 patients there were 243 single valve replacements (89.33 per cent) and 29 multiple valve replacements (10.67 per cent). In the single replacement group, 147 patients (60.49 per cent) received mitral valves, 88 patients (36.21 per cent) aortic valves and eight patients (3.29 per cent) tricuspid valves (*Table 7.1*). Of the 29 patients with multiple replacements 22 had mitral and aortic valves, five had mitral and tricuspid and two patients received mitral, aortic and tricuspid valve replacement. At the beginning of our experience six

TABLE 7.1
Type of valve lesions in 243 patients with isolated mitral,
aortic and tricuspid valve replacement

Type of valve lesion	*Mitral—147 patients*			*Aortic—88 patients*			*Tricuspid—8 patients*		
	M	F	Total (per cent)	M	F	Total (per cent)	M	F	Total (per cent)
Stenosis	5	2	7 (4.76)	9	3	12 (13.63)	–	–	–
Regurgitation	22	31	53 (36.06)	40	12	52 (59.10)	4	4	8 (100)
Combined disease	21	38	59 (40.14)	13	5	18 (20.46)	–	–	–
Thromboembolism of previous prosthetic valves	9	19	28 (19.04)	3	1	4 (4.54)	–	–	–
Previously inserted aortic allograft valves	–	–	–	2	–	2 (2.27)	–	–	–

M = males, F = females

patients received a combination of dura mater allografts and Starr ball valve prostheses, as shown in *Table 7.2.* The total number of dura mater valves inserted in this series of patients is, therefore, 297.

The age of patients ranged from 6–67 years and the mean age was 34.1 years. For the mitral group, the ages ranged from 9–67 years (mean 33.6); for the aortic group from 6–65 years (mean 34.9); for the tricuspid group from 6–52

TABLE 7.2
Age and sex incidence of 272 patients having heart valve
replacement with dura mater allografts

Age groups (years)	*Mitral*		*Aortic*		*Tricuspid*		*Mitral and aortic* *		*Mitral and tricuspid* †		*Mitral, aortic and tricuspid* ‡		*Total*	
	M	F	M	F	M	F	M	F	M	F	M	F	M	F
5–10	2	–	–	1	1	–	–	–	–	–	–	–	3	1
11–15	1	2	1	–	–	–	–	–	1	–	–	–	3	2
16–20	5	13	15	2	2	–	1	2	–	2	–	–	23	19
21–30	16	30	14	4	–	2	1	2	–	1	–	1	31	40
31–40	14	20	15	6	1	1	2	4	–	1	1	–	33	32
41–50	11	16	13	4	–	–	6	2	–	–	–	–	30	22
51–60	8	8	4	4	–	1	1	1	–	–	–	–	13	14
61–70	–	1	3	2	–	–	–	–	–	–	–	–	3	3
Total	57	90	65	23	4	4	11	11	1	4	1	1	139	133

M = males, F = females
* Four patients had Starr prostheses in the aortic position
†One patient had Starr prosthesis in the tricuspid position
‡One patient had Starr prosthesis in the aortic position

(mean 27); and for the multiple valve replacement group the ages ranged from 14–53 (mean 33.9). There were 139 males and 133 females. Men predominated in the aortic group (65 patients–73.86 per cent) and women in the mitral group (90 patients–61.2 per cent). Both sexes were equally represented in patients submitted to tricuspid or multiple valvular replacement.

Rheumatic fever was the most frequent cause of valvular disease in this series. Pre-operatively the patients were assessed according to the New York Heart Association (NYHA) classification. *Table 7.3* shows that before the operation 15 patients (5.25 per cent) were in class I, 64 patients (23.52 per cent) in class II, 137 patients (50.37 per cent) in class III and 56 patients (20.5 per cent) in class IV. The group of 15 patients belonging to class I had Starr ball valve prostheses and presented with recurrent thromboembolic episodes.

TABLE 7.3
Pre-operative functional classification of 272 patients subjected to heart valve replacement with dura mater allografts

NYHA class	Mitral	Aortic	Tricuspid	Mitral and aortic	Mitral and tricuspid	Mitral, aortic and tricuspid
I	12	2	–	1	–	–
II	26	36	–	2	–	–
III	77	37	6	12	4	1
IV	32	13	2	7	1	1

NYHA = New York Heart Association

TABLE 7.4
Patients lost to follow-up during the period of observation

Valve replacement	Patients operated upon		Patients lost to follow-up	
	Number	Per cent	Number	Per cent
Mitral	147	54.05	13	8.84
Aortic	88	32.35	6	6.80
Tricuspid	8	2.94	1	12.50
Multiple replacements	29	10.66	1	3.40

Table 7.4 shows that from the total of 272 patients operated upon 21 patients (7.72 per cent) were not available for evaluation during the last six months and were therefore considered lost to follow-up.

High risk patients, or patients with severely depressed myocardial function, were not denied open heart surgery for valvular replacement.

Only the first 42 patients operated upon received anticoagulant therapy for a period of four weeks following valve replacement. No post-operative anticoagulation was used in the subsequent 230 patients.

Mortality and complications were described as early if they occurred within the first 30 post-operative days, and as late if they occurred beyond the first post-operative month. Infective endocarditis was considered as an early post-operative complication when it occurred during the first three months following surgery.

Late post-operative evaluation was based on uniform clinical and laboratory criteria. The survival rate and the incidence of complications were analysed by the actuarial method[2].

CONCEPTS AND TECHNIQUE OF CONSTRUCTION AND SURGICAL IMPLANTATION OF THE DURA MATER ALLOGRAFT VALVE

Anatomy and histology of the dura mater

Dura mater is the most external of the three meninges enveloping the brain. It is a resistant yellowish membrane with a limited distensibility which contains the pressure variations inside the skull[28]. The external aspect of the dura mater is attached to the bone surface by fibrous and vascular connections. The adhesion of the dura mater to the skull is very strong in children and elderly persons; at the frontal and occipital regions; near to the sutures of the cranial bones; and at the base of the skull. On the other hand, dura mater is less firmly attached at the temporal regions, the so-called easily detachable area, well known to the neurosurgeons. This detachable area is limited cranially by a line going from the falx cerebri to the lesser wings of the sphenoid bone and to the superior border of the petrous part of the temporal bone. Laterally its margins come from the apophysis of Ingrassia to the internal occipital protuberance[52].

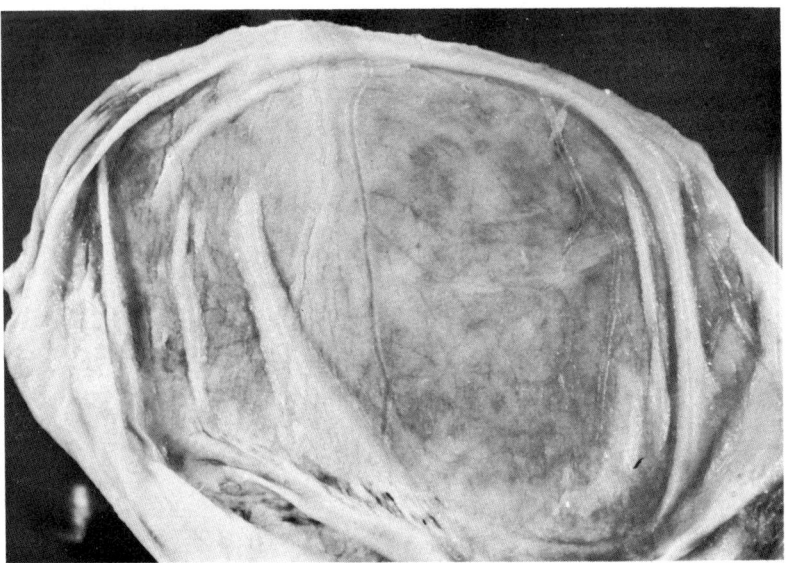

Figure 7.1 Macroscopic appearance of human dura mater showing the principal meningeal vessels and the 'avascular' areas in between

The external aspect of the dura mater has a smooth and shining surface. Its internal aspect is covered by the delicate arachnoidal layer of endothelial cells. At the level of the sutures of the cranial bones, dura mater is thickened by fibrous tissue and larger meningeal blood vessels[34]. In the great majority of cases, at the easily detachable area, dura mater has a reduced vasculature and uniform thickness, resistance and flexibility (*Figure 7.1*). The cranial dura mater consists of fibrous tissue, elastic fibres, lacunar spaces and blood vessels. There are two layers of fibrous tissue, an outer or endosteal and an inner or meningeal. The outer layer contains collagenous fibres arranged in different directions. The inner layer, which is thinner, has the collagenous fibres arranged in approximately the same way. The two layers are firmly united by collagenous fibres and both contain a few scattered fibroblasts and elastic fibres. Until 24 h after death the collagenous fibres maintain their normal appearance (*Figure 7.2*) and the number and aspect of fibroblasts and endothelial cells remain unchanged, without pyknosis of the nuclei. Under the electron microscope the collagenous fibres show a disposition at right angles (*Figure 7.3*).

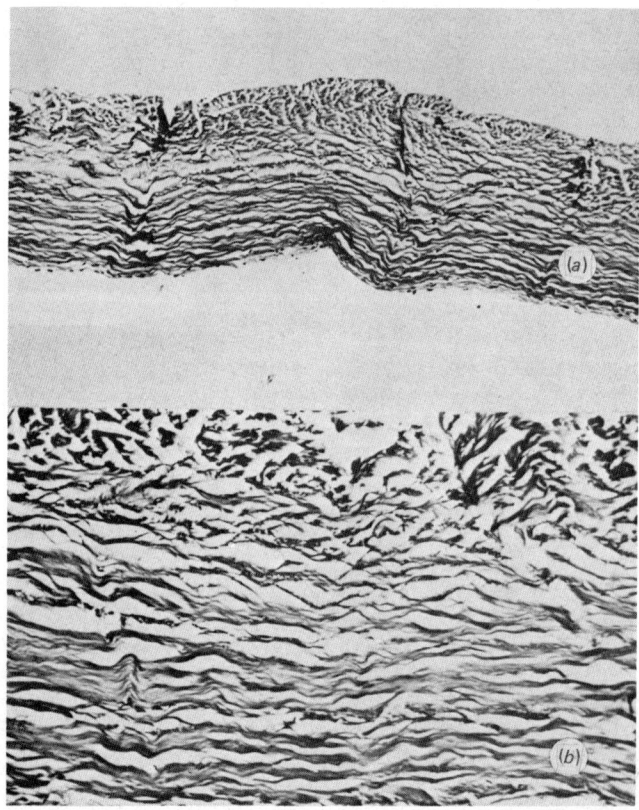

Figure 7.2 Microscopic appearance of dura mater fixed and stored in glycerol showing good preservation of the collagen matrix. (Verhoeff stain: magnification, (*a*) × 54, reduced by 20% in printing; (*b*) × 200, reduced by 20% in printing)

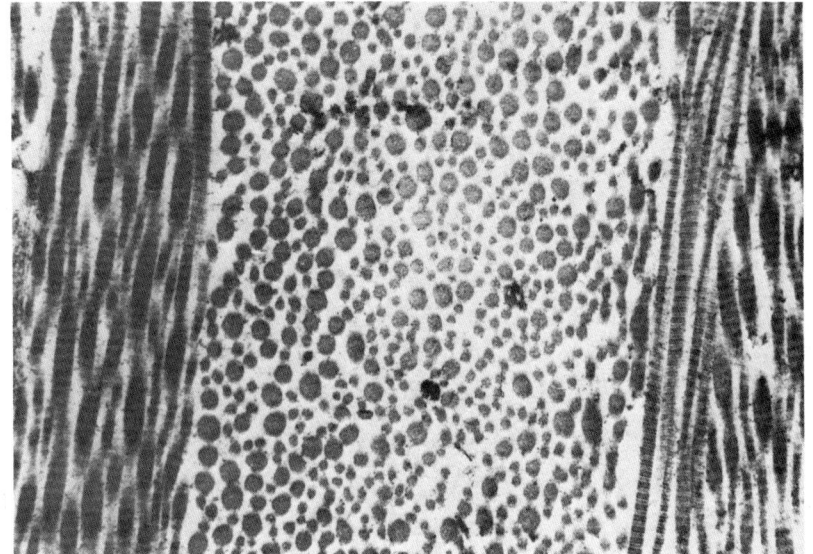

Figure 7.3 Electron micrograph of dura mater preserved in glycerol showing the right angle disposition of the fibrillary pattern. (Magnification × 28 500)

Removal and preservation of the dura mater

Dura mater was obtained from human cadavers of persons within an age range of 10–50 years. The collection was performed within 20 h from death. Cases of infective or degenerative diseases, as well as neoplasia, were excluded.

The dura mater was removed during necropsy using sterile gloves and instruments. The skull was exposed by a posterior transverse incision of the scalp between the mastoid apophyses. The bone was incompletely sawn in order to avoid the exposure and contamination of the dura mater. The opening of the skull was completed by percussion. The dura mater was removed and thoroughly washed with a continuous flow of water for 1–2 h. Following this the dura mater was placed in a sterile container filled with 98 per cent glycerol[32], for preservation at room temperature, for a period of 10–20 days. At the end of this period of time a piece of dura mater was removed and used for sterility control. Aerobic and anaerobic bacteria, as well as fungi, were searched for by appropriate laboratory techniques.

In our experience 18.7 per cent of the early samples of dura mater were found to be contaminated and were discarded. Gram positive bacilli, particularly *Bacillus subtilis* were the predominant organisms found (87.5 per cent). The following bacteria were also identified: *Streptococcus faecalis*, *Streptococcus* alpha-haemolitic, *Streptococcus* beta-haemolitic, *Staphylococcus* and *Micrococcus*. Gram negative bacteria were found in two specimens, while fungi have never been identified.

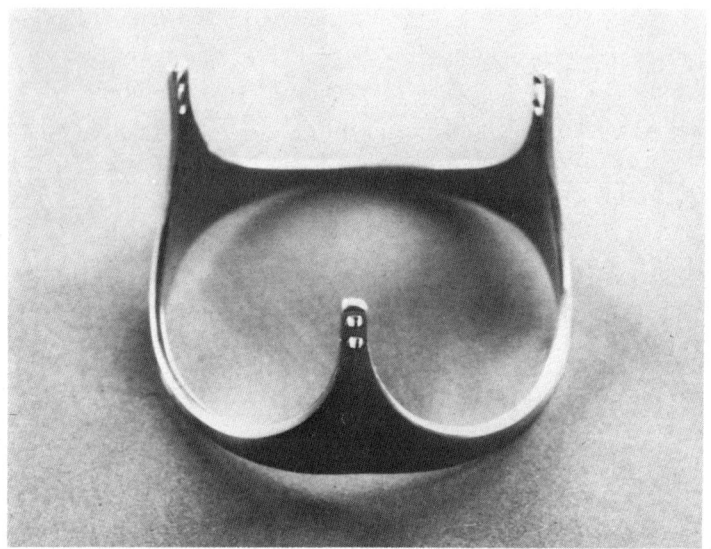

Figure 7.4 The stainless steel frame for the support of the dura mater allograft

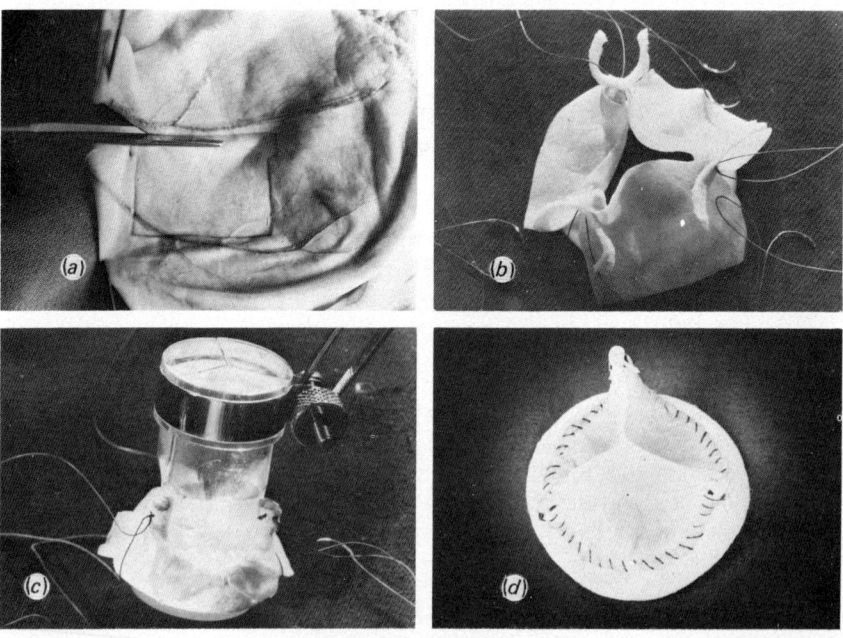

Figure 7.5 (*a*) An individual dura mater cusp is being tailored from an area between meningeal vessels; (*b*) The attachment of the three cusps to the support frame began with a suture passed through the two holes at the top of the struts. This suture was tied over a small, tape-shaped, piece of Dacron fabric or dura mater tissue; (*c*) The pieces of plastic mould are firmly kept in position by a metal ring to avoid movement of the cusps during suturing; (*d*) A dura mater allograft valve ready for implantation showing perfect coaptation of the cusps (seen from its outflow aspect)

Construction of the dura mater valve

The valve was made of three similarly shaped dura mater leaflets sutured onto a Dacron velour covered stainless steel support frame[38] (*Figure 7.4*). The manufacture of the valve was based on the procedure described by Ionescu and colleagues for the construction of fascia lata[25] and pericardial xenografts[26]. A few modifications were introduced in the course of our experience in order to correct the distribution of haemodynamic stress at the free margins of the leaflets as observed in the pulse duplicator.

The valve construction took place in an aseptic environment. The dura mater was removed from the glycerol container and rehydrated in sterile physiological solution for 5–10 min, until it acquired its normal aspect. Three 'avascular' areas, with similar thickness and pliability were selected for the tailoring of the valve cusps. The leaflets were separately cut from the dura mater and individually shaped according to the dimensions of metallic templates (*Figure 7.5a* and *Table 7.5*). The shape and sizes of the stainless steel support frame are shown in *Table 7.6*. The three pieces of dura mater were attached to the top of the support frame prongs with sutures tied over strips of Dacron fabric (*Figure 7.5b*). During the next step of valve construction an apparatus was used to hold in place and mould into shape the three leaflets. The apparatus consisted of a basal support placed underneath the frame and three corresponding moulds made in the shape of the aortic valve. When mounted, the apparatus held the dura mater cusps in position for their final suture attachment to the Dacron covered support frame (*Figure 7.5c*).

The dura mater valve is manufactured in a variety of sizes for aortic and atrioventricular valve replacements (*Figure 7.5d*). The sizes of the valve relate to

TABLE 7.5
Correlation between the stainless steel template dimensions
and the internal diameter of the support frame

Inside diameter of support frame (mm)	Dimensions of the template (mm)		
	S	*L*	*I*
18	26	19	22
20	28	21	24
22	30	23	26
24	32	25	28
26	34	27	30
28	36	29	32
30	38	31	34

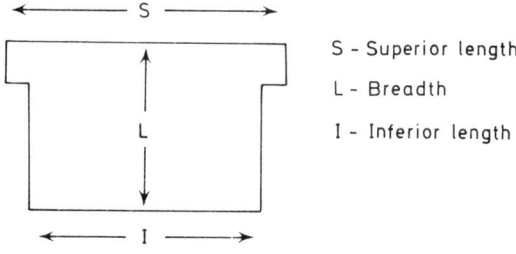

S – Superior length

L – Breadth

I – Inferior length

TABLE 7.6
Dimensions of the metal support frame

Internal diameter (mm) (d)	Thickness (mm) (t)	Height (mm) (h)	Breadth (mm) (l)
18	0.6	10	1.4
20	0.6	12.5	1.5
22	0.6	14	1.6
24	0.8	15	1.8
26	0.8	16	1.8
28	0.8	17	1.8
30	0.8	18	1.8

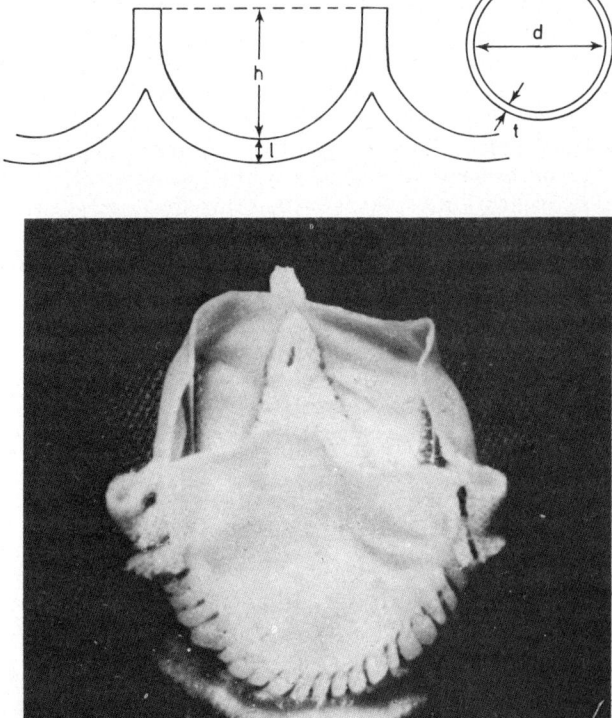

Figure 7.6 The completely free inner aspect of the strut is seen through the retracted cusps. The attachment of the cusps by a commissural suture placed at the very top of the struts permits a wider opening of the valve

the inside diameter (in millimetres) of the metal frame. The completed valves are replaced for storage in sterile, individual containers with glycerol.

Initially the leaflets were attached around the supporting prongs by a mattress suture, which produced an area of stress, probably responsible for the rupture of the dura mater at the commissure, as described in this chapter. Since 1975 the

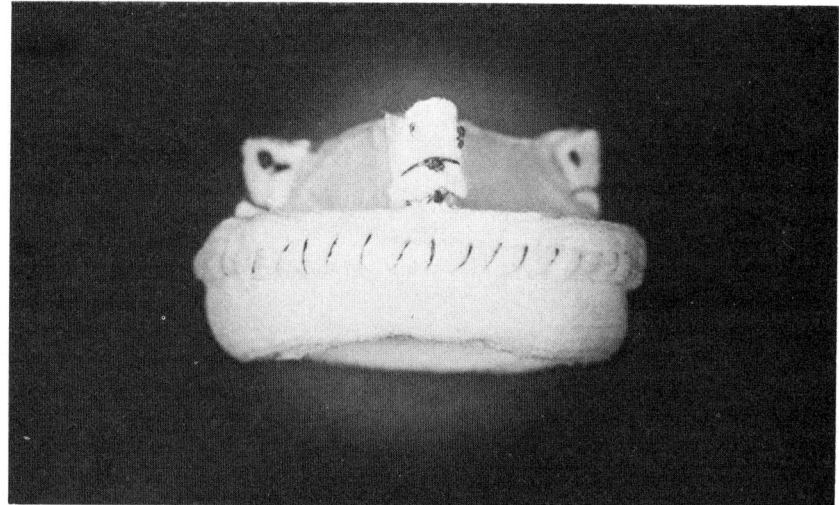

Figure 7.7 The dura mater allograft especially made for mitral valve replacement in cases of atrioventricularis communis. An additional sewing rim was placed around the valve in order to prevent protrusion into the left ventricular outflow tract. The valve is seated mostly into the left atrium

way of attaching the dura mater to the top of the prongs has been altered and the cusps were made somewhat redundant in order to reduce the haemodynamic stress at the commissures and to enlarge the effective valve opening (*Figure 7.6*). We are investigating, at present, the possibility of using a flexible polypropylene support frame on the assumption that it may contribute to the prevention of cusp rupture.

For the replacement of the mitral valve in cases of atrioventricularis communis a special dura mater valve was constructed. This valve was mounted with an additional sewing rim in such a way as to reduce the protrusion of the valve inside the left ventricular cavity and to prevent obstruction to ventricular emptying (*Figure 7.7*).

For surgical insertion, the valves were selected for a particular patient 24–48 h prior to operation and placed, under sterile conditions in physiological electrolyte solution, to which 1 g of cephalothin, 300 mg of rifampicin and 5 mg of amphotericin B were added. The containers with the reconstitution solution and valve were kept at 4 °C. If the prepared valves were not used for that particular patient, they were returned to the glycerol container.

Operative technique

The basilic or cephalic veins were cannulated for drug administration and a separate catheter was advanced into the superior vena cava for central venous pressure monitoring. The arterial pressure was monitored through a catheter in the radial artery and the inferior vena caval pressure through another catheter introduced through the saphenous vein. Extracorporeal perfusion was performed by cannulation of the ascending aorta or the common femoral artery.

A median sternotomy was used for aortic valve replacement, for combined

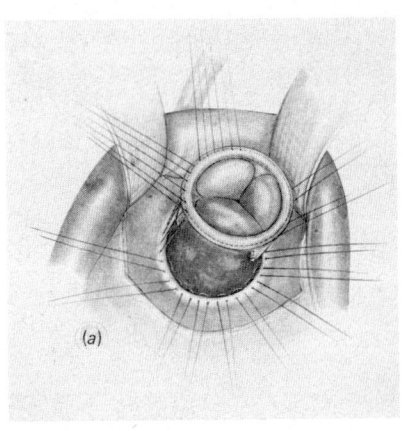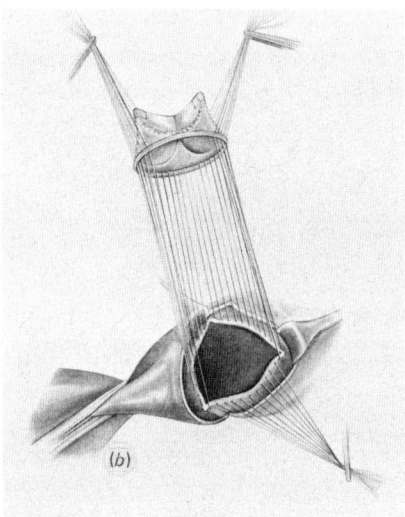

Figure 7.8 (*a*) Artist's view of the technique of implantation of the dura mater valve in the mitral position using multiple interrupted mattress sutures; (*b*) Artist's view of the insertion of the dura mater allograft in the aortic position with multiple interrupted sutures. Anoxic cardiac arrest, without coronary perfusion, was used for valve replacement

TABLE 7.7
Correlation between the type of heart valve lesion and the size of the dura mater
allograft valve inserted

Type of valve lesion	Size of the dura mater valve inserted inside diameter of the metal support frame (mm)					
	18	*20*	*22*	*24*	*26*	*28*
MITRAL						
Regurgitation	–	–	1	1	29	34
Stenosis	–	–	1	–	7	–
Combined disease	–	–	–	2	63	9
Thromboembolism of previous prostheses	–	–	–	–	28	1
AORTIC						
Regurgitation	1	17	44	–	–	–
Stenosis	–	6	7	–	–	–
Combined disease	–	12	13	–	–	–
Thromboembolism of previous prostheses	–	3	2	–	–	–
Previously inserted aortic allografts	–	–	2	–	–	–
TRICUSPID						
Regurgitation	–	–	–	–	2	12

mitral and aortic valve replacement and for re-operation on the mitral valve. A right anterolateral thoracotomy in the fourth intercostal space was preferred for isolated or combined replacement of the mitral and tricuspid valves.

Venous return to the heart–lung machine was obtained by cannulation of both venae cavae through the right atrium. Euthermic perfusion was used for mitral valve replacement, while moderate hypothermia at 28–30 °C was employed for aortic or multiple valve replacement procedures. Coronary artery perfusion has not been used. Anoxic arrest was induced by cross-clamping the aorta for mitral and aortic valve replacement. During the anoxic arrest, surface hypothermia was achieved by irrigation of the pericardial sac with 4 °C Ringer's lactate solution. Frequently, the tricuspid valve was replaced with the heart beating. Blood substitutes were usually employed.

Following excision of the diseased valves, the dura mater allografts were attached to the heart valve annuli with multiple interrupted 2–0 polyester mattress sutures (*Figure 7.8a* and *b*). The valves in the mitral and tricuspid positions were tested for competence and freedom of movement of all three cusps as soon as the heart had resumed rhythmic contraction. This manoeuvre may identify valve incompetence induced by misplaced sutures around the supporting prongs. The valve sizes implanted in the patients reported herein are shown in *Table 7.7*. *Table 7.8* details the duration of cardiopulmonary bypass and of anoxic cardiac arrest.

TABLE 7.8
Duration of cardiopulmonary bypass and of the period of anoxic cardiac arrest

Valves replaced	Duration of heart–lung bypass (min)		Duration of anoxic arrest (min)	
	Range	Mean	Range	Mean
Mitral	38–128	64.5	27–92	45.2
Aortic	48–150	66.7	33–103	54.4
Tricuspid	26–53	28.5	11–25	17.1
Mitral and aortic	60–170	121.1	47–124	84.0
Mitral and tricuspid	70–150	111.6	23–65	46.8

Prophylactic antibiotic treatment

Pre-operatively all patients were carefully investigated to detect bacteria and fungi by direct search and culture of sputum and swabs from the mouth, genital organs and skin. Special precipitin tests for *Candida* and *Aspergillus* were also performed. Patients presenting positive mycological tests were submitted to local treatment with amphotericin B. All patients received 1 g of cephalothin and 0.5 g of streptomycin 4 h prior to operation. During the procedure 1 g of cephalothin was added to the priming solution of the heart–lung machine. The same antibiotic combination used before the operation was continued during the first three post-operative days.

RESULTS

The late clinical and laboratory evaluation of this series of patients has shown that the great majority were asymptomatic at the latest examination, without digitalis treatment and have returned to active employment, according to their age group. None of the patients are treated with anticoagulants. The late follow-up group is comprised of 209 patients who were recently evaluated. The follow-up period totals 11 747 patient months.

The results from each individual valve replacement group are described separately.

Mitral valve replacement

Early mortality

There were 19 deaths in the immediate post-operative period (12.9 per cent). Myocardial failure was the most frequent cause of early mortality and occurred in ten patients (52.6 per cent). Rupture of the left ventricle, as a complication of mitral valve replacement, and fungal endocarditis occurred in one patient each and were considered as causes of death directly related to the use of the dura mater valve. The number of patients and the causes of early deaths are shown in *Table 7.9*.

TABLE 7.9
Early mortality in 147 patients subjected to mitral valve
replacement with dura mater allografts

Cause of death	Number of patients
Myocardial failure	10
Arrhythmia	2
Hepatic insufficiency	2
Renal failure	1
Left ventricle rupture	1
Myocardial infarction	1
Gastrointestinal haemorrhage	1
Fungal endocarditis	1
Total	19

Follow-up

Thirteen patients (6.80 per cent) could not be re-evaluated during the last six months and were considered lost to follow-up. There were 115 patients observed over a period of 51–78 months (mean 56.9) for a total of 6261 patient months.

Late mortality

Nineteen patients died during the late post-operative period (16.5 per cent). The causes of death are outlined in *Table 7.10*. Heart failure was the most frequent cause of death and was encountered in seven patients (36.8 per cent). Bacterial

TABLE 7.10
Late mortality in 115 hospital survivors having mitral valve replacement with
dura mater allografts*

Causes of death	Number of patients	Time of death (months post-op)
Heart failure	7	2, 3, 25, 25, 34, 35, 46
Sudden death	3	1, 39, 44
Bacterial endocarditis	3	45, 60, 65
Bronchopneumonia	2	24, 46
Arrhythmia	1	3
Pulmonary hypertension	1	47
Haemoperitoneum	1	2
Acute abdominal disorder	1	13

*From the total of 128 hospital survivors 13 had been lost to follow-up

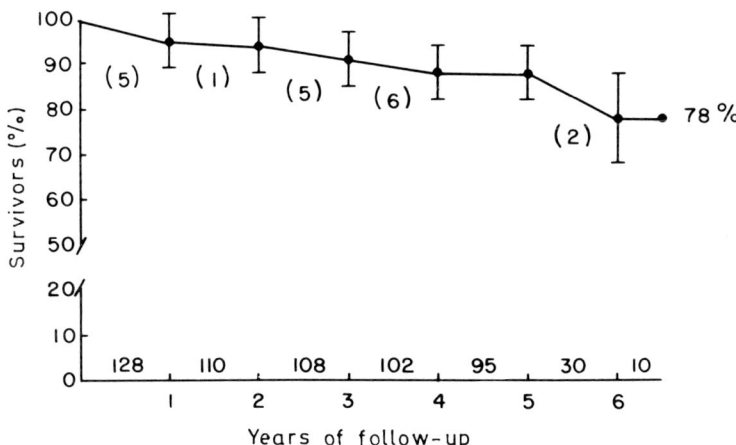

Figure 7.9 Actuarial analysis of survival rates in patients having mitral valve replacement with dura mater allografts. The figures above the horizontal axis show the number of patients at risk at the beginning of each year of follow-up. The figures in parentheses indicate the number of late deaths

endocarditis caused three deaths and occurred at 45, 60 and 65 months following the operation. A nine year old boy lived for 47 months after mitral replacement when he died from severe pulmonary hypertension, confirmed by haemodynamic studies.

Figure 7.9 shows the actuarial curve for survival rate. At one year 95 per cent of patients are expected to be alive; at four years and five years 88 per cent; and beyond six years post-operatively 78 per cent of patients.

Endocarditis

Fungal endocarditis, produced by *Aspergillus fumigatus*, occurred in the immediate post-operative period in one patient (0.68 per cent). Bacterial endocarditis developed in three patients at 45, 60 and 65 months after the operation respectively and the complication was fatal in all cases. The endocarditis occurred following an infected abortion in one patient. The second patient had rheumatic fever and bacterial endocarditis produced by *Staphylococcus albus.* The third patient was admitted to hospital in a poor condition and it was impossible to control the infection.

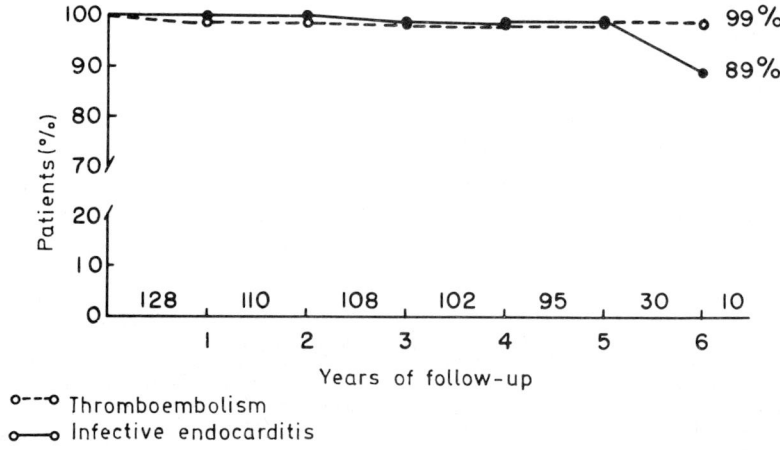

Figure 7.10 Actuarial representation of event-free curves for patients having mitral valve replacement with dura mater allografts. Analysis of infective endocarditis and thromboembolism

Figure 7.10 shows the actuarial event-free curve for infective endocarditis. At five years following valve replacement 99 per cent of patients are predicted to be free from bacterial endocarditis and at six years post-operatively 89 per cent of patients.

Thromboembolism

In this series anticoagulation was not used, except for 22 patients, at the beginning of the experience, who received anticoagulant drugs for four weeks following the operation. Thromboembolic episodes were observed in two patients (1.73 per cent or 0.85 embolic episodes/100 patient years). One patient had an embolus to the lower limb 30 days following the operation and recovered after embolectomy. The second patient, a 50 year old female had a mild and transient cerebral embolic episode six months after surgery. Both patients had atrial fibrillation with grossly enlarged left atria. No anticoagulants were administered, even after the occurrence of thromboembolic complications and no other episodes occurred.

The actuarial analysis predicts that 99 per cent of patients with mitral valve replacement should be free from late thromboembolic complications at six years post-operatively (*Figure 7.10*).

Valve dysfunction

During the early post-operative period, nine patients (6.1 per cent) developed a mild or moderate systolic murmur. In three of these patients the intensity of the murmur increased and they became progressively and severely symptomatic. All three required re-operation. One patient was re-operated upon early after valve insertion and was found to have perivalvular leak (0.6 per cent). Two patients (1.3 per cent) had mitral regurgitation produced by rupture of the dura mater cusps caused by a misplaced suture which was tied around a prong. The remaining six patients (4.0 per cent) were followed up for a period of four years and the intensity and quality of the systolic murmurs remained unchanged with the exception of one patient whose murmur disappeared with the passage of time. Haemodynamic investigations performed in this patient showed that the dura mater valve was competent. Two patients, from this group with unchanged systolic murmurs, were subjected to haemodynamic studies and the valves were found to be competent.

A minor amount of central regurgitation through the valve was observed at the time of the operation when the valves were assessed with the heart beating. This was observed in three patients, none of whom had systolic murmurs at the late clinical evaluation. The central regurgitation could be attributed to imperfect manufacture of the valve cusps.

Five patients (4.3 per cent) developed trivial or mild systolic murmurs late after the operation and two of them were re-operated upon.

Actuarial analysis of the event-free curve shows 92 per cent of the patients to be free of systolic murmurs six years following valve replacement (*Figure 7.11*).

Cusp rupture

Two patients with systolic murmurs of late occurrence were re-operated upon 35 and 45 months respectively, following the first operation. Both valves showed rupture of the cusps at the commissures.

The actuarial curve shows that 97 per cent of the patients are expected to be free from cusp rupture at six years after valve replacement (*Figure 7.11*).

Re-operation

Five patients underwent re-operation and all survived the procedure. The first patient (0.6 per cent) developed a systolic murmur early after valve replacement and re-operation was performed one month following valve insertion. A perivalvular leak was found and obliterated with additional sutures. Two other patients (1.3 per cent) developed systolic murmurs and progressive clinical deterioration. They required re-operation at five and 19 months respectively after the original operation. In both cases there was mitral regurgitation produced by ruptured cusps due to misplaced sutures which were tied around the valve prongs. Two further patients developed systolic murmurs at 32 and 37 months respectively after valve replacement. They were re-operated upon during the 35th and 45th post-operative months, respectively, with satisfactory recovery.

Both valves had ruptured cusps in the commissural area. The substance of the dura mater had normal flexibility without fibrosis and there was neither calcification nor retraction of the tissue.

Actuarial analysis shows that 95 per cent of the patients are expected to be free from re-operation at six years following mitral valve replacement (*Figure 7.11*).

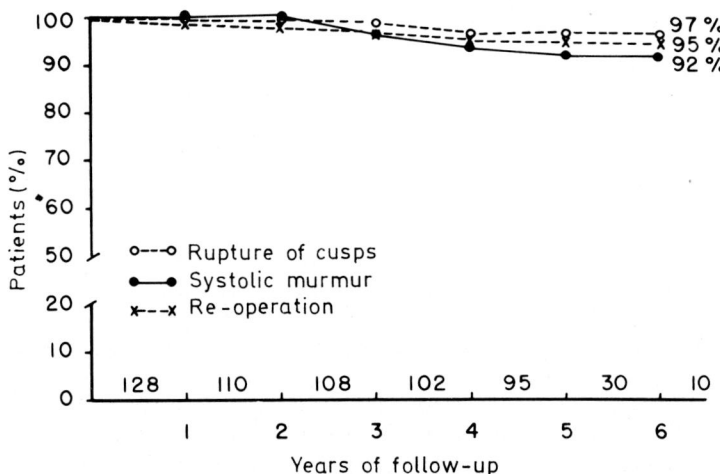

Figure 7.11 Actuarial representation of event-free curves for patients having mitral valve replacement with dura mater allografts. Analysis of cusp rupture, systolic murmur and re-operation

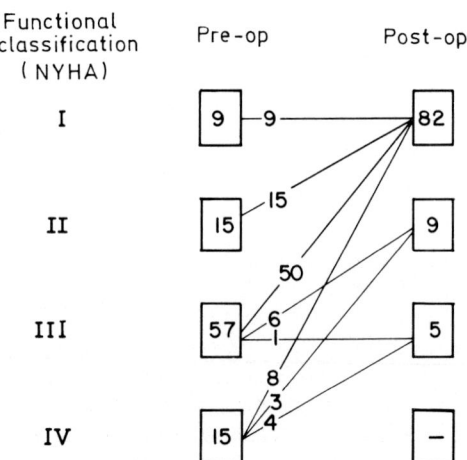

Figure 7.12 Diagrammatic representation of the pre- and post-operative clinical condition based on the NYHA classification. This evaluation comprises 96 patients subjected to mitral valve replacement with dura mater allografts

TABLE 7.11
Post-operative haemodynamic data from 21 patients having mitral valve replacement with dura mater allografts*

Patient No.	Inside diameter of the metal support frame† (mm)	Time of investigation (months post-op)	Pulmonary artery systolic pressure (mmHg)	Mean pulmonary wedge pressure (mmHg)	Left ventricular end diastolic pressure (mmHg)	Mean diastolic gradient (mmHg)
1	24	4	16	5	0	6.3
2	26	4	30	8	8	4.2
3	28	28	16	2	2	3.8
4	28	6	48	8	2	4.0
5	26	37	24	11	8	6.1
6	28	43	25	12	12	1.0
7	26	7	78	25	25	5.9
8	28	7	37	15	11	4.9
9	28	24	28	6	6	6.3
10	28	1	20	3	1	3.0
11	28	10	33	9	7	2.5
12	26	6	23	9	9	2.2
13	26	5	19	3	3	1.2
14	28	5	30	10	9	3.0
15	26	2	35	20	12	9.7
16	26	37	40	17	17	5.1
17	28	31	26	15	20	4.0
18	26	20	18	8	2	4.5
19	28	30	18	7	3	6.1
20	26	21	30	13	8	7.0
21	26	8	21	2	2	5.5
Mean values		16.00	29.29	9.90	7.48	4.59
± standard deviation		±13.59	±13.99	± 6.03	± 6.01	±2.08

*Data recorded at rest
†The annulus (sewing) diameter of the valves is 10 mm larger than the inside diameter of the metal frame

TABLE 7.12
Post-operative haemodynamic data at rest and during exercise from 11 patients with mitral dura mater allografts

Patient No.	Inside diameter of the metal support frame* (mm)	Time of investigation (months post-op)	Mean left atrial pressure (mmHg) R	E	Left ventricular end diastolic pressure (mmHg) R	E	Mean diastolic gradient (mmHg) R	E	Cardiac index (ℓ/min/m²) R	E
1	28	24	2	3	2	0	1.9	8.2	3.11	11.90
2	28	36	12	8	12	8	1.3	4.4	2.70	11.70
3	28	48	5	5	5	3	2.5	2.8	2.66	11.90
4	28	25	7	9	7	5	3.5	3.8	2.31	7.70
5	28	48	17	15	17	15	1.7	5.2	2.54	8.80
6	26	30	18	15	18	15	3.5	7.0	3.12	7.70
7	26	37	18	18	18	16	5.1	6.3	2.48	9.30
8	26	34	6	7	2	4	2.8	3.2	2.40	5.00
9	26	33	9	6	9	2	2.0	9.0	3.38	10.40
10	26	50	12	9	6	9	2.2	2.5	4.42	11.84
11	28	54	9	9	4	9	8.7	8.7	2.52	8.88
Mean values		35.36	10.45	9.45	9.09	11.00	3.20	5.53	2.88	9.56
± standard deviation		±14.21	±5.47	±4.66	±6.22	±6.00	±2.11	±2.44	±0.66	±2.24

*The annulus (sewing) diameter of the valves is 10 mm larger than the inside diameter of the metal frame

R = rest, E = exercise

Clinical condition

Ninety-six patients were followed-up during a period from 51–78 months. Twenty-eight patients (29.1 per cent) still receive digitalis and 68 are asymptomatic without medication.

As assessed pre-operatively, the great majority of the patients were in class III (NYHA). The post-operative clinical evolution has been satisfactory and 82 patients (85.4 per cent) were asymptomatic at the latest assessment (*Figure 7.12*).

Haemodynamic investigations

Two different groups of patients were subjected to haemodynamic investigations during the late post-operative period. The first group consists of 21 patients who

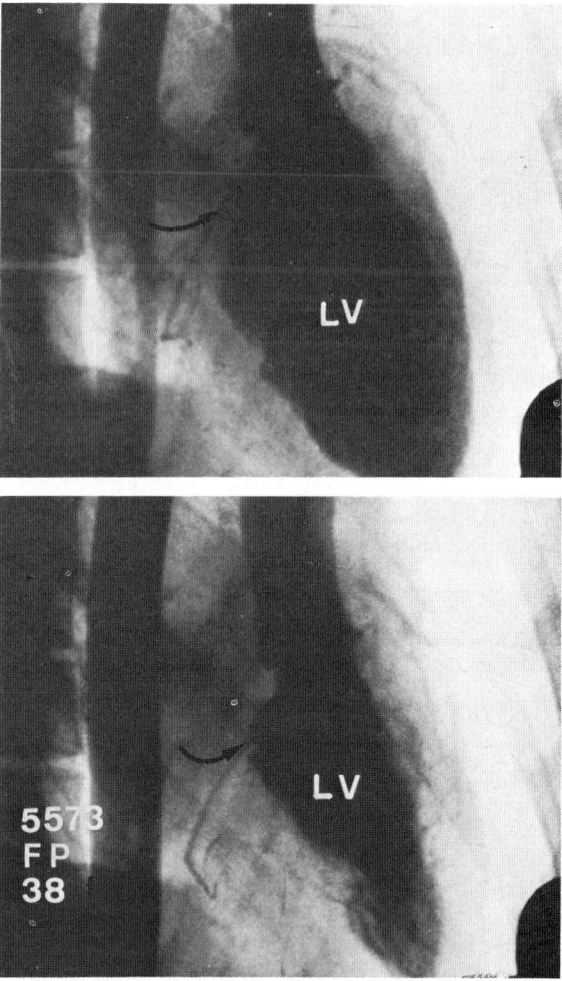

Figure 7.13 Left ventriculogram in diastole (above) and systole (below) demonstrating a competent dura mater valve in the mitral position and mild left ventricular hypokinesia.
LV = left ventricle

were studied at rest at a mean post-operative duration of 16 months (range 1-43 months). The second group contains 11 patients who were subjected to haemodynamic investigations at rest and during exercise at a mean post-operative duration of 35.36 months (range 24-54 months) (*Tables 7.11* and *7.12*).

There was no mitral regurgitation in any of the patients studied, not even in the three patients with systolic murmurs (*Figure 7.13*).

In the group of patients studied at rest the mitral diastolic gradients ranged from 1.0-9.7 mmHg (mean 4.59 ± 2.08 standard deviation) (*Table 7.11*).

In the group of 11 patients subjected to haemodynamic investigations at rest and during exercise, the diastolic gradient ranged from 1.3-8.7 mmHg (3.20 ± 2.11) at rest and from 2.5-9.0 mmHg (5.53 ± 2.44) during exercise (*Table 7.12*).

Aortic valve replacement

Eighty-eight patients in this series were subjected to aortic valve replacement with dura mater allograft valves.

Early mortality

Ten patients (11.3 per cent) died in the immediate post-operative period. Myocardial failure was the most frequent cause of early death and occurred in four patients. One death was caused by bacterial endocarditis and this was the only valve related early death in the aortic valve replacement group of patients (*Table 7.13*).

TABLE 7.13
Early mortality in 88 patients subjected to aortic
valve replacement with dura mater allografts

Cause of death	Number of patients
Myocardial failure	4
Cardiac tamponade	2
Systemic calcific embolization	1
Renal failure	1
Coagulopathy	1
Bacterial endocarditis	1
Total	10

Follow-up

Six patients could not be re-assessed during the last six months (6.8 per cent) and were considered lost to follow-up. The remaining 72 patients were observed for a period of 51-78 months, completing a total of 4203 (mean 60) months.

Late mortality

Five patients died during the late post-operative period. Two patients died suddenly at four and 48 months after the operation, respectively. One patient was re-operated upon 12 months following the first operation to correct a valvular insufficiency and did not recover from surgery. One other patient died

TABLE 7.14
Late mortality in 72 hospital survivors having aortic valve
replacement with dura mater allografts*

Cause of death	Number of patients	Time of death (months post-op)
Sudden death	2	4, 48
Myocardial failure	1	12
Fungal endocarditis	1	5
Undetermined	1	60

[1] From the total of 78 hospital survivors, six had been lost to follow-up

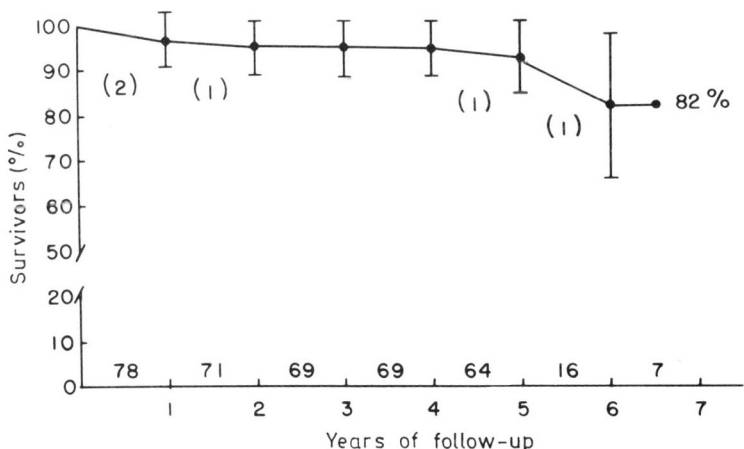

Figure 7.14 Actuarial analysis of survival rates in patients having aortic valve replacement with dura mater allografts. The figures above the horizontal axis show the number of patients at risk at the beginning of each year of follow-up. The figures in parentheses indicate the number of late deaths

60 months following valve insertion and the cause of death could not be established. Fungal endocarditis due to *Aspergillus fumigatus* produced the only valve related death which occurred five months post-operatively (Table 7.14).

Actuarial analysis showed an expected survival rate of 97 per cent at one year, 95 per cent at two and four years, 93 per cent at five years and 82 per cent from six years onwards (*Figure 7.14*).

Infective endocarditis

One patient (1.1 per cent) developed bacterial endocarditis 15 days following valve replacement and died shortly thereafter. Two patients (2.7 per cent) developed bacterial endocarditis during the late post-operative period and were re-operated on at 39 and 41 months after the first operation, respectively. Both valves were found to have perforations and rupture of the cusps and were removed and replaced. Both patients recovered from surgery. These two patients had episodes of pyrexia 40 days and ten months, respectively, prior to the first valve replacement operation.

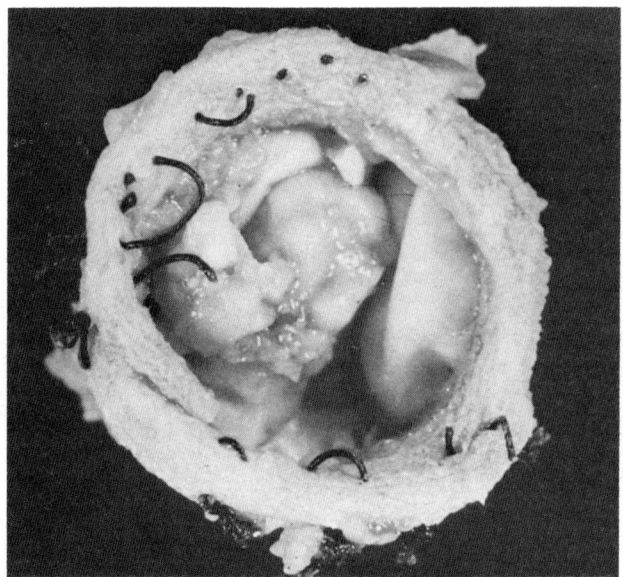

Figure 7.15 A dura mater allograft affected by fungal endocarditis (*Aspergillus fumigatus*). The fungi produced exuberant vegetations on the support frame and valve cusps

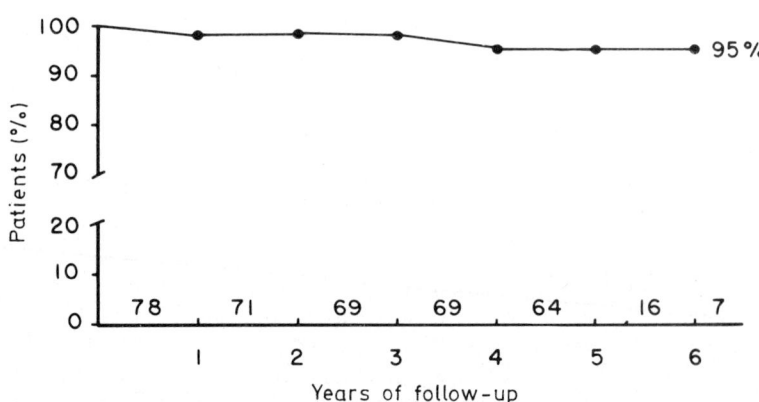

Figure 7.16 Actuarial representation of the event-free curve for patients having aortic valve replacement with dura mater allografts. Analysis of infective endocarditis

One patient developed infective endocarditis seven years following the replacement of his aortic valve with an aortic allograft valve. The allograft which was damaged by retraction, calcification and vegetations of the cusps, was removed and replaced with a dura mater valve. The process of infective endocarditis recurred five months after dura mater valve replacement. The patient died and the responsible organism was *Aspergillus fumigatus* which was cultured from the dura mater valve cusps (*Figure 7.15*).

The actuarial event-free curve for infective endocarditis showed that 98 per cent of patients are predicted to be free from endocarditis at the end of the first year and 95 per cent at six years after valve replacement (*Figure 7.16*).

Thromboembolism

There have not been any thromboembolic complications in the aortic valve replacement group during the late post-operative period.

Valve dysfunction

During the early post-operative period, four patients (4.5 per cent) developed mild or moderate aortic early diastolic murmurs. The patients were re-operated upon and it was found that two patients had perivalvular leaks while the other two patients had rupture of the valve cusps. The first patient with perivalvular leak was re-operated upon early post-operatively and the dura mater valve was removed and replaced by a Starr prosthesis. The patient did not survive re-operation. The second patient was observed until clinical deterioration occurred and he was re-operated upon at 26 months following valve insertion and the leak was successfully obliterated. The other two patients showed progression of the early diastolic murmur during ten and 45 months post-operatively, and were re-operated upon at 12 and 46 months following the original operation. Both

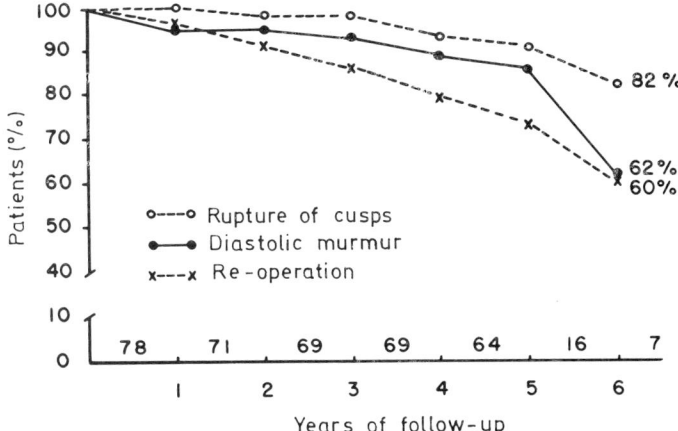

Figure 7.17 Actuarial representation of event-free curves for patients having aortic valve replacement with dura mater allografts. Analysis of cusp rupture, early diastolic murmur and re-operation

patients had rupture of the cusps at the commissures and the valves were removed and replaced with dura mater valves. One of these two patients died of myocardial failure following re-operation.

During the late follow-up, nine patients (12.5 per cent) developed early diastolic murmurs, which were recognized between 20 and 72 months (mean 54) following the operation. In three patients the murmur was first heard at 61, 67 and 70 months respectively after the operation. They were in class II (NYHA) and were maintained under clinical control. Six patients were re-operated upon and were asymptomatic at the latest examination. Five of these patients had sustained rupture of the valve cusps and one a perivalvular leak.

The actuarial event-free curve showed that 85 per cent of the patients are expected to be free from diastolic murmurs at five years, and 62 per cent at six years post-operatively (*Figure 7.17*).

Cusp rupture

Laceration of the cusps occurred in seven patients. The earliest case of this complication was observed at ten months after the operation and the latest one occurred at 72 months post-operatively. In two patients subjected to re-operation early after valve replacement, the dura mater valve was found to be incompetent due to a manufacturing defect which resulted in a shorter leaflet. In all the patients with cusp rupture the laceration occurred at the commissural area. The substance of the dura mater had a normal appearance.

The actuarial event free curve showed that 90 per cent of the patients are expected to be free from this complication at five years and 82 per cent at six years following the operation (*Figure 7.17*).

Re-operation

Twelve patients were subjected to re-operation; one early post-operatively and 11 during a period from 12–75 months from the original operation (*Table 7.15*). Rupture of the cusps was found in seven patients, perivalvular leak in three and mechanical damage produced by bacterial endocarditis in two patients. In all cases of cusp rupture, the tears occurred near the commissural area. In two patients the perivalvular leaks were successfully obliterated by additional sutures, but one of these patients developed recurrence of the leak.

The patients with bacterial endocarditis were treated with antibiotics initially and subjected to valve replacement after the infection was controlled by medical means.

The actuarial event-free curve showed that 73 per cent of the patients are expected to be free from re-operation at five years and 60 per cent at, and beyond, six years post-operatively (*Figure 7.17*).

Clinical condition

Sixty-seven patients were followed-up for a period of 51–78 months. Sixteen patients (23.8 per cent) are currently receiving digitalis treatment. Before the operation, 59 patients (88 per cent) were in class II or III; at the latest post-operative evaluation 60 patients (89 per cent) were in class I (NYHA) (*Figure 7.18*).

TABLE 7.15

Details of re-operation in 12 patients with aortic valve replacement

Patient No.	Age (years)	Sex	Time between surgery and appearance of symptoms (months)	Surgical findings	Time of re-operation (months post-op)	Results
1	20	M	72	Rupture of cusp	75	Asymptomatic
2	54	F	64	Rupture of cusp	66	Asymptomatic
3	35	F	54	Rupture of cusp	63	Asymptomatic
4	40	M	Immediate	Rupture of cusp	46	Asymptomatic
5	34	M	43	Rupture of cusp	45	Asymptomatic
6	34	M	36	Rupture of cusp	38	Asymptomatic
7	19	M	Immediate	Rupture of cusp	12	Died, myocardial failure
8	31	F	40	Bacterial endocarditis	41	Asymptomatic
9	34	M	38	Bacterial endocarditis	39	Asymptomatic
10	19	M	Immediate	Perivalvular leak	1	Died, myocardial failure
11	25	F	20	Perivalvular leak	22	Recurrence of leak
12	23	M	Immediate	Perivalvular leak	14	Asymptomatic

M = male; F = female

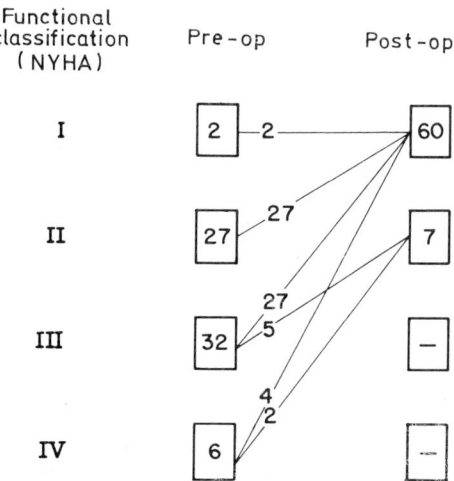

Functional classification (NYHA) | Pre-op | Post-op

	Pre-op	Post-op
I	2 —2	60
II	27 / 27	7
III	32 / 27 / 5	—
IV	6 / 4 / 2	—

Figure 7.18 Diagrammatic representation of the pre- and post-operative clinical condition based on the NYHA classification. The evaluation comprises 67 patients subjected to aortic valve replacement with dura mater allografts

TABLE 7.16
Post-operative haemodynamic data from 15 patients having aortic valve replacement with dura mater allografts*

Patient No.	Inside diameter of the metal support frame† (mm)	Time of investigation (months post-op)	Left ventricular systolic pressure (mmHg)	Aortic systolic pressure (mmHg)	Peak systolic gradient (mmHg)
1	22	2	126	101	25
2	22	7	100	100	0
3	22	8	114	97	17
4	22	5	122	112	10
5	22	6	113	100	13
6	22	6	138	120	18
7	22	4	131	117	14
8	22	4	118	116	2
9	22	4	103	101	2
10	22	14	152	124	28
11	22	4	134	134	0
12	22	2	138	128	10
13	22	3	222	222	0
14	22	23	170	170	0
15	20	5	129	110	19
Mean values		6.47	134.00	123.47	10.53
± standard deviation		±5.44	±30.30	±32.99	±9.60

*Data recorded at rest
†The annulus (sewing) diameter of the valve is 5 mm larger than the inside diameter of the metal frame

Haemodynamic investigation

Fifteen patients underwent haemodynamic investigations at rest, at a mean post-operative interval of 6.47 months (range 2–23 months) (*Figure 7.19*). Fourteen patients in this group had valves with 22 mm internal diameter and one had a valve with 20 mm diameter. Transvalvular gradients ranged from 0–28 mmHg (mean 10.53 ± 9.60 standard deviation) (*Table 7.16*).

Five patients had aortic regurgitation. In two patients perivalvular leaks were demonstrated but there were no clinical signs of aortic incompetence. The remaining three patients were subjected to re-operation. In two of them the regurgitation was produced by perivalvular leak, while in the third the regurgitation was through an imperfectly constructed valve.

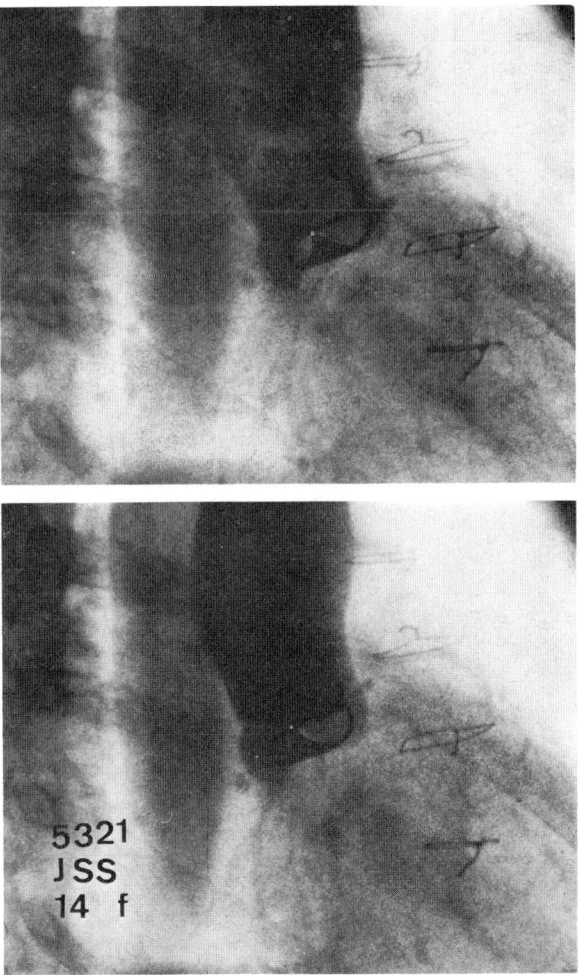

Figure 7.19 Aortic root angiogram in systole (above) and diastole (below) demonstrating a competent dura mater valve in the aortic position

Tricuspid valve replacement

Eight patients underwent isolated tricuspid valve replacement.

Early mortality

Three patients (37.5 per cent) died in the immediate post-operative period. Myocardial failure was the cause of death in two patients and renal failure in one.

Follow-up

One patient (12.5 per cent) was lost to follow-up. Four patients were observed over a period of 51–76 months for a total of 238 months (mean 59.5).

Late mortality

There were no deaths during the period of observation.

Complications

One patient with Ebstein's anomaly of the tricuspid valve developed complete heart block requiring the insertion of a permanent pacemaker at 30 months following tricuspid valve replacement. This patient was well at the latest examination, 58 months after the operation.

There were no incidents of valvular dysfunction, endocarditis or re-operation in this small series.

Clinical condition

Pre-operatively three patients were in class III and one in class IV (NYHA). At the latest post-operative assessment three patients were in class I and one in class II (NYHA).

Haemodynamic investigations

Two patients were subjected to haemodynamic investigations at rest, at one and seven months following the operation respectively. The internal diameter of the valves was 28 mm. Diastolic gradients of 1.4 mmHg and 4.7 mmHg were observed. Both valves were competent.

Multiple valve replacement

Twenty-nine patients were subjected to multiple valve replacement.

Early mortality

Ten patients (34.4 per cent) died in the immediate post-operative period. Myocardial failure was the most frequent cause of death and occurred in five patients with mitral and aortic valve replacement. Two deaths were caused by infective endocarditis, one bacterial and one fungal (*Table 7.17*).

TABLE 7.17
Early mortality in 29 patients having multiple valve replacement
with dura mater allografts

Causes of death	Valves replaced	Number of patients
Myocardial failure	Mitral and aortic	5
Air embolism	Mitral and aortic	1
Bacterial endocarditis	Mitral and aortic	1
Fungal endocarditis	Mitral and aortic	1
Coagulopathy	Mitral and aortic	1
Coagulopathy	Mitral and tricuspid	1

Follow-up

One patient (3.4 per cent) was lost to follow-up. Eighteen patients were observed over a period of 51–75 months for a total of 1045 months (mean 58).

Late mortality

Two patients died during the late post-operative period and the causes of death were not directly related to the implanted valve (*Table 7.18*). One patient died from a carcinoma of the colon and the mitral and tricuspid dura mater valves were found to be well preserved. The second patient died from heart failure.

TABLE 7.18
Late mortality in 18 hospital survivors having multiple valve replacement
with dura mater allografts*

Causes of death	Valves replaced	Number of patients	Time of death (months post-op)
Heart failure	Mitral and aortic	1	56
Neoplasm	Mitral and tricuspid	1	18

*From the total of 19 hospital survivors one patient had been lost to follow-up

Infective endocarditis

This complication was observed in two instances. It was produced by bacteria in one patient and by *Aspergillus fumigatus* in the second.

Thromboembolism and re-operation

Thromboembolic complications have not occurred in this group of patients and none required re-operation.

Valve dysfunction

A moderate amount of regurgitation was observed in one patient through the mitral valve during the operation while the heart was beating. However, no clinical or auscultatory signs of mitral regurgitation have been detected during the period of follow-up. In a second patient a mitral systolic murmur of moderate intensity was noted at 52 months after the operation but the patient continued to remain in a satisfactory clinical condition. Aortic or tricuspid valve dysfunction was not observed in patients with multiple valve replacement.

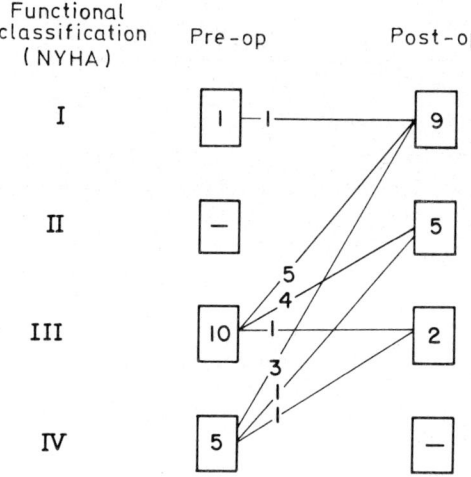

Figure 7.20 Diagrammatic representation of the pre- and post-operative clinical condition based on the NYHA classification. The study comprises 16 patients subjected to multiple valve replacement with dura mater allografts

Clinical condition

Sixteen patients were observed during a period of 51–74 months post-operatively. Eleven patients (68.7 per cent) are currently receiving digitalis treatment. Prior to the operation, all the patients in this group were in class III and IV (NYHA) except one who was in class I. This patient underwent re-operation for replacement of a Starr valve prosthesis which produced repeated emboli. Nine patients (58.2 per cent) were asymptomatic at the latest evaluation (*Figure 7.20*).

Haemodynamic investigations

Two patients had haemodynamic studies at rest. One patient with mitral, aortic and tricuspid valve replacement and another one with mitral and tricuspid replacement. The investigations were performed at eight and 24 months following the operation, respectively. In the first patient the internal diameter of the valve frames was 26, 20 and 28 mm and the transvalvular gradients were 5.5, 17 and 4.7 mmHg, respectively, for the mitral, aortic and tricuspid valves. In the second patient both dura mater valves had 28 mm internal frame diameter and the gradients were 6.5 and 4.0 mmHg, respectively, in the mitral and tricuspid positions. All five valves proved to be competent (*Figure 7.21*).

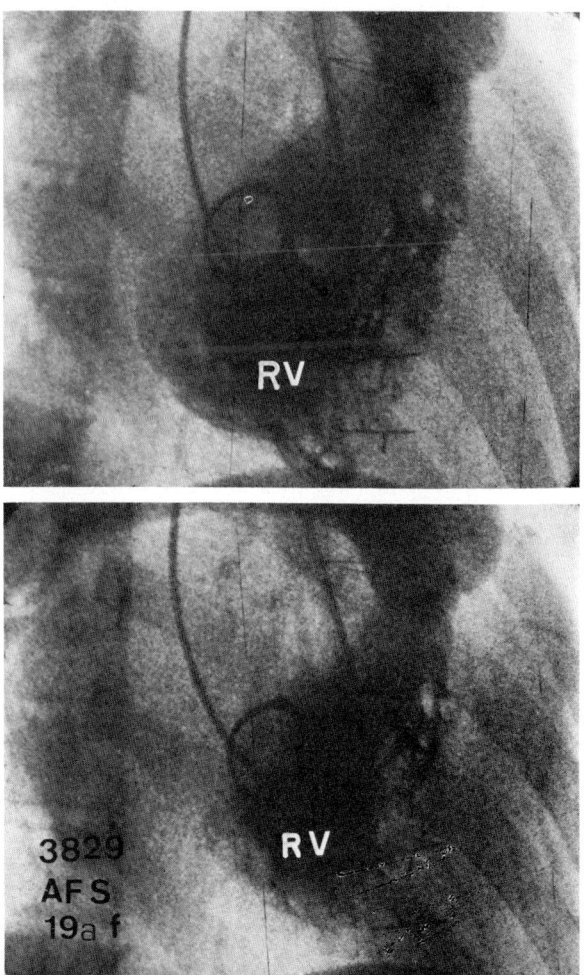

Figure 7.21 Right ventriculogram performed 24 months following mitral and tricuspid valve replacement with dura mater allografts. The valve in the tricuspid position is competent (above–diastole; below–systole; RV = right ventricle)

TABLE 7.19

Pathology of dura mater allografts

Patient No.	Age (years)	Valve replaced	Duration of valve in situ (months post-op)	Retrieval of the valve	Macroscopic aspect	Histology
1	16	Mitral	2.5	Autopsy	Normal appearance	
2	28	Mitral	5.0	Re-operation	Misplaced suture, pliability and thickness preserved, no retraction or calcification	
3	40	Mitral	19.0	Re-operation	Misplaced suture, pliability and thickness preserved, no retraction or calcification	
4	39	Mitral	34.0	Autopsy	Small commissural detachment of a cusp, one leaflet slightly thickened near to the base, pliability satisfactory	Normal histological appearance of the valves examined
5	23	Mitral	35.0	Re-operation	Cusp tear, pliability and thickness preserved, no retraction or calcification	
6	51	Mitral	40.0	Re-operation	Cusp tear, pliability and thickness preserved, no retraction or calcification	
7	16	Mitral	46.0	Autopsy	Focal calcification, thickness preserved, reduced pliability, no retraction	
8	19	Aortic	1.2	Re-operation	Perivalvular leak, normal appearance	
9	19	Aortic	12.0	Re-operation	Cusp tear, pliability and thickness preserved, no retraction or calcification	
10	40	Aortic	46.0	Re-operation	Cusp tear, pliability and thickness preserved, no retraction or calcification	
11	35	Aortic	63.0	Re-operation	Cusp tear, pliability and thickness preserved, no retraction or calcification	
12	54	Aortic	66.0	Re-operation	Cusp tear, pliability and thickness preserved, no retraction or calcification	
13	19	Aortic	75.0	Re-operation	Cusp tear, pliability and thickness preserved, no retraction, calcification present at the edge of the tear.	

PATHOLOGY OF THE DURA MATER ALLOGRAFT

The present study was performed at the Department of Pathology of the University of São Paulo Medical School by Dr Kiyoshi Iriya and Dr Antonio Sesso.

Thirteen dura mater valves were available for examination. The valves were removed from the patients at post-operative intervals varying from 37 days to 75 months. Ten valves were recovered at re-operation and three during post-mortem examination. Seven dura mater valves had been inserted in the mitral and six in the aortic position (*Table 7.19*). The valves were examined with particular regard to tissue thickness, pliability, retraction, rupture, calcification and presence of thrombus. For microscopic examination the dura mater was stained with haematoxylin-eosin, Verhoeff, Perdran, periodic acid-Schiff and phosphotungstic and haematoxylin stains.

In all the specimens a thin layer of autogenous tissue was found to cover the Dacron velour sewing rim of the valve. This layer extended 1–3 mm over the base of the dura mater cusps, and imperceptibly merged into the atrial and ventricular endocardium or into the aortic intima.

The causes of death or re-operation and the pathological findings were as follows:

Case 1. Death due to heart failure at 75 days following the operation. Normal aspect of the mitral valve. Microscopic texture of the dura mater well preserved.

Case 2. Re-operation for mitral valve regurgitation five months after the original operation. Two sutures had been misplaced around the support prongs of the valve and produced rupture of the dura mater cusps. The thickness and pliability of the dura mater tissue were preserved. The microscopic appearance of the cusps was normal (*Figure 7.22*).

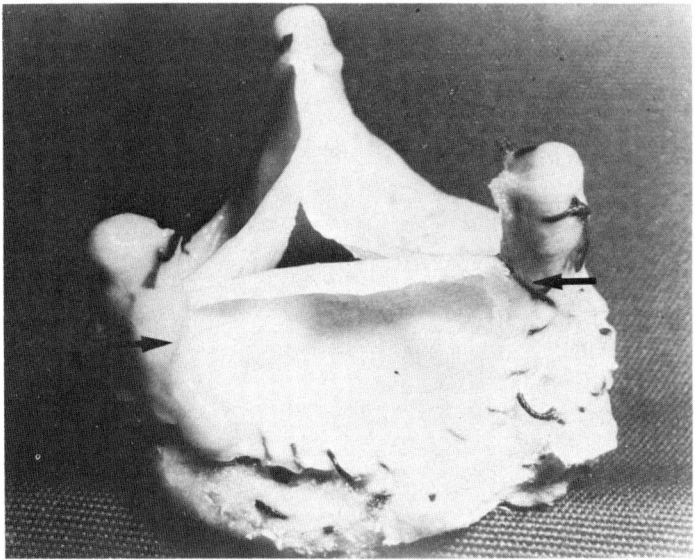

Figure 7.22 A dura mater valve removed from the mitral position (Case 2). Two sutures were inadvertently tied around the prongs of the valve (arrows). The cusps were rendered incompetent and eventually ruptured. Microscopically there was no degeneration of the dura mater tissue. (Reproduced from Puig, L. B. *et al.*[39], by courtsey of *Journal of thoracic and cardiovascular Surgery*)

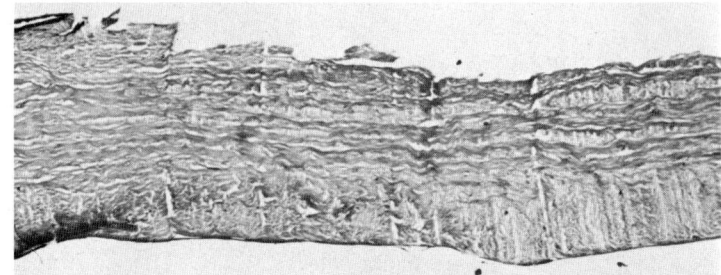

Figure 7.23 Histology of the dura mater 19 months following implantation. The collagenous and elastic tissues show a normal appearance. (Verhoeff stain, magnification × 54, reduced by 20% in printing)

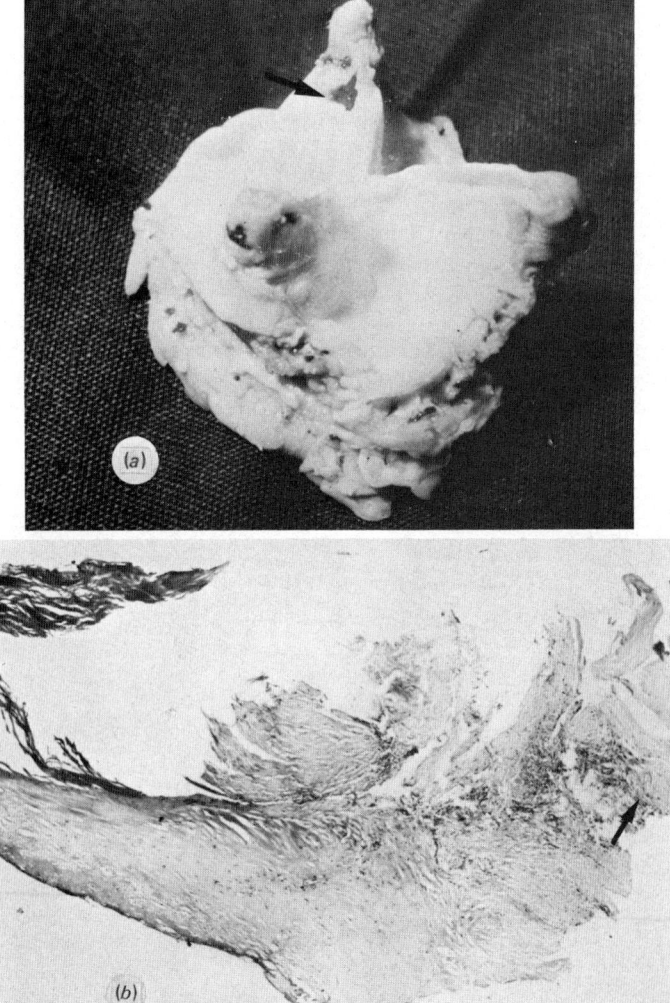

Figure 7.24 (*a*) A dura mater valve removed from the mitral position 35 months after its implantation (Case 5). The suture line at the top of the commissure is indicated by the arrow. The cusps have a normal aspect; (*b*) Microscopy section across the base of a cusp showing infiltration with lymphocytes, plasma cells, fibroblasts and a fragment of a suture (arrow). (Haematoxylin and eosin stain, magnification × 54, reduced by 20% in printing)

Case 3. Re-operation for mitral regurgitation 19 months after the original operation. One misplaced suture, as in the previous case, had cut a cusp. The histological aspect of the dura mater was normal (*Figure 7.23*).

Case 4. Sudden death at 34 months post-operatively. One cusp was loose and thickened at the commissure but the pliability of the dura mater was satisfactory and its microscopic aspect was normal.

Case 5. Re-operation for mitral regurgitation 35 months after surgery. There was rupture of a cusp at the commissure. The pliability and thickness of the dura mater were preserved. Microscopically the dura mater was normal and the collagen matrix was preserved. Birefringent material was observed near the cusp rupture suggesting the presence of suture material (*Figure 7.24*).

Case 6. Re-operation for mitral regurgitation 40 months after valve implantation. Rupture of a cusp near to the commissure was the main finding. The pliability and thickness of the dura mater were preserved and the histological aspect was normal.

Case 7. Death due to bronchopneumonia at 46 months following mitral valve replacement. Isolated yellowish areas were present on the ventricular aspect of one cusp. Except for those areas, the thickness of the cusps was normal, but the pliability of the dura mater was reduced. Histological examination showed

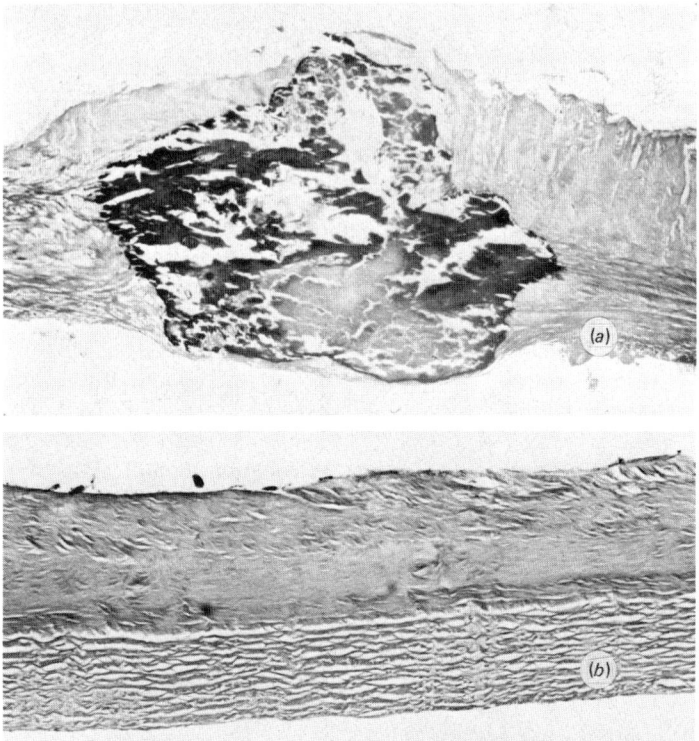

Figure 7.25 (*a*) Microscopic section through a small area of calcification of the dura mater without surrounding cellular reaction, observed at 46 months following valve insertion (Case 7). Haematoxylin and eosin stain, magnification × 54, reduced by 20% in printing; (*b*) Microscopic examination of the same specimen away from the calcified area shows preservation of the fibrillary structure of the dura mater tissue. Verhoeff stain, magnification × 54, reduced by 20% in printing

calcification circumscribed around the yellow focal areas. With the exception of the calcified areas the histological aspect of the valve was normal (*Figure 7.25*).

Case 8. Re-operation for aortic perivalvular leak 37 days post-operatively. The macroscopic and microscopic aspects of the dura mater valve were normal.

Case 9. Re-operation for aortic regurgitation 12 months after valve replacement. Two cusps showed rupture adjacent to the commissures. Histologically the dura mater was well preserved.

Case 10. Re-operation for aortic regurgitation 46 months after the original operation. There was rupture of one cusp in the commissural area. The dura mater was normal.

Case 11. Re-operation for aortic regurgitation 63 months following valve replacement. Two cusps had been ruptured near the commissural area. Histologically the dura mater was normal (*Figure 7.26*).

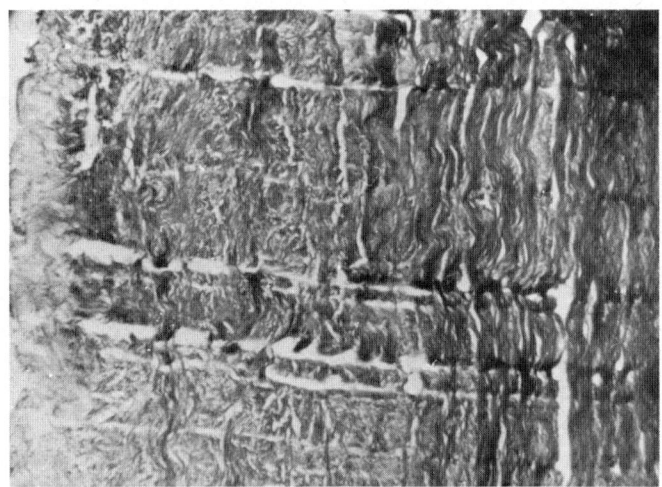

Figure 7.26   Case 11. Microscopic appearance of a dura mater cusp 63 months following its implantation. The fibrillary structure of the dura mater is well preserved. Verhoeff stain, magnification × 250, reduced by 20% in printing

Case 12. Re-operation for aortic regurgitation 66 months after valve replacement. One leaflet was ruptured near to the commissure. The dura mater was normal.

Case 13. Re-operation for aortic regurgitation 75 months after valve implantation. All three cusps were ruptured near to the commissures. At one cusp rupture, microscopy demonstrated calcification of the tissue. Except in this area the dura mater had preserved its thickness, pliability and its microscopic aspect (*Figure 7.27*).

HAEMOLYSIS

There were no clinical signs of haemolysis in the entire series. Laboratory studies for the detection of chronic intravascular haemolysis were carried out in 19 unselected patients more than one year after valve replacement. The following tests were performed: red cell count, haemoglobin estimation, reticulocyte

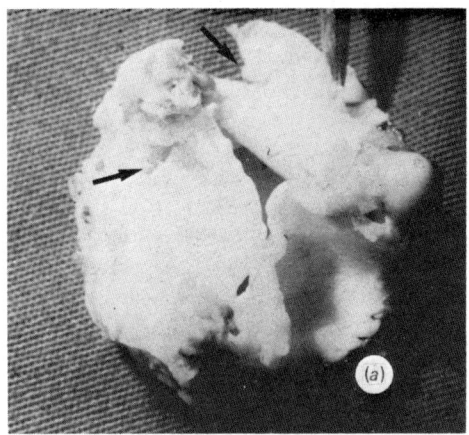

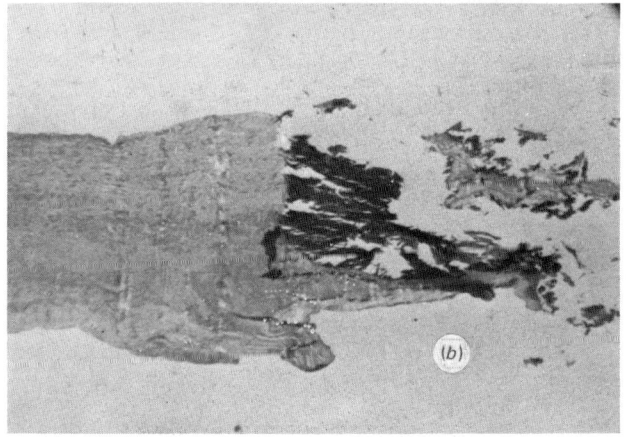

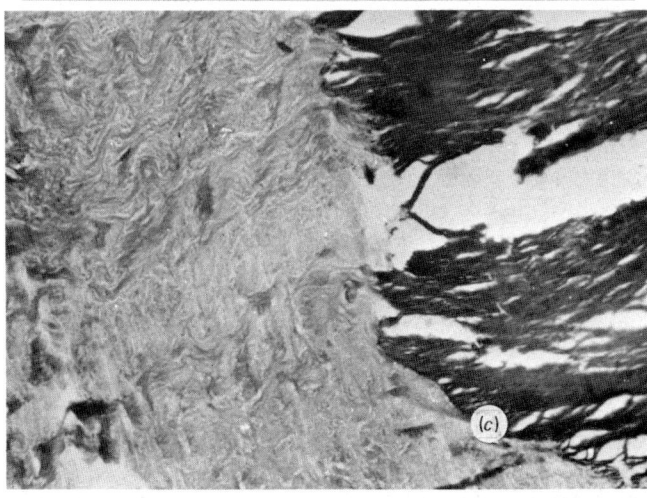

Figure 7.27 (a) A dura mater valve removed from the aortic position 75 months following its implantation. The cusps are ruptured at the commissure (arrows); (b) Microscopy shows a small and limited area of calcification without surrounding inflammatory reaction. Haematoxylin and eosin stain, magnification × 54, reduced by 20% in printing; (c) In the same area there is preservation of the normal structure of the dura mater. Haematoxylin and eosin stain, magnification × 250, reduced by 20% in printing

count, total and fractional bilirubin levels, haptoglobin, lactic dehydrogenase, serum iron and total and free haemosiderin determinations in the plasma and direct Coombs' test.

All patients investigated for haemolysis were in a satisfactory clinical condition. One patient with mitral valve replacement had a moderate systolic murmur of mitral origin. The laboratory investigation showed a certain degree of intravascular haemolysis with an increase in the reticulocyte count, bilirubin and lactic dehydrogenase levels and a low level of haptoglobin. The Coombs test was negative. In the remaining patients the laboratory tests for haemolysis were essentially normal.

PREGNANCY IN PATIENTS WITH DURA MATER VALVES

Ten patients became pregnant following valve replacement with dura mater allografts. Six patients had mitral valve replacement, two had aortic replacement and one patient each had isolated tricuspid replacement and combined mitral and tricuspid valve replacement.

The functional classification (NYHA) of these patients during their pregnancy was as follows: class I, five patients; class II, three patients; class III, two patients. The period of time between valve replacement and the end of the pregnancy varied from 24–68 months. Five patients had a normal delivery, four patients had Caesarian section and two patients had forceps delivery. One patient had two pregnancies. As none of these patients was treated with anticoagulants there were no episodes of bleeding. Thromboembolic complications were not encountered and the babies did not present any abnormalities.

DISCUSSIONS

The persistent demand for an improved cardiac valve substitute has encouraged clinical and laboratory research and investigations for the perfection of either prostheses or tissue valves.

A variety of non-cardiac tissues have been used for the manufacture of heart valve substitutes such as: fascia lata[50], pericardium[26], peritoneum[19], reaction tissue to implanted Silastic[21], vena cava[45] and dura mater[36]. The clinical experience with peritoneum, vena cava and reaction tissue valves is limited and inconclusive. The late results with fascia lata cardiac valves were sub-optimal due to the degeneration of the implanted tissue and, therefore, the use of fascial valves for mitral and tricuspid replacement was discontinued. On the other hand, xenogeneic pericardium and allogeneic dura mater valves have been implanted for seven years with satisfactory results.

The allogeneic dura mater has the necessary qualities for use in the preparation of artificial cardiac valves. It has an almost uniform thickness and pliability in the 'avascular' areas. Its tensile strength is satisfactory and uniform for a particular area. This is due to the arrangement of the collagenous fibres in different directions. The dura mater consists basically of two layers of fibrous tissue with dense collagenous texture, which give the tissue a great tensile resistance.

The preparation of the dura mater valve is simple, economical and standardized. The preservation and sterilization in 98 per cent glycerol has been efficient. The glycerol seems to reduce the antigenic potential of the dura mater and to preclude the denaturation of the collagen[32]. Under these circumstances, the durability of the valve does not depend upon regeneration of the tissue by host cells, but rather upon the stability of the pre-treated biological material[26].

The antibiotic solution was used as an additional protection of the valve against contamination during its preparation. Cephalothin has demonstrated its activity over Gram positive and Gram negative bacteria. Amphotericin B is an antifungal agent. Considering the importance and the difficulty of protecting the patients against fungal contamination, more active antifungal drugs, such as 5-fluorocytosine should be used. Unfortunately, this drug is not available in solution for the purpose of sterilization of the dura mater. Another acceptable association would be the use of amphotericin B which has its effect on the wall of the cells and rifampicin which acts directly on the cell proteins[29,30]. Similarly the association of penicillin and some aminoglycosides was found useful in the treatment of infections produced by *Enterococcus*.

The operative technique for the insertion of dura mater valves is similar to that employed for prosthetic valves.

In our experience, valvular incompetence has been produced either by imperfect manufacture of the valve with misaligned cusps leading to insufficient apposition or by misplaced sutures around the top of the prongs supporting the commissures at the time of valve insertion. This latter situation produced valve incompetence by tying the suture over the free margin of the cusps and finally causing cusp rupture. Perivalvular leak was another cause of regurgitation.

The regurgitation which occurred immediately post-operatively, through a defective valve, usually increased and lead to rupture of the cusps at the commissure area. The incidence of imperfect manufacture of the valve has decreased with the passage of time and increased experience. Until recently a step in the construction of the valve was to tie together two cusps, near to the top of the prong supporting the commissures, with a thin polypropylene suture buttressed by a strip of braided Dacron. The suture was tied on the inflow aspect of the commissure, inside the frame. This technique produced a point of stress at the free margin of the cusps, which became more evident during ventricular systole. This haemodynamic stress was well identified in the pulse duplicator. The technique of suturing the cusps was modified and the incidence of cusp rupture at the commissures has diminished. Moreover, we believe that the use of a flexible polypropylene support frame could further improve the haemodynamic performance of the dura mater allograft.

An iatrogenic cause of valve incompetence was the misplaced suture which looped around a valve prong and was tied in such a position. At the beginning of our experience this complication occurred in two patients who were reoperated upon. The cusps were found to be restricted in their mobility and eventually ruptured under the tension of the suture. This complication has not been observed any more following the introduction of a routine procedure for testing the competence and mobility of the valve cusps, with the heart beating, at the completion of valve insertion. The cause of a mild systolic murmur could not always be defined. One patient in this series, for example, developed a mild mitral systolic murmur immediately after valve replacement but the murmur disappeared within one year.

The late results of this series of patients having valve replacement with dura mater allografts are satisfactory and encouraging, considering the number of patients observed and the duration of the follow-up period. The mean follow-up duration was 56.9 months for patients with mitral valve replacement, 60.0 months for patients with aortic valve replacement, 59.5 months for those with tricuspid and 58.0 months for patients with multiple valve replacement. The late results showed that a great number of patients became asymptomatic following the operation and did not require specific anti-failure medication. In addition, the incidence of thromboembolism, as well as valvular dysfunction of the dura mater allograft in the mitral position, was extremely low when compared with the high incidence of such complications associated with the use of prosthetic devices in the mitral position.

The incidence of infective endocarditis in this series was comparable to that encountered following the use of other types of artificial valves[14,54]. During the immediate post-operative period the occurrence of infective endocarditis was infrequent. This proved the protective effect of glycerol and antibiotics used for the preservation of the dura mater allografts. Since amphotericin B was added to the preservative solution fungal endocarditis has no longer been encountered.

Although anticoagulant therapy was not used in this series, the incidence of thromboembolic complications was insignificant in the mitral replacement group and absent in patients with aortic or tricuspid valve replacement. Moreover, in the patients with mitral replacement and thromboembolic complications the implanted valve was not the only source of thromboembolism. Other factors could be responsible such as the age of the patient, previous surgery, left atrial enlargement, and above all, the presence of atrial fibrillation and the degree of functional disability of the patient[56].

A number of patients required re-operation. In the cases of dura mater valve incompetence, re-operation was performed as a precaution, in order to prevent progressive deterioration and severe cardiac failure. One patient refused re-operation and her clinical and haemodynamic conditions remained stable for a period of nine months when the second operation was performed. Re-operation did not present any particular technical difficulty despite the pericardial adhesions. Yet, the necessary duration of anoxic cardiac arrest was prolonged in two patients and both failed to survive. The remaining patients who underwent re-operations had a satisfactory outcome.

The analysis of post-operative haemodynamic data showed satisfactory results. The studies performed at rest and on exercise in patients following mitral valve replacement showed an insignificant mean diastolic gradient across the valve[41,42]. During exercise, the increase in cardiac output was accompanied by a slight increase in the diastolic gradient[20]. It was expected to find significant gradients during exercise in patients having artificial valves with rigid rings, considering the parabolic correlation between pressure and flow in such valves. The tissue valves with central flow are expected to have haemodynamic characteristics closer to the normal natural valves. The three-cusps valves, mounted on a rigid frame, do not produce a physiological flow pattern and, therefore, could cause endocardial 'jet lesions' in the left ventricle or dyskinesia interfering with the pump function of the ventricle[48]. Although an abnormal jet flow toward the apex of the left ventricle could be observed with the dura mater valve, these deleterious phenomena were not encountered in this series. The systolic gradients across the aortic dura mater valves at rest were mild when considering the high pressure, high velocity pattern of the left ventricular aortic flow[44].

Mild haemolysis was observed in one patient with a systolic murmur suggesting that haemolysis was produced by the mechanical turbulence through the valve[17,51]. The Coombs test was negative and this excluded an autoimmune process.

Anticoagulation was not used in this series of patients. This advantage was particularly manifest during pregnancy. A large proportion of pregnant women with prosthetic valves and receiving anticoagulant drugs are reported to have had abortion[11,22,57]. This complication was not present in our patients.

The study of 13 dura mater allografts recovered from patients during a period of from 37 days to 75 months following valve insertion showed preservation of the reticular structure of the dura mater with normal appearance of the collagenous and elastic tissue. The pliability of the dura mater was normal and there was no significant retraction of the cusps. A thin layer of autogenous tissue in continuity with the endocardium covered the sutures, the sewing rim and the base of the cusps. This tissue covered the surface but did not penetrate into the substance of the dura mater. An inflammatory reaction was found around the suture line where birefringent material with the characteristics of suture material remnants was observed[16]. Small scattered areas of dystrophy and calcification were observed in two studied specimens. The importance and prognostic significance of calcification depend on its frequency, magnitude and extension[9]. These findings associated with the mechanical stress in the commissural area could explain the occurrence of cusp rupture observed in this series, before the technique of valve manufacture was improved.

GENERAL CONSIDERATIONS

After 16 years of clinical experience with heart valve replacement and an impressive amount of intensive and imaginative work performed by many investigators, the ideal heart valve substitute is far from being a reality.

The major complications associated with the use of artificial heart valves are the thromboembolic episodes, more frequently related to prostheses, and the potential fatigue or degeneration of the tissue valves.

With the experience gained so far in the field of heart valve replacement surgery, it is obvious that for the evaluation of any valve substitute a period of clinical follow-up of at least five years is necessary in order to formulate valid conclusions.

At the present time we believe that the tissue valves have advantages over the prosthetic devices especially with respect to their low thromboembolic rate without the use of prothrombin depressants. Even if the durability of tissue valves may not prove to be indefinite, the tissue valve failure is a slow and progressive phenomenon allowing sufficient time for a planned, safe re-operation. Like the manufacture of any implant device, tissue heart valves require great care and exactitude in their construction. At present, the technical aspects of tissue valve construction, availability and choice of size are no longer limiting factors in their clinical use.

SUMMARY

The clinical use of dura mater allografts started at our institution in January of 1971 and until June 1977, 1593 consecutive patients were subjected to heart valve replacements with dura mater allografts. This chapter deals with a limited series of 272 patients operated upon before April 1973 and followed-up for late evaluation of the results. This series comprised 147 patients with mitral valve replacement, 88 patients with aortic replacement, eight with tricuspid and 29 patients with multiple valve replacement. Twenty-one patients (7.72 per cent) were not available for evaluation during the last six months and were, therefore, considered lost to follow-up. The survivors were observed for a period of 51–78 months.

Dura mater was obtained from cadavers ranging from 10–50 years of age, up to 20 h after death and was preserved in 98 per cent glycerol at room temperature.

The hospital mortality was 12.9 per cent in patients with mitral replacement, 11.3 per cent in patients with aortic replacement, 37.5 per cent in patients with tricuspid replacement and 34.4 per cent in those with multiple valve replacement. The late mortality for the same groups of patients was 16.5, 6.9, zero and 11.1 per cent, respectively.

Infective endocarditis was encountered in two patients in the early post-operative period and in eight patients during the late follow-up.

Cusp rupture occurred during the late post-operative period in two patients subjected to mitral valve replacement and in seven patients following aortic valve replacement.

Thromboembolism occurred in two patients with mitral valve replacement. No anticoagulant drugs were used in the entire series.

The long-term clinical and laboratory results have been satisfactory. The majority of patients operated upon were asymptomatic, without anti-failure treatment and were fully employed, at the latest evaluation. Haemodynamic studies at rest and during exercise demonstrated no significant gradient across the valves. Thirteen dura mater allografts were removed from patients at re-operation or post-mortem examination and microscopy showed preservation of the reticular structure of the dura mater with normal appearance of the collagenous and elastic tissue. The pliability of the cusps was normal and there was no significant retraction of the dura mater tissue.

Acknowledgement

We should like to thank the editor of this book for the invitation to contribute this chapter.

REFERENCES

[1] Allen, W. B., Karp, R. B. and Kouchoukos, N. T. 'Mitral valve replacement', *Archives of Surgery*, 109, 642 (1974)
[2] Anderson, R. P., Bonchek, L. I., Grunkermeier, G. L., Lambert, L. E. and Starr, A. 'The analysis and presentation of surgical results by actuarial methods', *Journal of surgical Research*, 16, 224 (1974)
[3] Aris, A., Fast, A. J., Tector, A. J., Flemma, R. J. and Lepley, D. A. 'A comparative study of ball and disc prosthesis in mitral replacement', *Journal of thoracic and cardiovascular Surgery*, 68, 335 (1974)
[4] Ben-Zvi, J., Hildner, F. J., Chandraratna, A. P. and Samet, P. 'Thrombosis on Björk–Shiley aortic valve prosthesis: Clinical, arteriographic, echocardiographic and therapeutic observations in seven cases', *Journal of Cardiology*, 34, 538 (1974)

[5] Björk, V. O. 'The central flow tilting disc valve prosthesis (Björk–Shiley) for mitral valve replacement', *Scandinavian Journal of thoracic and cardiovascular Surgery*, 4, 15 (1970)

[6] Björk, V. O. and Henze, A. 'Encapsulation of the Björk–Shiley aortic valve prosthesis caused by the lack of anticoagulant treatment', *Scandinavian Journal of thoracic and cardiovascular Surgery*, 7, 17 (1973)

[7] Bonchek, L. J. and Starr, A. 'Ball valve prosthesis: current appraisal of late results', *American Journal of Cardiology*, 35, 843 (1975)

[8] Braun, L. O., Kincaid, O. W. and Morrow, A. G. 'Pathologic anatomy of cardiac valve replacement. A study of 224 necropsy patients', *Progress in cardiovascular Disease*, 13, 343 (1973)

[9] Braunwald, N. S. and Detmer, D. E. 'Un analysis critico de las valvulas protesicas y de los homoinjertos', *Progressos em enfermidades Cardiovasculares*, 9, 125 (1969)

[10] Brawley, R. K., Donahoo, J. S. and Gott, V. C. 'Current status of the Beall, Björk–Shiley, Braunwald–Cutter, Lillehei–Kaster and Smellof–Cutter cardiac valve prostheses', *American Journal of Cardiology*, 35, 855 (1975)

[11] Buxbaum, A., Aygen, M. M., Shahin, W., Levy, M. J. and Ekerling, B. 'Pregnancy in patients with prosthetic heart valves', *Chest*, 59, 639 (1971)

[12] Carpentier, A., Blondeau, P., Laurens, P., Hay, A., Laurent, D. and Dubost, C. 'Mitral and tricuspid valve replacement with frame mounted aortic heterografts', *Journal of thoracic and cardiovascular Surgery*, 56, 368 (1968)

[13] Christo, M. C., Sousa, J. M., Stortini, M. J., Figueroa, C. S. and Santana F°, G. P. 'Próteses pivotantes de disco de Lillehei–Kaster em substituicões valvares. Resultados iniciais', *Arquivo Brasileiro de Cardiologia*, 29, 379 (1976)

[14] Clarkson, P. M. and Barratt-Boyes, B. C. 'Bacterial endocarditis following homograft replacement of the aortic valve', *Circulation*, 42, 987 (1970)

[15] Cokkinos, D. V., Voridis, E., Bakoulas, G., Theodossiou, A. and Skalkeas, G. D. 'Thrombosis of two high-flow prosthetic valves', *Journal of thoracic and cardiovascular Surgery*, 62, 947 (1971)

[16] Conceicao, A. N., Puig, L. B., Verginelli, G., Iryia, K., Bittencourt, D. and Zerbini, E. J. 'Homologous dura mater cardiac valves. Structural aspect of eight implanted valves', *Journal of thoracic and cardiovascular Surgery*, 70, 499 (1975)

[17] De Cesare, W., Rath, C. and Hufnagel, C. 'Haemolytic anemia of mechanical origin with aortic valve prosthesis', *New England Journal of Medicine*, 272, 1045 (1965)

[18] Duvoisin, G. E., Brandenburg, R. O. and McGoon, D. C. 'Factors affecting thromboembolism associated with prosthetic heart valves', *Circulation*, 35/36 (*Suppl. 1*), 70 (1967)

[19] Fadali, A. M., Ramos, M. D., Topaz, S. R. and Gott, V. L. 'The use of autogenous peritoneum for heart valve replacement', *Journal of thoracic and cardiovascular Surgery*, 60, 188 (1970)

[20] Garcia, D. P., Macruz, R., Pileggi, F., Arie, S., Galiano, N., Puig, L. B. and Décourt, L. V. 'Avaliação hemodinâmica em pórtadores de protese de dura mater em posição mitral', *Arquivo Brasileiro de Cardiologia*, 30, 29 (1977)

[21] Geha, A. S., Salaymel, M. T., Davis, G. L. and Baue, A. E. 'Replacement of the aortic valve with molded autogenous grafts grown in response to implanted silastic', *Journal of thoracic and cardiovascular Surgery*, 60, 661 (1970)

[22] Gilbert, C. S., Sullivan, G. J. and Laughein, J. J. 'Heart disease in pregnancy: ten years' report from the Lewis Memorial Maternity Hospital', *Obstetrics and Gynecology*, 9, 58 (1957)

[23] Gray, L. A. Jr., Fulton, R. L., Srivastava, T. N. and Flowers, N. C. 'Surgical treatment of thrombosed Björk–Shiley aortic valve prostheses', *Journal of thoracic and cardiovascular Surgery*, 71, 429 (1976)

[24] Hannah, H. III and Reis, R. L. 'Current status of porcine heterograft prostheses: a 5-year appraisal', *Circulation*, 51–52 (*Suppl. 2*), 30 (1975)

[25] Ionescu, M. I. and Ross, D. N. 'Heart valve replacement with autologous fascia lata', *Lancet*, 2, 335 (1969)

[26] Ionescu, M. I., Tandon, A. P., Mary, D. A. S. and Abid, A. 'Heart valve replacement with the Ionescu–Shiley pericardial xenograft', *Journal of thoracic and cardiovascular Surgery*, 73, 31 (1977)

[27] Isom, O. W., Williams, C. D., Falk, E. A., Glasman, E. and Spencer, F. C. 'Long-term evaluation of cloth-covered metallic ball prostheses', *Journal of thoracic and cardiovascular Surgery*, 64, 354 (1972)

²⁸ Maximow, A. A. and Bloom, W. *Tratado de Histologia*, p. 174. Buenos Aires; Labor (1947)

²⁹ Medoff, G., Kuvan, C. N. and Schlesinger, D. 'Potentiation of rifampicin and 5-fluorocytosin as antifungal antibiotics by amphotericin B', *Proceedings of the National Academy of Science of the USA*, 69, 196 (1972)

³⁰ Medoff, G. and Koabayashi, G. S. 'Amphotericin B. Old drug, new therapy', *Journal of the American medical Association*, 232, 619 (1975)

³¹ Mitha, A. S., Matisonn, R. E., Roux, B. T. and Chesler, E. 'Clinical experience with the Lillehei–Kaster cardiac valve prosthesis', *Journal of thoracic and cardiovascular Surgery*, 72, 401 (1976)

³² Pigossi, N. 'A glicerina na conservação de dura máter: estudo experimental'. Thesis, Faculdade de Medicina da Universidade de São Paulo. São Paulo (1967)

³³ Pluth, J. R. and McGoon, D. C. 'Estado actual del reemplazo de valvulas cardiacas', *Conceptos Modernos en Enfermedades Cardiovasculares*, 43, 1 (1974)

³⁴ Popa, G. T. 'Mechanostruktur und Mechanofunktion der Dura Mater der Menschen', *Morphologisches Jahrbuch*, 78, 85 (1936)

³⁵ Puig, L. B. and Verginelli, G. 'Válvulas cardíacas de dura máter homóloga', *Revista Paulista de Medicina*, 78, 33 (1971)

³⁶ Puig, L. B., Verginelli, G., Bellotti, G., Kawabe, L., Frack, C. C. R., Pileggi, F., Décourt, L. V. and Zerbini, E. J. 'Homologous dura mater cardiac valves. Preliminary study of 30 cases', *Journal of thoracic and cardiovascular Surgery*, 64, 154 (1972)

³⁷ Puig, L. B., Verginelli, G., Bellotti, G., Kawabe, L., Sosa, E., Pileggi, F., Décourt, L. V. and Zerbini, E. J. 'Substituição da valva aórtica por valva de dura máter homóloga', *Revista do Hospital das Clinicas da Universidade de São Paulo*, 29, 119 (1974)

³⁸ Puig, L. B., Verginelli, G., Kawabe, L. and Zerbini, E. J. 'Valva cardíaca de dura máter homólga. Método de preparação da valva', *Revista do Hospital das Clinicas da Faculdade de Medicina da Unversidade de São Paulo*, 29, 85 (1974)

³⁹ Puig, L. B., Verginelli, G., Bellotti, G., Iryia, K., Kawabe, L., Sosa, E. A., Pileggi, F. and Zerbini, E. J. 'Homologous dura mater cardiac valves. Study of 533 surgical cases', *Journal of thoracic and cardiovascular Surgery*, 69, 722 (1975)

⁴⁰ Puig, L. B. 'Substituição de valva mitral por valva de dura máter homóloga. Resultados tardios'. Thesis, Faculdade de Medicina da Universidade de São Paulo, São Paulo (1976)

⁴¹ Puig, L. B., Verginelli, G., Santana, G. P., Sosa, E. A., Castro, A. M., Pileggi, F. and Zerbini, E. J. 'Triplice troca por valva de dura máter. Relato de um caso', *Arquivo Brasileiro de Cardiologia*, 29, 59 (1976)

⁴² Puig, L. B., Verginelli, G., Sosa, E. A., Roma, L. S. L., Garcia, D. P., Conceição, A. N., Zerbini, E. J. and Pileggi, F. 'Avaliação hemodinâmica da valva de dura máter mitral e tricúspide', *Arquivo Brasileiro de Cardiologia*, 29, 297 (1976)

⁴³ Puig, L. B., Verginelli, G., Kawabe, L., Melo, R., Conceição, A., Bittencourt, D. and Zerbini, E. J. 'Four years' experience with dura mater cardiac valve', *Journal of cardiovascular Surgery*, 18, 247 (1977)

⁴⁴ Puig, L. B., Verginelli, G., Sosa, E., Roma, L. S. L., Garcia, D. P., Conceicão, A. N., Zerbini, E. J. and Pileggi, F. 'Avaliação hemodinâmica da valva de dura máter em posição aórtica', *Arquivo Brasileiro de Cardiologia*, 30, 59 (1977)

⁴⁵ Ramos, G., Aspeitia, D., Romero, E. G., Castillo-Olivares, J. L. and Figuera, D. 'Evaluation of physical properties of biological tissues that can be used for reconstruction of cardiac valves. An experimental study', *Journal of thoracic and cardiovascular Surgery*, 65, 359 (1973)

⁴⁶ Roberts, W. C., Bulkley, B. H. and Morrow, A. G. 'Pathologic anatomy of cardiac valve replacement. A study of 224 necropsy patients', *Progress in cardiovascular Diseases*, 13, 343 (1973)

⁴⁷ Roberts, W. C., Fishbein, M. C. and Golden, A. 'Cardiac pathology after valve replacement by disc prosthesis. A study of 61 necropsy patients', *American Journal of Cardiology*, 35, 740 (1975)

⁴⁸ Ross, D. N. 'Biologic valves. Their performance and prospects', *Circulation*, 45, 1259 (1972)

⁴⁹ Ross, D. N. and Parker, D. J. 'Current aspects of valve replacement'. In *Progress in Cardiology*. Ed. by P. N. Yu and J. F. Goodwin, p. 253. Philadelphia; Lea and Febiger (1974)

⁵⁰ Senning, A. 'Fascia lata replacement of aortic valve', *Journal of thoracic and cardiovascular Surgery*, 54, 465 (1967)

51 Sigler, A. T., Forman, E. N., Zinkhan, W. H. and Neill, C. A. 'Severe intravascular hemolysis following surgical repair of endocardial cushion defects', *American Journal of Medicine,* **35**, 467 (1963)

52 Starr, A., Herr, R. H. and Wood, J. A. 'Mitral replacement: review of six years' experience', *Journal of thoracic and cardiovascular Surgery,* **54**, 333 (1967)

53 Testut, L. and Jacob, O. *Anatomia Topografica.* p. 57. Barcelona; Salvat (1956)

54 Verginelli, G., Barbero-Marcial, M., Puig, L. B., Lemos, P. C. P., Sosa, E., Bittencourt, D. and Zerbini, E. J. 'Substituição da valva aórtica pela prótese de Starr–Edwards: experiência em 332 operados'. *Arquivo Brasileiro de Cardiologia,* **24**, 15 (1971)

55 Verginelli, G. 'Substituição de valva atrioventricular por valva de dura máter'. Thesis, Faculdade de Medicina da Universidade de São Paulo, São Paulo (1972)

56 Wersk, J. J., Ludington, L. G., Walker, W. J., Mundall, S. and Brewer, L. A. 'The occurrence and management of left atrial thrombi in mitral valve surgery', *Journal of cardiovascular Surgery,* **15**, 516 (1974)

57 Xavier, P. M., Devis, C. D. and Escudero, J. 'Fatal risks with the use of coumarin anticoagulants in pregnant patients with intracardiac ball valve prosthesis', *American Journal of Cardiology,* **24**, 853 (1969)

58 Zerbini, E. J. 'Results of replacement of cardiac valves by homologous dura mater valves', *Chest,* **67**, 706 (1975)

8

The Use of Valved Conduits in the Surgical Treatment of Congenital Heart Disease

Robert J. Szarnicki
Jaroslav Stark and
Marc R. de Leval

Le temps mûrit toutes choses; par temps toutes choses viennent en évidence; le temps est père de vérité.

François Rabelais (1494–1553)

INTRODUCTION

The use of valved conduits has permitted correction of cardiac lesions which, in the past, were considered uncorrectable. Continued research in the design and materials used in the construction of valved conduits employed today will hopefully reduce the incidence of complications related to the prosthesis itself.

HISTORICAL BACKGROUND

As early as 1913, Jeger[28] experimented in dogs with methods for the bypass of stenotic valves using an external cardiac conduit constructed from the jugular vein. He bypassed a stenotic aortic valve by anastomosing the vein proximally to a small left ventriculotomy and distally by end-to-end suture of the vein to the divided innominate artery. The animal survived four days and the conduit was seen to be patent at post-mortem examination. In 1948 Herwitt[26] inserted a pre-bent polyethylene tube between the right ventricle and the main pulmonary artery, using an experimental model in cats. Three of six animals survived surgery and two survived for 36 and 46 days respectively. At autopsy all prostheses were found to be occluded with thrombus. These experiments showed that a prosthesis could technically be used to restore ventricular to pulmonary artery continuity. Further work has been performed by Donovan[19] who used a vein segment with intact valves and a plastic ring at its proximal end to avoid anastomotic stenosis. In time, these conduits were all noted to shrink and become occluded by dense mediastinal scarring and vein wall thickening. In 1951 Donovan, Hufnagel and Eastcott[20] demonstrated that long-term patency was achieved by using conduits constructed from venous-lined plastic tubing. Gilbert, Corness and Cooper[24] were the first to experiment with a totally synthetic external cardiac conduit. Using a valveless Edwards–Tapp woven Teflon tube with a polyethylene sleeve at the ventricular anastomosis they demonstrated patency for 90 days or more in six of 15 conduits used experimentally. Haemodynamic studies revealed moderate elevations of right ventricular pressures and increase in the resting heart rate in these animals who were otherwise well. These changes were considered to be due to regurgitation through the valveless conduit. Glatzer and Herwitt[25] described a technique similar to that currently employed in which the pulmonary valve is bypassed. Following creation of an elliptical defect in the right ventricular wall, a woven Dacron tube with an obliquely cut proximal end was anastomosed to the ventricle, and the distal end to the pulmonary artery, following ligation of the main pulmonary artery.

The first successful clinical application of the use of an external conduit was reported by Rastelli and colleagues in 1965[48] in a six and a half year old child with pulmonary atresia, ventricular septal defect and coronary artery to pulmonary artery fistula with a functioning aortopulmonary shunt anastomosis. The repair was achieved by closing the ventricular septal defect with a Teflon patch. Right ventricular to pulmonary artery continuity was achieved with the insertion of a valveless conduit constructed from autogeneic pericardium. In 1965, Arai *et al.*[5] reported experiments using fresh aortic root allografts for the construction of conduits from the right ventricle to the pulmonary artery, and from the left ventricle to the pulmonary artery or to the aorta. This work suggested that the presence of a valved conduit would be preferable to a valveless tube. Cooley and Hallman[17] were the first to attempt the incorporation of a prosthetic valve in a conduit in two patients in order to restore right ventricular to pulmonary artery continuity. In 1966, Ross and Somerville[51] reported the first successful clinical use of an aortic root allograft in a patient with pulmonary atresia. The anterior leaflet of the mitral valve provided a gusset for enlarging the outflow tract of the right ventricle. After this initial clinical success, numerous centres began working on the techniques of preserving the aortic root allograft. Formaldehyde preservation, freeze-drying, ethylene oxide sterilization and irradiation sterilization were used. The discussion between the advocates of 'fresh viable' and 'preserved' allografts continues[27,35,52,60,64,66]. The fresh antibiotic preserved allograft (antibiotic sterilization and storage in a nutrient medium at $4\,^{\circ}$C) advocated by Ross continues to give satisfactory clinical results[2,8,23,42,43].

The major disadvantage of the fresh aortic allograft is its limited availability. Because of this, there is a growing interest in the field of preserved xenograft valves. The pioneering work of Carpentier[14] using the porcine xenograft led to the development of the stabilized glutaraldehyde preservation procedure which renders the valve inert and adds strength to the valve tissues by enhancing cross-linkage between collagen fibrils. The incorporation of a xenograft into a woven Dacron tube[12] has proved to be adaptable to most patients requiring the reconstruction of an outflow tract in either the pulmonary or systemic circulations.

Two types of external conduits were used in our first patients operated upon. One type consisted of a composite conduit incorporating an allograft aortic valve mounted inside a short segment of knitted Dacron tube which was extended proximally with a woven Dacron tube[13]. The second preparation was the Hancock composite xenograft aortic valve in a woven Dacron prosthetic tube.

TECHNIQUE OF CONDUIT INSERTION

When either the xenograft valved conduit or the fresh, antibiotic preserved, allograft is used, a number of fundamental technical points must be borne in mind in order to avoid anastomotic gradients and sternal compression of the conduit. Care must be taken to create the largest possible distal anastomosis while avoiding any distortion to the frequently small and friable pulmonary arteries. An appropriately tailored distal end of the conduit will usually suffice to extend the anastomosis beyond the bifurcation either to the right, or more often to the left pulmonary artery. To avoid distortion of the conduit valve annulus, the distal end of the conduit should be cut as short as possible to enable the valve annulus to sit near to the pulmonary artery bifurcation, and well away from the anterior chest wall. We frequently resect the thymus gland, particularly in small infants, to further reduce the risk of compression of the distal anastomosis.

The length of the conduit depends on the features of the particular anatomy. We estimate the length after completion of the distal anastomosis and with the aorta unclamped. When the heart regains its tone and starts contracting, the distance from the posterior wall of the conduit to the uppermost point of the ventriculotomy is assessed. The conduit is then cut to this point. Final trimming is illustrated in *Figure 8.1*. The trimming of the prosthesis follows the principles used in vascular surgery and thus secures a wide anastomosis to the ventricle. In

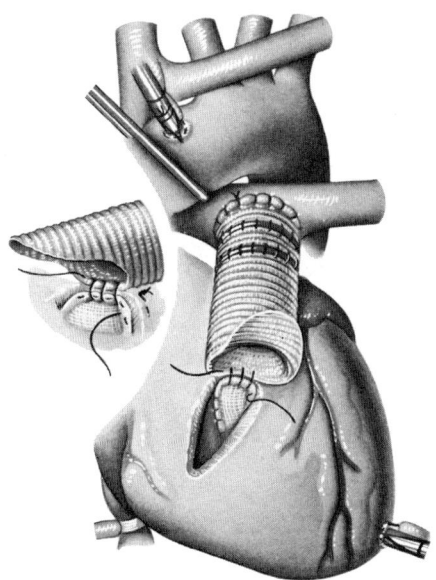

Figure 8.1 Trimming of the proximal end of the conduit which provides a very wide anastomosis. (Reproduced from Stark, J. 'Transposition of the great arteries. "The Rastelli Operation"'. In *Operative Surgery*, 3rd Edition. *Cardiothoracic Surgery*, Ed. by John W. Jackson, p. 130 (1978) by courtesy of Butterworths, London)

some defects, particularly truncus arteriosus and transposition of the great arteries, the ventricular septal defect patch extends to the superior aspect of the ventriculotomy to create a wide intraventricular tunnel. This avoids left ventricular outflow tract obstruction and also provides firm material for attachment of the conduit to the ventricle. Sutures are passed through the superior margin of the ventricular septal defect patch and then through the heel of the conduit bevel (*Figure 8.1*). This manoeuvre ensures haemostasis in the area which is difficult to achieve once the proximal anastomosis has been completed. The conduit is anastomosed to the margins of the ventriculotomy incision without excision of a button of muscle. If the anterior wall of the right ventricle is excessively thick, it can be thinned.

Appropriate positioning of the conduit is critical to avoid its anterior compression by the sternum. We endeavour to place the conduit in such a way as not to cross over the midline. The conduit usually lies to the left of the aorta. If compression of the conduit by the anterior chest wall is suspected, the pericardium is opened longitudinally posterior to the left phrenic nerve. The heart is then rotated posteriorly and to the left, moving the conduit away from the sternum[21]. This manoeuvre is particularly useful in small infants.

INDICATIONS

Valved conduits are currently used to establish continuity between cardiac chambers and the pulmonary circulation (cardiopulmonary conduits) or between the systemic ventricle and aorta. The insertion of cardiopulmonary conduits is indicated in: (i) complex forms of transposition of the great arteries (TGA); (ii) double outlet ventricles; (iii) single arterial trunk; (iv) absence of one atrioventricular valve; (v) coronary artery distribution incompatible with relief of valvar or subvalvar pulmonary stenosis; (vi) cases of atrioventricular discordance and univentricular hearts in which an intracardiac repair could damage the conduction system; (vii) patients in whom attempts to relieve pulmonary valve stenosis would produce pulmonary valve insufficiency in the presence of pulmonary hypertension.

The use of conduits between the systemic ventricle and the aorta is indicated for the relief of left ventricular outflow tract obstruction (LVOTO) not amenable to standard surgical techniques.

I. Transposition of the great arteries

The main indications for the use of external valved conduits in this group of patients is for either those with transposition of the great arteries (TGA) with ventricular septal defect (VSD) and left ventricular outflow tract obstruction (LVOTO) or for those with TGA, LVOTO and with intact ventricular septum.

(a) TGA with VSD and LVOTO

Early attempts to repair TGA in the presence of a VSD and severe LVOTO were associated with a high mortality rate. This was primarily related to the inability to adequately relieve the obstruction without damage to the adjacent structures. In 1969, Rastelli, McGoon and Wallace[47] conceived a new technique for the anatomic repair of this combination of anomalies based on the redirection of ventricular outflows. An intracardiac channel is constructed to connect the left ventricle to the aorta and an external valved conduit is inserted to establish continuity between the right ventricle and the pulmonary artery.

If present, a patent ductus arteriosus, or a surgically created systemic-pulmonary shunt, is controlled in the standard fashion when cardiopulmonary bypass is instituted. A wide ventriculotomy is then made from about the midpoint of the anterior wall of the right ventricle to the base of the heart towards the origin of the pulmonary artery (*Figure 8.2a*) and the intraventricular anatomy is assessed. The VSD should be enlarged if its diameter is smaller than that of the root of the aorta. The enlargement is carried out anteriorly and superiorly in order to avoid the conduction system and the attachment of the tricuspid valve.

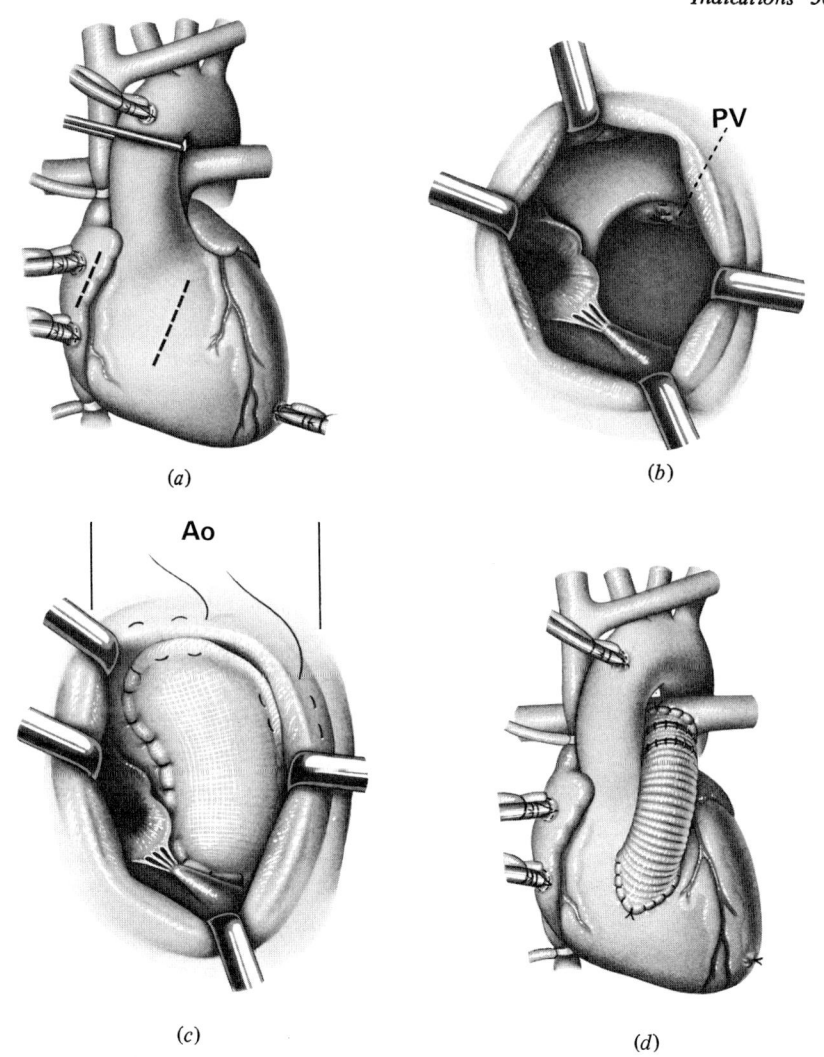

Figure 8.2 (*a*) The Rastelli Operation. The dotted line indicates the site of the right ventriculotomy. (Reproduced from Stark, J. 'Transposition of the great arteries. "The Rastelli Operation"'. In *Operative Surgery*, 3rd Edition. *Cardiothoracic Surgery*, Ed. by John. W. Jackson, p. 130 (1978) by courtesy of Butterworths, London)

(*b*) The Rastelli Operation. The pulmonary valve was closed by approximating its cusps through the ventricular septal defect. (Reproduced from Stark, J. 'Transposition of the great arteries. "The Rastelli Operation"'. In *Operative Surgery*, 3rd Edition. *Cardiothoracic Surgery*, Ed. by John W. Jackson p. 130 (1978) by courtesy of Butterworths, London)

(*c*) The Rastelli Operation. The intraventricular tunnel is completed by attaching the cephalad end of the patch to the upper margin of the ventriculotomy. (Reproduced from Stark, J. 'Transposition of the great arteries. 'The Rastelli Operation"'. In *Operative Surgery*, 3rd Edition. *Cardiothoracic Surgery*, Ed. by John W. Jackson, p. 130 (1978) by courtesy of Butterworths, London)

(*d*) The Rastelli Operation completed. The composite valved conduit, was sutured directly to the pulmonary artery and proximally to the right ventriculotomy. (Reproduced from Stark, J. 'Transposition of the great arteries. "The Rastelli Operation"'. In *Operative Surgery*, 3rd Edition. *Cardiothoracic Surgery*, Ed. by John W. Jackson, p. 130 (1978) by courtesy of Butterworths, London)

If accessible through the VSD, the pulmonary valve is closed by approximating the cusps with a running stitch (*Figure 8.2b*). A tunnel is then constructed from the left ventricle to the aorta by means of a prosthetic patch, the cephalad end of which is anchored to the upper end of the ventriculotomy (*Figure 8.2c*). The pulmonary artery is doubly ligated above the pulmonary valve and continuity between the right ventricle and the pulmonary artery is then established with a valved conduit (*Figure 8.2d*). Alternatively, the pulmonary artery can be divided, the proximal ventricular end oversewn and an end-to-end anastomosis performed between the distal ends of the pulmonary artery and the conduit.

Although insertion of an external valved conduit is technically possible in infancy, we still prefer to postpone the Rastelli operation until the age of three to five years, and to perform a systemic to pulmonary artery shunt in infants and small children who need surgery before that age as the risk of a shunt operation is low in this group of children. At a later date, i.e. at the age of three to five years, an adult size valved conduit can be used.

The concept of the Rastelli operation has also been applied to patients with TGA and large VSDs who have undergone pulmonary artery banding. When the intraventricular anatomy is suitable, we prefer to carry out a Rastelli operation rather than the combination of the Mustard procedure, closure of the VSD and debanding of the pulmonary artery.

(b) TGA with LVOTO and intact ventricular septum

Pressure gradients across the left ventricular outflow tract are common in infants with simple TGA. In the majority of children, it is believed that the gradients are functional because of the excessive blood flow through this area[18,56]. This gradient is usually abolished following redirection of the venous inflow. Various anatomic types of outflow tract obstruction have been described in patients with TGA[55,56,63]. They include: (i) subvalvar membrane; (ii) abnormal attachment of the anterior leaflet of the mitral valve; (iii) bulging of the muscular interventricular septum; (iv) fibromuscular tunnel; (v) valvar and supravalvar stenosis; (vi) aneurysm of the membranous septum. Apart from the rare cases of aneurysms or diaphragms which can be resected, and the cases of pulmonary valve stenosis, the surgical relief of these obstructions is difficult because of the risk of injury to the mitral valve and the conduction system. The presence of the left circumflex coronary artery traversing this region anterior to the pulmonary artery precludes surgical widening of the LVOTO.

Patients with TGA tolerate mild to moderate gradient across the left ventricular outflow tract quite well following the Mustard operation. We, therefore, accept left ventricular pressures up to systemic levels as long as the pulmonary artery pressure remains normal, or near normal. In those children in whom the left ventricular pressure is at suprasystemic levels, a valved external conduit, connecting the apex of the left ventricle and the pulmonary artery, is inserted following the Mustard operation[38,57]. A short apical ventriculotomy is first performed parallel to the left anterior descending coronary artery. The incision is then extended once the papillary muscles of the mitral valve have been visualized. The conduit is bevelled and sutured to the left ventriculotomy. For this suture line we prefer to buttress the stitches with two strips of Teflon felt. The posterior pericardium is opened to allow the conduit to lie to the left and behind the heart. The proximal anastomosis to the pulmonary artery is then performed.

In 1976, McGoon[38] suggested the use of biventricular conduits from the right ventricle to the pulmonary artery, and from the left ventricle to the aorta, as an alternative repair. More data will be required in order to assess the performance and the clinical results with both the left ventricle to pulmonary artery conduits and the biventricular conduits.

II. Double outlet ventricles

The double outlet situation can be defined as that in which more than one and a half great arteries arise from the same ventricular chamber. Double outlet ventricles can exist with atrioventricular concordance or atrioventricular discordance. We will consider here only patients with atrioventricular concordance. Patients with atrioventricular discordance will be discussed in Section VI of this Chapter.

(a) Double outlet right ventricle (DORV)

Numerous anatomic variants of DORV can be encountered according to the position of the aorta and pulmonary artery, the location of the VSD and the presence, or absence of pulmonary stenosis. The main indications to use extracardiac valved conduits in DORV are for the following anatomic situations:

(i) DORV with subpulmonic VSD in which an internal baffle connecting the left ventricle to the aorta through the VSD is constructed and an external conduit is used to connect the right ventricle and the pulmonary artery. Alternatively, the repair may consist of an internal baffle connecting the left ventricle to the pulmonary artery through the VSD followed by a Mustard procedure.

(ii) DORV with doubly committed VSD and with or without pulmonary stenosis can be managed with an internal baffle from the VSD to the aorta, closure of the pulmonary artery and placement of an external conduit from the right ventricle to the pulmonary artery.

(iii) DORV with non-committed VSD and with or without pulmonary stenosis can also be treated with an external conduit or by using an intraventricular repair[32].

(b) Double outlet left ventricle (DOLV)

This anatomic entity is a rare malformation. The precise spatial interrelations between the semilunar valves and the VSD have to be assessed before deciding on the type of repair. A rerouting of the ventricular outflow tracts has been described in patients without associated pulmonary stenosis[54]. However, in most reported cases, external valved conduits have been used between the right ventricle and the pulmonary artery[45].

III. Single arterial trunk

In this section we include patients with persistent truncus arteriosus and patients with pulmonary atresia and VSD.

(a) Persistent truncus arteriosus

This is a rare condition which accounts for less than 3 per cent of all congenital heart defects[29]. We define persistent truncus arteriosus as that condition in which a single arterial trunk leaves the heart via a single semilunar valve and which gives rise directly to the coronary, systemic and one or both pulmonary arteries. The pulmonary arteries may originate from a short pulmonary trunk or separately from the persistent truncus. Wide separation (Collett and Edwards, Type III)[15] may cause technical problems during repair. Patients with Collett and Edwards Type IV[15] truncus arteriosus, in whom the lungs are supplied from the systemic arteries, should be grouped with patients having pulmonary atresia. The crucial factors influencing surgical results in this group of patients are the early development of pulmonary vascular disease and the presence of truncal

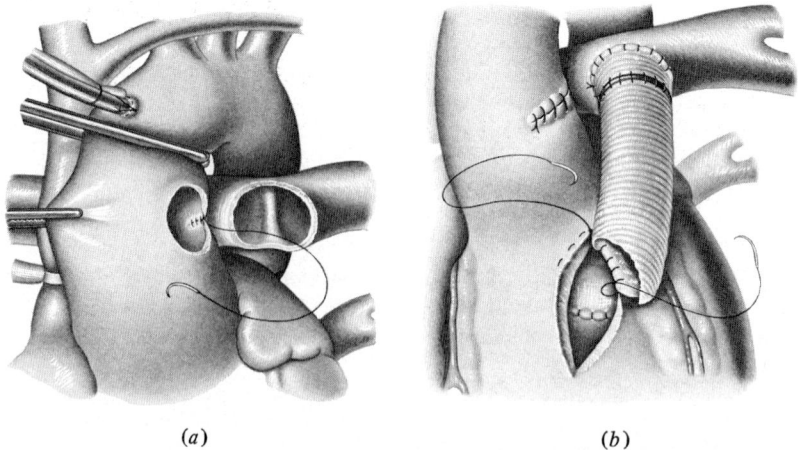

(a)   (b)

Figure 8.3 (a) Surgical repair of persistent truncus arteriosus. Following the detachment of the pulmonary arteries from the truncus, the defect into the aorta is closed with a continuous suture line. (Reproduced from de Leval, M. R. 'Persistent truncus arteriosus'. In *Operative Surgery,* 3rd Edition. *Cardiothoracic Surgery,* Ed. by John W. Jackson, p. 142 (1978) by courtesy of Butterworths, London)

(b) Surgical repair of persistent truncus arteriosus. The correction is completed by the proximal anastomosis. The external valved conduit is being sutured to the right ventriculotomy. (Reproduced from de Leval, M. R. 'Persistent truncus arteriosus'. In *Operative Surgery*, 3rd Edition. *Cardiothoracic Surgery,* Ed. by John W. Jackson, p. 142 (1978) by courtesy of Butterworths, London)

valve incompetence. Prior to successful attempts at complete correction in infancy, pulmonary artery banding has been recommended as palliation to enable delay of corrective surgery until the children were four to five years old. Until recently, the corrective operation was performed in older children, usually after the age of five years. Pulmonary artery banding used to be the only surgical technique available in infancy. Because of the high risk with this procedure[46,59] and the fact that without operation most patients either died or developed severe pulmonary vascular obstructive disease, correction of persistent truncus arteriosus in infancy has been suggested[3,7,21,57,58,61,62]. The pulmonary arteries are excised from the truncus and the defect thus created is closed by direct suture (*Figure 8.3a*). A vertical incision is then performed in the anterior wall of the right ventricle at a sufficient distance from the level of the truncal valve and the left anterior descending coronary artery. The VSD is closed with a Dacron patch so that the left ventricle empties into the aorta. The patch is attached superiorly to the upper margin of the ventriculotomy, the distal end of the valved conduit attached to the pulmonary artery and the proximal end anastomosed to the margins of the ventriculotomy to complete the repair (*Figure 8.3b*).

(b) Pulmonary atresia with VSD

The anatomy in pulmonary atresia may consist of pulmonary valve atresia only, atresia of the main pulmonary artery, or the so-called absence of one or both pulmonary arteries. The anatomy of the vessels providing pulmonary blood supply is established by aortography and by multiple selective injections of contrast medium into the aortopulmonary anastomosis or the pulmonary arteries[34]. The central pulmonary arteries (derived from the embryological sixth aortic arch) may be supplied via a persistent ductus arteriosus, a surgical systemic to pulmonary shunt, major aortopulmonary collateral arteries or a combination of the above. According to the distribution of the pulmonary blood flow the patients can be divided into two groups:

(1) patients with unifocal pulmonary blood supply in whom the sixth aortic arch anastomosed with the systemic artery or arteries provides a single focus for all systemic sources of pulmonary blood supply, and
(2) patients with multifocal pulmonary blood supply in whom one or more aortopulmonary collateral arteries provide pulmonary blood supply independent of the sixth aortic arch.

Indications for operation must be carefully considered. A complete repair can be performed only in patients in whom the pulmonary vascular resistance is compatible with satisfactory right ventricular function. An increased pulmonary arteriolar resistance can be due to the development of pulmonary vascular disease or to the small size of these pulmonary arteries which sometimes only perfuse part of the lungs' parenchyma.

If the pulmonary vascular resistance is expected to be within normal limits, the surgical repair consists of careful control of all systemic to pulmonary connections, closure of the VSD so that the left ventricle empties into the aorta and connection of the right ventricle to the pulmonary artery with an outflow tract patch or an external valved conduit depending on the anatomy of the lesion. Large aortopulmonary collaterals can be ligated either through a midline sternotomy approach or through a separate lateral thoracotomy. If midline sternotomy is used the dissection is usually carried out on heart-lung bypass. If, on the other hand, the dissection of the collaterals is performed through a lateral thoracotomy this is done before the heart-lung bypass is instituted. In some patients we still prefer to dissect the collaterals from a separate thoracotomy. The vessels are dissected and encircled with ligatures which are not tied. The thoracotomy is closed, a midline sternotomy performed and the patient placed on cardiopulmonary bypass. The pleura is then opened widely, ligatures identified and collateral vessels safely ligated. The control of surgically created aortopulmonary shunts is performed in the usual way.

IV. Absence of one atrioventricular valve

(a) Tricuspid atresia

In 1971, Fontan and Baudet[23] described a new approach for the surgical treatment of tricuspid atresia in which the entire systemic venous return is rerouted into the lungs before entering the left side of the heart. This was achieved by closure of the atrial septal defect and conversion of the right atrium into a closed unidirectional pumping chamber using a valved conduit. The authors initially believed that in addition to the right atrial-pulmonary connection, both a superior vena cava–pulmonary anastomosis and a valve in the inferior vena cava were necessary. It has since been shown that the entire venous return from both cavae can be directed from the right atrium to the main pulmonary artery and that an atriocaval valve was not indispensable to prevent stasis and inadequate cardiac filling. Fontan now uses a valved conduit (aortic root allograft) to connect the right atrial appendage with the pulmonary artery in the treatment of tricuspid atresia with transposed great arteries (Type II). When the great arteries are normally related (Type I), a valveless Dacron conduit is interposed between the right atrium and the right ventricle. Bowman[11] uses an alternative approach in which the small right ventricular chamber is opened widely and, if necessary, the whole anterior wall incised. A valved conduit (Hancock composite bioprosthesis) is inserted between the right atrium and the widely opened right ventricle. The patient's pulmonary valve is thus preserved. Following this type of repair post-operative cardiac catheterization revealed ventricular pressure tracings within the conduit, distal to the valve. In patients with pulmonary valve stenosis, the distal end of the conduit can be extended as an outflow patch across the annulus into the main pulmonary artery. The factors to be emphasized in the selection of patients for this type of surgical treatment are the presence of normal pulmonary arteriolar resistance and normal left ventricular function. As far as the surgical technique is concerned, the following points are of particular importance. In order to avoid any impairment of the contractile function of the right atrium the venae cavae should be cannulated directly and the incision for the suture of the conduit should be limited to the right auricular appendage. Great care must be taken to completely close the atrial septal defect in order to eliminate any possibility of post-operative right-to-left shunting at atrial level. As large a conduit as possible should be used to eliminate gradients across the valve. At present, we prefer to use the aortic root allograft.

(b) Univentricular hearts

An extension of the technique described by Fontan and Baudet[23] for the repair of tricuspid atresia has permitted repair of certain forms of univentricular hearts. In this group of anomalies, the cases with right atrioventricular valve atresia seem to be the best indications for a Fontan type of repair. However, some surgeons have applied the same principle to treat univentricular hearts with two atrioventricular valves or a common atrioventricular valve. In those patients, the connection between the right-sided atrial chamber and the ventricular chamber has to be interrupted and closed with a patch. Right atrial hypertrophy, however, does not usually develop as much as in patients with tricuspid atresia. A superior vena cava–pulmonary anastomosis should be performed when the right atrial pressure is too high at the end of the operation.

V. Abnormal coronary arteries traversing the outflow tract

Abnormal distribution of coronary arteries, namely the left anterior descending branch originating from the right coronary artery and traversing the outflow tract of the right ventricle may preclude the use of outflow tract enlargement by a patch. Recognition of an abnormal location of the coronary arteries is imperative to avoid intraoperative injury. The vessel may be intramyocardial, and recognition by examination of the topical anatomy may be impossible. In cases where pericardial adhesions are anticipated because of previous intrapericardial surgical procedures, and also prior to corrective cardiac operations in infancy, pre-operative selective coronary angiography would seem warranted. In a series of 926 patients[41] with tetralogy of Fallot who underwent total correction, 23 patients were found to have anomalous coronary artery distribution. Twenty-two of these had the left anterior descending coronary artery arising from the right coronary artery and one patient had a right coronary artery arising from the anterior descending branch of the left coronary artery. Two patients in this series died of myocardial failure in the post-operative period because of injury to the anterior descending coronary artery.

In the majority of cases, an appropriate transverse or oblique ventriculotomy can be made to avoid injury to the abnormal vessels, and the repair can be carried out successfully through this approach. If the pulmonary annulus is hypoplastic, enlargement of this region by a patch is not possible without risk of injury to the coronary arteries. In those unusual situations, a valved conduit from an appropriately placed right ventriculotomy to the pulmonary artery should be used.

VI. Anatomy of the conduction system

Surgical relief of subvalvar pulmonary stenosis in cases of atrioventricular discordance and septation of univentricular hearts carries a significant risk of producing complete atrioventricular block. This is related to the peculiar anatomy of the conduction system in these conditions[1,4,65].

(a) Defects with atrioventricular discordance

An anterior atrioventricular node located at the junction of the right auricular appendage with the anterior interatrial septum has been identified[4]. This node connects with the atrioventricular bundle near to the right anterior aspect of the pulmonary valve annulus. In patients with VSD, the bundle was noted to follow a course along the superior margin of the septal defect. Avoidance of this area during surgical closure of the defect is mandatory if the occurrence of complete heart block is to be prevented. The presence of pulmonary stenosis presents an additional hazard during operative correction. When a subvalvar obstruction is present, the insertion of a valved conduit from the morphologic left ventricle to the pulmonary artery will decrease the risks of complete heart block.

(b) The conduction tissue in univentricular hearts with an outlet chamber

This is also usually situated anteriorly at the base of the heart between the semilunar valves[65]. When pulmonary stenosis is present, the intraventricular septation patch should be placed to the right side of the semilunar valves and a valved conduit is then used to connect the pulmonary ventricle with the pulmonary artery. For cases without pulmonary stenosis, the intracardiac repair alone could be tried. Because of the danger of injury to the conduction system while placing the sutures between the two semilunar valves, it may be preferable to use a conduit even in patients who do not have pulmonary stenosis[40].

VII. Pulmonary valve incompetence in patients with pulmonary hypertension

Pulmonary valve incompetence and pulmonary hypertension may result from patch enlargement of the right ventricular outflow tract across the pulmonary valve annulus in the following circumstances:

(1) pulmonary vascular obstructive disease following systemic to pulmonary artery shunt,
(2) absence of one pulmonary artery,
(3) abnormal origin of one pulmonary artery from the ascending aorta with pulmonary vascular obstructive disease in the lung supplied by that pulmonary artery,
(4) hypoplastic pulmonary arteries.

Pulmonary incompetence which may lead to severe right ventricular failure can be avoided by either the insertion of a valved conduit between the right ventricle and the pulmonary artery therefore providing a competent pulmonary valve, or by insertion of an allograft or a xenograft valve in the pulmonary position together with an outflow tract patch.

Left ventricle to aorta conduits

Various causes of obstruction of the left ventricular outflow tract are encountered. Direct relief of the obstruction is preferable, but significant residual gradients
were observed in some patients following such techniques. Frustrated by many
of the direct approach techniques for the relief of LVOTO, Sarnoff, Donovan
and Case[54] demonstrated, in 1955, that bypassing the aortic outflow tract by
means of a shunt from the apex of the left ventricle to the descending aorta
was feasible. In 1962, Templeton was the first to apply this technique clinically
using a rigid lucite tube. Although his work has never been published, one
patient apparently survived 13 years with the prosthesis in place. In 1975,
Bernard, Poirier and LaFarge[10] implanted a stainless steel tube connected to a
conduit containing a Hancock porcine xenograft valve in a 20 year old patient
with congenital aortic stenosis and hypoplasia of the ascending aorta. The
patient's post-operative course was uneventful and at follow-up eight weeks
post-operatively he was in excellent condition. More recently Cooley[16] reported
the successful use of a curved semi-rigid apical conduit connected to a Hancock
bioprosthesis in 15 patients. He placed the conduit between the left ventricular
apex and the abdominal aorta, proximal to the coeliac vessels. The application of
this technique to a number of congenital lesions causing obstruction to left
ventricular ejection is appealing and the initial results with its use are encouraging.

Very limited experience is available with this approach in small infants. An
alternative approach for the relief of severe LVOTO has been described by
Konno and colleagues[32] and Rastan and Konez[49]. Such a technique involves an
incision through the aortic annulus, the right ventricle and interventricular
septum. A patch is then inserted into the septum, right ventricle and ascending
aorta in such a way as to widen the outflow from the left ventricle to the aorta.
The aortic valve is replaced with a larger valve substitute, that would have fitted
prior to this procedure. Further experience with this technique as well as with
the left ventricle to aorta conduits will be needed for better evaluation of the
results.

RESULTS

It would be most valuable, in reviewing results of these operations, if we were
able to assess the results for each individual category of lesions for which the
technique was employed. A complete review of the available data, however,
makes this almost impossible and we shall briefly review only the results published from a few cardiac centres.

The Mayo Clinic group recently reported the early and late results of the
Rastelli operation[36] and the results of the surgical repair of truncus arteriosus[37].
From July 1968 to September 1975, 59 consecutive patients underwent Rastelli
operation at the Mayo Clinic. In this group of patients the operative mortality
was 19 per cent and the late mortality 13 per cent. Re-operation was required in
11 patients. Stenosis of the aortic allograft became severe enough to require re-
operation in eight patients. Two patients were re-operated upon for recurrent
ventricular septal defect and one patient for subaortic stenosis. The high incidence of re-operation for stenosis of the aortic allograft conduit (eight out of 25

patients) is perhaps related to the position of the conduit which, in transposition of the great arteries, often crosses the midline and might be compressed by the sternum. This would perhaps explain the difference between the higher incidence of conduit stenosis in patients with transposition of the great arteries when compared with the lower one encountered in patients having conduit repair for truncus arteriosus (two out of 39 patients), or for pulmonary atresia (two out of 13 patients) also reported from the Mayo Clinic. Between 1967 and 1975, 92 patients had corrective operations for truncus arteriosus at the Mayo Clinic. The overall hospital mortality in this entire series was 25 per cent but the more recent mortality rate for the last 33 operations was only 9 per cent and the overall late mortality was also 9 per cent. The age distribution of the patients reported is of some interest since only six were less than two years of age. The presence of significant truncal valve regurgitation increased the technical difficulty of the operation, but did not appear to represent a substantial early risk factor in that series. The degree of pulmonary vascular obstructive disease increases the operative mortality and the probability of poor late results or late deaths.

Behrendt *et al.*[9] reported 12 cases of truncus arteriosus Types I and II with five deaths (41 per cent mortality). The age range in this series was six months to 16 years with a median age of eight years. In one patient an unsuccessful attempt was made to directly anastomose the proximal end of the pulmonary artery to the right ventricle. Four patients in this series were corrected with valveless conduits of Teflon or Dacron cloth. Three patients survived the operation and two remained well nine and 11 years post-operatively respectively. One of these three patients developed severe stenosis of the proximal anastomosis and had his Teflon tube replaced, one year following its insertion, with a fresh aortic root allograft. The remaining seven patients received antibiotic sterilized fresh aortic root allografts and five of them survived the operation. One patient died two years following operation, from a massive pulmonary embolus and four patients remained well one to five years post-operatively. Four of the survivors had systolic and diastolic murmurs post-operatively. One patient developed severe calcification of the allograft conduit and underwent successful replacement with a second allograft and was well one year later.

The Boston group[44] has recently reported its experience with valved conduits in 56 patients. The age range was 15 days to 33 years (median 11 years). The first four patients in this series received frozen irradiated aortic allografts and the remainder had Dacron conduits containing a porcine aortic valve (Hancock Laboratories) inserted. The spectrum of lesions treated in this series is shown in *Table 8.1*. It is interesting to note that the patients with tetralogy of Fallot represented 57 per cent of the total series of patients receiving conduits. We, as well as others[30], believe that outflow patch reconstruction remains the preferred treatment for this group of patients. In our own experience, from the total number of patients treated with valved conduits, only 3 per cent had tetralogy of Fallot. Late results from the Boston series[50] are very encouraging as shown in the actuarial survival rate curves (*Figure 8.4*). When hospital deaths are excluded from the analysis, the expected survival rate at 48 months' follow-up is in the region of 90 per cent.

Haemodynamic investigations of 16 patients who had valved conduits inserted at the Children's Hospital in Boston were carried out six months to five years post-operatively. All four patients who had frozen irradiated aortic allograft conduits demonstrated some degree of calcification and all had severe obstruction. However, none had evidence of pulmonary insufficiency.

TABLE 8.1
Distribution of congenital cardiac lesions repaired at Boston Children's Hospital

Lesion	Number of defects	Mortality	
		Hospital	Late
Tetralogy of Fallot	32	4	1
Pulmonary atresia	23*		
Single pulmonary artery	10		
Double outlet RV	2	–	–
TGA (S, D, D)	9		
VSD and PS	7	–	1
HRV and OTV†	1	1	–
Single ventricle	1	1	–
TGA (S, L, L), VSD and PS∮	2	–	1
Tricuspid atresia†	2	1	–
Truncus arteriosus communis	8	4	–
Pulmonary atresia and IVS†	1	1	–
Total	56	12 (21%)	3 (7%)

*One patient had both pulmonary atresia and single pulmonary artery
†Conduit interposed between RA and PA
∮Conduit interposed between LV and PA

TGA = transposition of the great arteries, VSD = ventricular septal defect, PS = sub-pulmonic stenosis, HRV = hypoplastic right ventricle, OTV = overriding tricuspid valve, IVS = intact ventricular septum, RV = right ventricle, PA = pulmonary artery, RA = right atrium, LV = left ventricle

(Reproduced from Norwood et al.[44], by courtesy of Annals of thoracic Surgery)

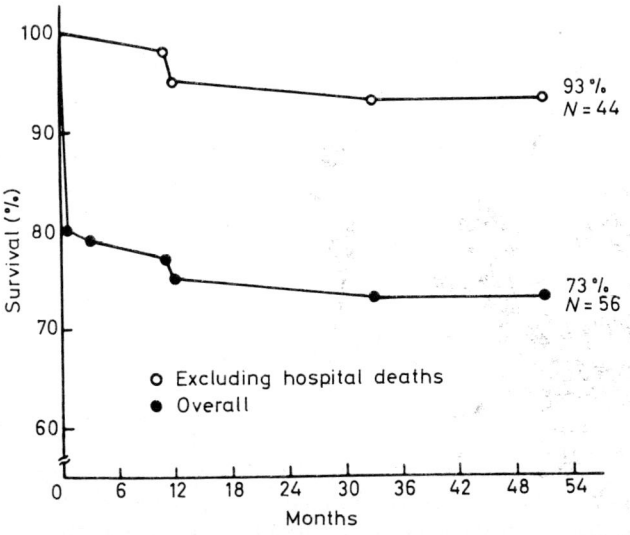

Figure 8.4 Actuarial survival curves for patients having corrective surgery with cardio-pulmonary valved conduits at Boston Children's Hospital. (Reproduced from Norwood, W. I. et al.[44], by courtesy of Annals of Thoracic Surgery)

In 12 patients having Hancock conduits, pressure gradients were measured between the body of the right ventricle and the pulmonary arteries. Selective pressure recordings made along the course of the conduit revealed three sites of obstruction: at the proximal anastomosis, at valve level and at the distal anastomosis. Six of 12 patients investigated had mild to severe pressure gradients at the site of the proximal anastomosis (range 9–60 mmHg). We consider that these gradients are completely avoidable by careful tailoring of the conduit to ensure the largest possible anastomosis and by creating an acute angular take-off from the ventricle to avoid kinking. Careful placement of the conduit to prevent sternal compression will also help to avoid this problem. Four patients demonstrated pressure gradients at the level of the porcine valve (range 11–42 mmHg). Two of these patients received size 16 conduits, while the remaining two had sizes 18 and 20. The specific cause of valvular gradients is currently believed to be due to the presence of the septal muscle which supports the base of the right coronary cusp of the porcine valve. This muscle bar limits the mobility of the right coronary cusp and therefore reduces the effective opening of the valve. This haemodynamic drawback increases progressively as the valve sizes decrease. Evaluation of a modified porcine valve is currently in progress. In this new preparation the right coronary cusp and attached septal muscle has been removed and replaced with a non-muscular cusp from another porcine valve. The durability of this newer bioprosthesis remains unknown at this time.

Eight of the 12 patients investigated were found to have pressure gradients at the distal anastomosis (range 3–62 mmHg). The most common cause of distal gradient was considered to be the presence of small, deformed pulmonary arteries secondary to previous systemic to pulmonary shunts. Varying degrees of hypoplasia of peripheral pulmonary arteries was also believed to be a contributing factor. These findings emphasize the importance of a meticulous surgical technique for the creation of the distal anastomosis and for the reconstruction of pulmonary arteries whose anatomy has been altered by previous palliative surgical procedures. Careful positioning of the conduit must also be emphasized as this will avoid any distortion of the distal anastomosis which can easily occur when pulmonary arteries are small and friable. We also consider that thymectomy is frequently a helpful adjunct in these patients in avoiding external compression of the distal anastomosis.

At the University of Alabama[6] 85 patients have survived operation with insertion of a valved conduit. Follow-up data (mean follow-up time 27.7 months) was available for 83 patients. In the first half of this series, 35 patients received a valved conduit constructed of frozen, irradiated allograft aortic roots. In the remaining 48 patients, Hancock xenograft conduits were used.

Seven of 83 patients have required re-operation for obstructive complications. In five patients, sternal compression was the primary cause of obstruction. Actuarial analysis of this group reveals that the proportion of patients requiring re-operation is 4.0 ± 2.8 per cent at two years, 12.9 ± 5.5 per cent at three and a half years and 30.4 ± 12.1 per cent at five years' follow-up (*Figure 8.5*). An analysis of patients exposed to the risk of re-operation for conduit compression is shown in *Figure 8.6*. The comparison of results by actuarial analysis of patients with allograft conduits and Hancock conduits suggests no significant difference in the incidence of obstructive complications with either type of conduit (*Figure 8.7*). The long-term survival in this series is similar to that reported by the Boston group at 24 and 36 months post-operatively (91.5 per cent and 86.7 per

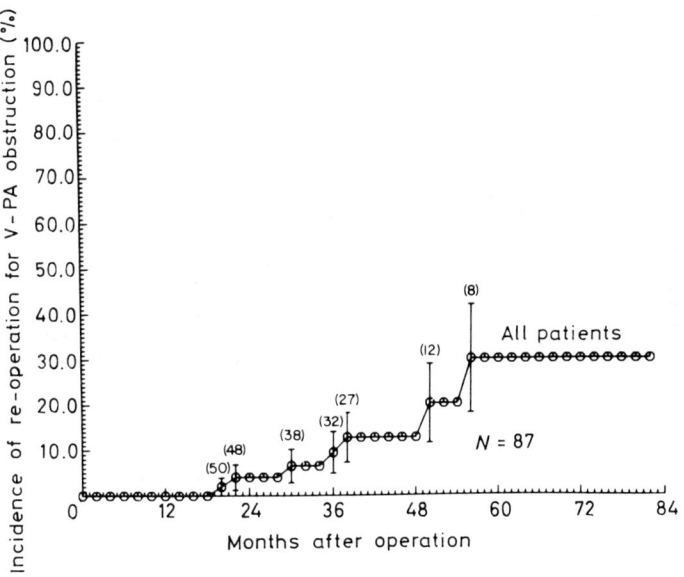

Figure 8.5 Actuarial incidence of obstruction requiring re-operation after restoration of ventricle to pulmonary artery continuity using valved conduits. (Reproduced from Bailey, W. W. *et al.*[6], by courtesy of *Circulation*)

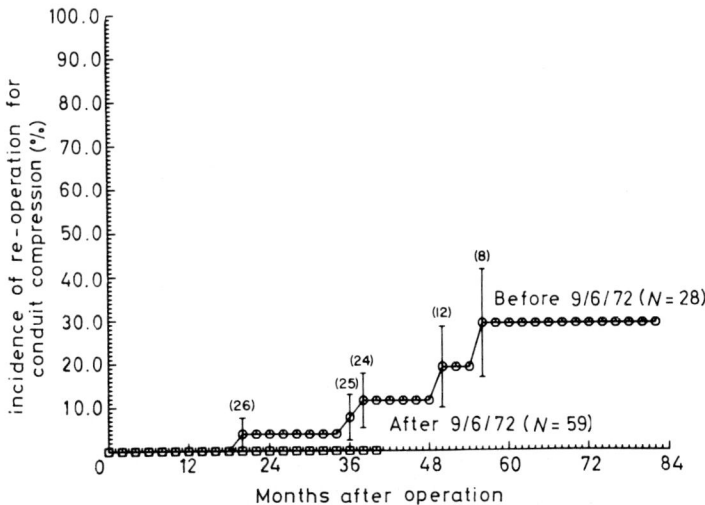

Figure 8.6 Actuarial incidence of re-operation for conduit compression. Comparison of two groups of patients: those operated upon prior to 6 September 1972 (○) and those operated upon after September 1972 (□). (Reproduced from Bailey, W. W. *et al.*[6], by courtesy of *Circulation*)

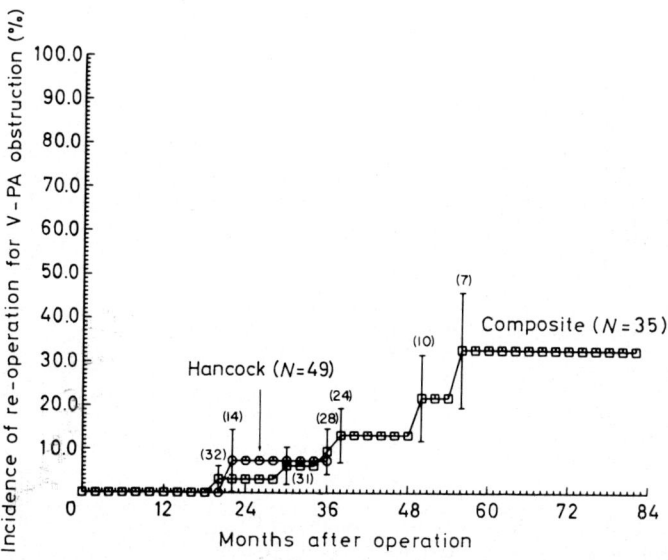

Figure 8.7 Actuarial incidence of ventriculopulmonary conduit obstruction requiring re-operation. Comparison of two types of conduits: Hancock bioprosthesis (○) and composite Dacron allograft valved conduit (□). (Reproduced from Bailey, W. W. *et al.*[6], by courtesy of *Circulation*)

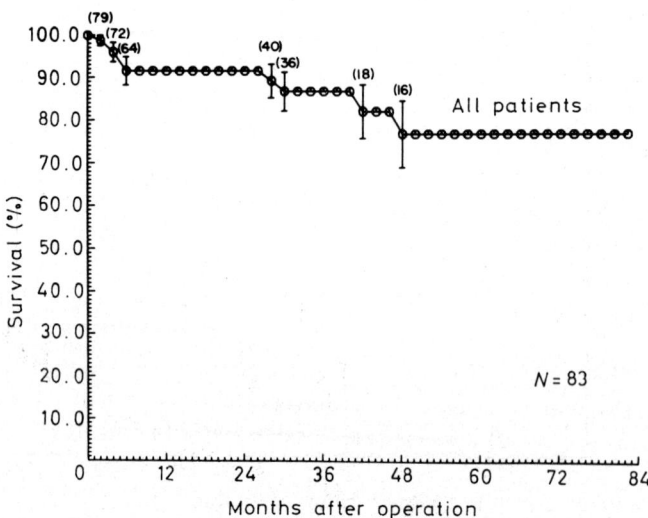

Figure 8.8 Actuarial survival curve of all patients who had cardiopulmonary conduits inserted at the University of Alabama Medical Center. (Reproduced from Bailey, W. W. *et al.*[6], by courtesy of *Circulation*)

cent respectively) (*Figure 8.8*). The five-year survival rate is 76.7 per cent. Again, no difference was noted between the allograft group and the group receiving Hancock bioprostheses.

During a period of ten years' experience with valved conduits for the correction of congenital heart defects, Malm and Bowman[11], at Columbia University, employed this technique in 69 patients (*Table 8.2*). The first 22 patients in their series received frozen, irradiated aortic allografts and the remaining 47 patients received Hancock porcine conduits. Their first patient, operated upon in March 1967, had an allograft inserted and he remains well more than ten years postoperatively. The conduit is calcified, there is mild valvular insufficiency with a pressure gradient of 20 mmHg across the valve, but he remains completely asymptomatic with no exercise limitation. In May 1971, Bowman inserted the first Hancock bioprosthesis in an eight year old child with ventricular septal defect and pulmonary atresia. Follow-up shows that he remains well with an insignificant pressure gradient across the porcine valve.

The age range in this group was seven weeks to 41 years. The spectrum of lesions encountered in this series is detailed in *Table 8.2*. Thirty-three of the survivors were restudied after operation. Significant obstruction was found in four patients with aortic allografts (one was re-operated upon, one died suddenly and two are well but with pressure gradients across the allografts measuring 60 and 100 mmHg).

TABLE 8.2
Restoration of right ventricular–pulmonary artery continuity with valved conduits at Columbia Presbyterian Medical Center, 1967–1977

Diagnosis of lesions	*Patients*	*Previous shunts*	*Mortality*	
			Hospital	*Late*
VSD and pulmonary atresia	12 (5)	8 (3)	1 –	2 (1)
Tetralogy of Fallot	3 (5)	2 (4)	– –	– (1)
Absent pulmonary valve	– (2)	– –	– –	– –
'Hermitruncus'	1 (1)	1 –	1 –	– –
Truncus arteriosus				
Types I to III	8 (3)	– –	2 –	– (1)
Type IV	2 (1)	– –	– (1)	– –
Transposition of the great arteries with VSO and PS	9 –	4 –	– –	– –
Corrected transposition with VSP and PS	6 (3)	1 (1)	– –	– (1)
Pulmonary atresia with IVS	2 (1)	2 (1)	– –	– –
Miscellaneous	4 (1)	1 (1)	2 (1)	– –
Total	47 (22) = 69	19 (10) = 29	6 (2) = 8	2 (4) = 6
Per cent	100	42	12	8.6

Figures without parentheses denote patients with Hancock conduits
Figures in parentheses denote patients with aortic allograft conduits

By courtesy of Dr. F. O. Bowman, Columbia Presbyterian Medical Center, New York.
(Personal communication)

Moderate to severe pulmonary incompetence was noted in four patients who received allografts. In the xenograft group no obstruction has so far been observed.

Ebert *et al.*[21] reported, in 1970, their experience with corrective surgery in ten infants less than six months of age. There were two deaths in the series. Five patients had truncus arteriosus and five had pulmonary atresia with either confluent or non-confluent pulmonary arteries. The indications for complete correction in truncus arteriosus are quite clear and this should be carried out at any time when there is continued deterioration despite maximal medical therapy. For pulmonary atresia, however, the debate continues. There remains a place for palliative systemic–pulmonary shunts which will permit growth of the pulmonary vessels to allow later correction with a larger conduit. Whether growth of the pulmonary arteries is more enhanced by the insertion of a conduit than by shunting remains to be demonstrated.

The current series at the University of California[22] includes 21 infants, less than six months of age, operated upon for truncus arteriosus. Of this group, there were 18 survivors with no late complications specifically related to the conduit used. Four of these infants received aortic allograft valves with Dacron tube extensions and the remainder had size 12 Hancock porcine conduits. Few patients have been restudied with cardiac catheterization, but those who had haemodynamic investigations up to three years post-operatively, have shown pressure gradients across the conduit of 30–40 mmHg. Although it is anticipated that with growth, these gradients will increase, necessitating re-operation and insertion of a larger conduit, none of these conduits has yet needed replacement.

At the Hospital for Sick Children (Great Ormond Street) 94 cardiopulmonary conduits were inserted for various complex congenital cardiac lesions between June 1971 and November 1977. The spectrum of lesions encountered in our series, together with hospital mortality, are listed in *Table 8.3*. Our choice

TABLE 8.3

Cardiopulmonary conduits inserted between July 1971 and November 1977 at the Hospital for Sick Children, Great Ormond Street

Diagnosis of lesions	Number of patients	Hospital mortality	
		Number	Per cent
TGA with VSD and LVOTO	33	5	15
TGA with IVS and LVOTO	5	3	60
Double outlet RV	3	1	33
Double outlet LV	1	1	100
Truncus arteriosus	27	11	40
Pulmonary atresia	10	2	20
Tricuspid atresia	4	–	–
Atrioventricular discordance	8	4	50
Tetralogy of Fallot	2	–	–
Anatomically corrected transposition	1	–	–
Total	94	27	28

TGA = transposition of the great arteries, VSD = ventricular septal defect, LVOTO = left ventricular outflow tract obstruction, IVS = intact ventricular septum, RV = right ventricle, LV = left ventricle

between the fresh antibiotic treated aortic root allograft and the xenograft conduit, was frequently determined by availability. Although the operative mortality for the Rastelli operation was fairly low, we had, in this group of patients, five late deaths. The overall mortality for truncus arteriosus was 40 per cent. We have now adopted a policy of early correction of truncus arteriosus because of the development of pulmonary vascular disease in the young age group. In our experience, the mortality has been high for those patients with increased pulmonary vascular resistance or for the very small infants, usually less than one month of age and in severe congestive heart failure. We currently think that an elective correction between six and 12 months of age might be indicated if one wants to improve the prognosis of the overall population of infants born with this anomaly. As previously mentioned, we have used valved conduits in only two cases of tetralogy of Fallot. In both cases, the indication was an abnormal distribution of the coronary arteries. As far as the anatomically corrected malposition is concerned, the indication for a cardiopulmonary conduit is again determined by the distribution of the right coronary artery which crosses the outflow tract of the pulmonary artery and does not permit patch enlargement of the pulmonary valve annulus.

SUMMARY

The ideal material for the construction of cardiopulmonary valved conduits has yet to be found. Although clinical results continue to improve with the conduits currently available, long-term durability of the tissue components continues to be a problem. The continuing search for the 'ideal' material, improved methods of sterilization and preservation, as well as refinements in design and construction of cardiac prostheses will ensure greater success in the future.

Since the first successful clinical use of an extracardiac conduit for restoration of right ventricular to pulmonary artery continuity, the indications for its use have been greatly expanded. Many children who otherwise were doomed to an early death are now alive and enjoying some of the fruits of a normal existence. Haemodynamic function has been excellent in most children during the relatively short follow-up period. Whether they will be able to continue to enjoy life and expect to survive into later years without further surgery will be determined by the life expectancy of the cardiopulmonary valved conduit.

REFERENCES

[1] Aberdeen, E. 'Transposition of the great arteries'. In *Surgery of the Chest*. Ed. by D. C. Sabiston, Jr. and F. C. Spencer, p. 1105. Philadelphia; W. B. Saunders (1976)

[2] Al-Janabi, N. and Ross, D. N. 'Enhanced viability of fresh aortic homografts stored in nutrient medium', *Cardiology Research*, 7, 817 (1973)

[3] Appelbaum, A., Bargeron, L. M., Pacifico, A. D. and Kirklin, J. W. 'Surgical treatment of truncus arteriosus with emphasis on infants and small children', *Journal of thoracic and cardiovascular Surgery*, 71, 436 (1976)

[4] Anderson, R. H., Arnold, R. and Wilkinson, J. L. 'The conducting system in congenitally corrected transposition', *Lancet*, 1, 1286 (1973)

[5] Arai, R., Tsuyki, Y., Nogi, M., Kurashiege, K., Koyanage, H., Nichida, H., Ikeda, Y. and Ichidawa, H. 'Experimental study on bypass between the right ventricle and pulmonary artery, left ventricle and pulmonary artery and left ventricle and aorta by means of homograft with valve', *Bulletin of the Heart Institute of Japan*, 9, 49 (1965)

[6] Bailey, W. W., Kirklin, J. W., Bargeron, L. M., Jr., Pacifico, A. D. and Kouchoukos, N. T. 'Late results with synthetic valved external conduits from venous ventricle to pulmonary arteries', *Circulation,* 56 *(Suppl. 2),* 73 (1977)

[7] Barratt-Boyes, B. G. 'Complete correction of cardiovascular malformations in the first two years of life using profound hypothermia'. In *Heart Disease in Infancy. Diagnosis and Surgical Treatment.* Ed. by B. G. Barratt-Boyes, J. M. Neutze and E. A. Harris, p. 25. Edinburgh/London; Churchill Livingstone (1973)

[8] Barratt-Boyes, B. G., Roche, A., Agnew, T. M., Cole, D., Kerr, A., Monroe, J. L., Lowe, J. B. and Branat, P. W. T. 'Homograft valves', *Medical Journal of Australia,* 2, 32 (1972)

[9] Behrendt, D. M., Kiesh, M. M., Stern, A., Segiuann, J., Perry, B. and Sloan, H. 'The surgical therapy for pulmonary artery ventricular discontinuity', *Annals of thoracic Surgery,* 18, 122 (1974)

[10] Bernhard, W. F., Poirier, V. and LaFarge, C. G. 'Relief of congenital obstruction to the left ventricular outflow with a ventricular-aortic prosthesis', *Journal of thoracic and cardiovascular Surgery,* 19, 223 (1975)

[11] Bowman, F. O. Personal communication (1977)

[12] Bowman, F. O., Hancock, W. D. and Malm, J. R. 'A valve containing Dacron prosthesis: Its use in restoring pulmonary artery–right ventricular continuity', *Archives of Surgery,* 107, 724 (1973)

[13] Breckenridge, I. M., Stark, J., Oelert, H. and Waterston, D. J. 'Transposition of the great arteries with ventricular septal defect and pulmonary stenosis treated by the Rastelli operation', *Zeitschrift für Kinderchirurgie und Grenzgebiete,* 11, 205 (1972)

[14] Carpentier, A., Lemaigre, G., Robert, L., Carpentier, S. and Dubost, C. 'Biological factors affecting long-term results of valvular heterografts', *Journal of thoracic and cardiovascular Surgery,* 58, 467 (1969)

[15] Collett, R. W. and Edwards, J. E. 'Persistent truncus arteriosus. A classification according to anatomic types', *Surgical Clinics of North America,* 29, 1245 (1949)

[16] Cooley, D. A. 'Double outlet to relieve left ventricular hypertension', *Hospital Practice,* 12, 60 (1977)

[17] Cooley, D. A. and Hallman, G. L. *Surgical Treatment of Congenital Heart Disease.* p. 185. Philadelphia; Lea and Febiger (1966)

[18] Deverall, P. B., Bargeron, L. M., Barcia, A. and Kirklin, J. W. 'Transposition of the great arteries and pulmonary stenosis. Surgical considerations'. In *The Natural History and Progress in the Treatment of Congenital Heart Defects.* Ed. by B. S. L. Kidd and J. D. Keith, p. 175. Springfield, Illinois; Charles C. Thomas (1971)

[19] Donovan, T. J. 'The experimental use of homologous vein grafts to circumvent the pulmonary valves', *Surgery, Gynecology and Obstetrics,* 90, 204 (1950)

[20] Donovan, T. J., Hufnagel, C. A. and Eastcott, H. H. G. 'Permanent ligation of the main pulmonary valve', *Surgical Forum,* 2, 229 (1951)

[21] Ebert, P. A., Robinson, S. J., Stanger, P. and Engle, M. A. 'Pulmonary artery conduits in infants younger than six months of age', *Journal of thoracic and cardiovascular Surgery,* 72, 351 (1976)

[22] Ebert, P. A. Personal communication (1977)

[23] Fontan, F. and Baudet, E. 'Surgical repair of tricuspid atresia', *Thorax,* 26, 240 (1971)

[24] Gilbert, J. W., Corness, W. P. and Cooper, T. 'An experimental study of pulmonary artery replacement', *Journal of thoracic and cardiovascular Surgery,* 40, 667 (1960)

[25] Glatzer, P. and Herwitt, E. S. 'Experimental infundibular bypass', *Journal of thoracic and cardiovascular Surgery,* 43, 234 (1962)

[26] Herwitt, E. S. 'An experimental approach to the problem of increasing the blood supply to the lungs: Preliminary observations on the use of plastics', *Surgery, Gynecology and Obstetrics,* 87, 313 (1948)

[27] Hudson, R. E. B. 'Pathology of the human aortic valve homograft', *British heart Journal,* 28, 291 (1966)

[28] Jeger, E. *Die Chirurgie der Blutgefässe und des Herzens.* p. 326. Berlin; Hirshwald (1913)

[29] Keith, J. D., Rowe, R. D. and Vlad, P. *Heart Disease in Infancy and Childhood.* New York; Macmillan Company (1967)

[30] Kirklin, J. W. and Bailey, W. W. 'Valved external conduits to pulmonary arteries', *Annals of thoracic Surgery,* 24, 202 (1977)

[31] Kirklin, J. W. and Castaneda, A. R. 'Surgical correction of double outlet right ventricle with noncommitted ventricular septal defect', *Journal of thoracic and cardiovascular Surgery,* 73, 399 (1977)

[32] Konno, S., Imai, Y., Iida, Y., Nakajama, M. and Tatsuno, K. 'A new method for prosthetic valve replacement in congenital aortic stenosis associated with hypoplasia of the aortic valve ring', *Journal of thoracic and cardiovascular Surgery*, 70, 909 (1975)

[33] Kouchoukos, N. T., Barcia, A., Bargeron, C. and Kirklin, J. W. 'Surgical treatment of congenital pulmonary atresia with ventricular septal defect', *Journal of thoracic and cardiovascular Surgery*, 61, 70 (1971)

[34] Macartney, F. J., Scott, O. and Deverall, P. B. 'Dynamic and anatomical characteristics of pulmonary blood supply in pulmonary atresia with ventricular septal defect including a case of persistent fifth aortic arch', *British heart Journal*, 36, 1049 (1974)

[35] Malm, J. R., Bowman, F. O., Harris, P. D. and Kowalik, A. T. W. 'An evaluation of aortic valve homografts sterilized by electron beam energy', *Journal of thoracic and cardiovascular Surgery*, 54, 471 (1967)

[36] Marcelletti, C., Mair, D. D., McGoon, D. C., Wallace, R. B. and Danielson, G. K. 'The Rastelli operation for transposition of the great arteries', *Journal of thoracic and cardiovascular Surgery*, 72, 427 (1976)

[37] Marcelletti, C., McGoon, D. C., Danielson, G. K., Wallace, R. B. and Mair, D. D. 'Early and late results of surgical repair of truncus arteriosus', *Circulation*, 55, 636 (1977)

[38] McGoon, D. C. 'Left ventricular and biventricular conduits', *Journal of thoracic and cardiovascular Surgery*, 72, 7 (1976)

[39] McGoon, D. C., Rastelli, G. C. and Ongley, P. A. 'An operation for the correction of truncus arteriosus defects', *Journal of the American medical Association*, 205, 69 (1968)

[40] McGoon, D. C., Danielson, G. K., Ritter, D. G., Wallace, R., Maloney, J. and Marcelletti, C. 'Corrections of the univentricular heart having two atrioventricular valves', *Journal of thoracic and cardiovascular Surgery*, 74, 218 (1977)

[41] Meyer, J., Chiariello, L., Hallman, G. L. and Cooley, D. A. 'Coronary artery anomalies in patients with tetralogy of Fallot', *Journal of thoracic and cardiovascular Surgery*, 69, 373 (1975)

[42] Moore, C. H., Martelli, V., Al-Janabi, N. and Ross, D. N. 'Analysis of homograft valve failure in 311 patients followed up to ten years', *Annals of thoracic Surgery*, 20, 274 (1975)

[43] Moore, C. H., Martelli, V., Ross, D. N. and Derrick, J. 'Reconstruction of right ventricular outflow tract with a valved conduit in 75 cases of congenital heart disease', *Journal of thoracic and cardiovascular Surgery*, 71, 11 (1976)

[44] Norwood, W. I., Freed, M. D., Rocchini, A. F., Bernhard, W. F. and Castaneda, A. R. 'Experience with valved conduits for repair of congenital cardiac lesions', *Annals of thoracic Surgery*, 24, 223 (1977)

[45] Pacifico, A., Kirklin, J. W., Bargeron, M. and Soto, B. 'Surgical treatment of double outlet left ventricle: report of 4 cases', *Circulation*, 47 and 48 (*Suppl. 3*) 19 (1973)

[46] Poirier, R. A., Berman, M. A. and Stansel, H. C. 'Current status of the surgical treatment of truncus arteriosus', *Journal of thoracic and cardiovascular Surgery*, 69, 169 (1975)

[47] Rastelli, G. C., McGoon, D. C. and Wallace, R. B. 'Anatomic correction of transposition of the great arteries with ventricular septal defect and subpulmonary stenosis', *Journal of thoracic and cardiovascular Surgery*, 58, 545 (1969)

[48] Rastelli, G. C., Ongley, P. A., Davis, G. D. and Kirklin, J. W. 'Surgical repair for pulmonary artery fistula: Report of a case', *Mayo Clinic Proceedings*, 40, 521 (1965)

[49] Rastan, H. and Konez, J. 'Aortoventriculoplasty. A new technique for the treatment of left ventricular outflow tract obstruction', *Journal of thoracic and cardiovascular Surgery*, 71, 920 (1976)

[50] Rocchini, A. P., Rosenthal, A., Keane, J. F., Castaneda, A. R. and Nadas, A. S. 'Haemodynamics after surgical repair with right ventricle to pulmonary artery conduit', *Circulation*, 54, 951 (1976)

[51] Ross, D. N. and Somerville, J. 'Correction of pulmonary atresia with homograft aortic valve', *Lancet*, 2, 1446 (1966)

[52] Ross, D. N. and Yacoub, M. H. 'Homograft replacement of the aortic valve: A critical review', *Progress in cardiovascular Disease*, 11, 275 (1969)

[53] Sakakibara, S., Takao, A., Arai, T. M., Hashimoto, A. and Nog, M. 'Both great vessels arising from the left ventricle', *Bulletin of the Heart Institute of Japan*, 66, 66 (1967)

[54] Sarnoff, S. J., Donovan, T. J. and Case, R. B. 'The surgical relief of aortic stenosis by means of apical-aortic valvular anastomosis', *Circulation*, 11, 564 (1955)

[55] Shrivastava, S., Tadavarthy, S. M., Fukuda, T. and Edwards, J. E. 'Anatomic causes of pulmonary stenosis in complete transposition', *Circulation*, 54, 154 (1976)

[56] Silove, E. D. and Taylor, J. F. N. 'Angiographic and anatomic features of sub-valvar left ventricular outflow obstruction in transposition of the great arteries. The possible role of the anterior mitral valve leaflet', *Pediatric Radiology,* 1, 87 (1973)

[57] Singh, A. K., Stark, J. and Taylor, J. F. N. 'Left ventricle to pulmonary artery conduit in treatment of transposition of the great arteries, restrictive ventricular septal defect and acquired pulmonary atresia', *British heart Journal,* 38, 1213 (1976)

[58] Singh, A. K., de Leval, M. and Stark, J. 'Total correction of Type I truncus arteriosus in a six-month-old infant'. *British heart Journal,* 37, 1314 (1975)

[59] Singh, A. K., de Leval, M. R., Pincott, J. R. and Stark, J. 'Pulmonary artery banding for truncus arteriosus in the first year of life', *Circulation,* 54 (*Suppl. 3*), 17 (1976)

[60] Smith, J. C. 'The pathology of human aortic valve homografts', *Thorax,* 22, 114 (1967)

[61] Stanger, P., Robinson, S. J., Engle, M. A. and Ebert, P. A. 'Corrective surgery for truncus arteriosus in the first year of life', *American Journal of Cardiology,* 39, 293 (1977)

[62] Sullivan, H., Sulayman, R., Replogle, R. and Arcilla, R. A. 'Surgical correction of truncus arteriosus in infancy', *American Journal of Cardiology,* 38, 113 (1976)

[63] Vidne, B. A., Subramanian, S. and Wagner, H. R. 'Aneurysm of the membranous ventricular septum in transposition of the great arteries', *Circulation,* 53, 157 (1976)

[64] Wallace, R. B. 'Tissue valves', *American Journal of Cardiology,* 35, 866 (1975)

[65] Wilkinson, J. L., Anderson, R. H., Arnold, R., Hamilton, D. I. and Smith, A. 'The conducting tissue in primitive ventricular hearts without an outlet chamber', *Circulation,* 53, 930 (1976)

[66] Yacoub, M. and Kittle, C. F. 'Sterilization of valve homografts by antibiotic solutions', *Circulation,* 41 (*Suppl. 2*), 29 (1970)

9

Right Ventricular Outflow Tract Reconstruction with Pericardial Monocusp Patch and Valved Conduit

Fergus J. Macartney
Anand P. Tandon and
Marian I. Ionescu

La vérité est un flambeau qui luit dans un brouillard sans le dissiper.
Claude Adrien Helvétius (1715–1771)

INTRODUCTION

The use of valved conduits between the heart and pulmonary artery is now standard practice, particularly in the management of complex congenital cardiac anomalies as detailed in Chapter 8.

Though there have been marked improvements in the performance of such conduits over the last few years there is still need for a reliable graft which is freely available in sizes appropriate for both adult and infant cardiac surgery and which does not stretch inordinately the resources available for health care. As is becoming increasingly clear, these resources are not limitless even in highly developed countries. In marked contrast to our previous experience with autogeneic fascia lata[4,11], the immediate and late results using glutaraldehyde stabilized xenogeneic pericardium have been much more encouraging[12]. The first operation of this type was carried out in May 1972, and this report concerns the entire series of patients operated on at the Leeds General Infirmary up until May 1977. Post-operative cardiac catheterizations were carried out either in the same hospital or at Killingbeck Hospital, Leeds.

MATERIAL AND METHODS

Patients

This series comprises 19 patients, of whom nine were male. Their ages at the time of definitive surgery ranged from seven to 32 years, and the mean was 18.8 ± 1.6 years (*Table 9.1*). The pre-operative congenital heart defects are

TABLE 9.1
Age and sex distribution of 19 patients with congenital cardiac anomalies

Sex	0-10	11-20	Age 21-30	31-40	Total
Male	1	3	5	–	9
Female	–	6	3	1	10
Total	1	9	8	1	19

listed in *Table 9.2*. Ten patients had had previous palliative operations, which were Blalock–Taussig shunt in eight, Potts in one and Waterston shunt in the other one. Furthermore, ten patients had had some type of previous intracardiac correction. In seven cases this had been fascia lata reconstruction of the right ventricular outlet which became complicated by graft stenosis[4] (*Table 9.3*).

TABLE 9.2
Pre-operative clinical diagnosis and sex distribution

Diagnosis	Male	Female	Total
Fallot's tetralogy	7	6	13
Fallot's tetralogy with bilateral pulmonary artery stenosis		1	1
Double outlet right ventricle with pulmonary stenosis (AV concordance)		2	2
Primitive ventricle, subaortic outlet chamber, subvalvular pulmonary stenosis	1		1
ASD with acquired pulmonary atresia	1	1	2
Total	9	10	19

ASD = atrial septal defect, AV = atrioventricular

TABLE 9.3
Previous cardiovascular operations performed in 19
patients with congenital cardiac anomalies

Surgical procedure	Number
Extracardiac shunts	10
Potts	1
Blalock–Taussig	8
Waterston	1
Intracardiac operations	
RVOT reconstruction with fascia lata	10
valved conduit	7
Other procedures	3
Total	20

RVOT = right ventricular outflow tract

Construction of pericardial monocusp patch and pericardial pulmonary valve conduit

Two preparations were used for enlargement and reconstruction of the right ventricular outflow tract.

Eighteen patients received a 'pericardial monocusp patch' made entirely from calf pericardium, stabilized with purified glutaraldehyde and sterilized and stored in formaldehyde, following the procedure detailed in Chapter 6. This preparation consists of a pericardial patch to which a pericardial monocusp valve mechanism is attached (*Figure 9.1*). Each preparation is made to closely defined standards, the measurements of the two components being determined by the overall size required.

One patient received a 'pericardial pulmonary valve conduit' consisting of a low porosity Dacron tube and a glutaraldehyde stabilized three-cusp pericardial xenograft valve. The conduit is constructed in such a way as to simulate the shape and function of the sinuses of Valsalva (*Figure 9.2*).

Both these preparations, the pericardial monocusp patch and the pericardial pulmonary valve conduit are now manufactured in a variety of sizes to cover the surgical requirements for all age groups*.

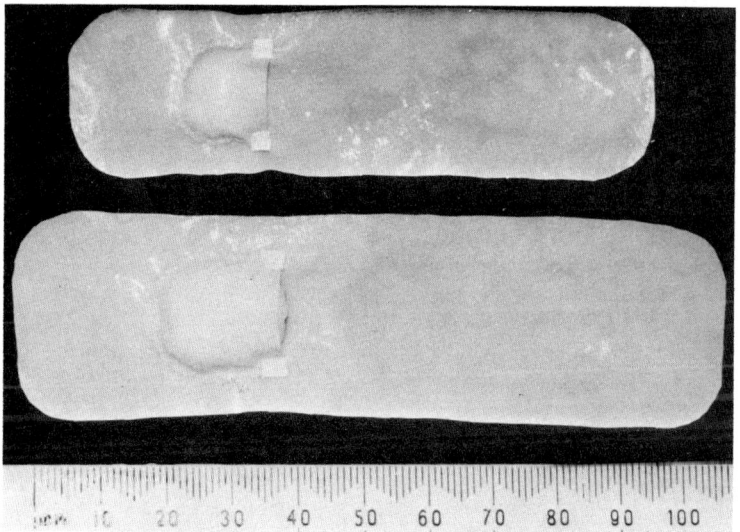

Figure 9.1 Pericardial monocusp patches for reconstruction of the right ventricular outflow tract with a valve mechanism. The entire preparation is made of xenogeneic pericardium stabilized with purified glutaraldehyde and stored in buffered formaldehyde. (Reproduced by courtesy of Shiley Laboratories Inc., Irvine, California)

Insertion of monocusp patch and valve conduit

In all patients there was continuity, if not communication between the right or primitive ventricle and the pulmonary artery. The method of insertion of the monocusp patch was similar to that previously described for the diamond shaped fascia lata grafts[3]. A short longitudinal incision was made in the outflow tract of the right ventricle and extended across the pulmonary annulus and valve as far into the pulmonary artery as necessary. Following the intracardiac repair (closure of ventricular septal defect, resection of infundibular obstruction, etc.) a monocusp patch of appropriate size was selected and rinsed as necessary to wash out the formaldehyde storage solution. The width of the pericardial patch was determined by the calculated circumference of the reconstructed pulmonary annulus.The pericardial patch was cut to match the

*Shiley Laboratories, Inc., Irvine, California

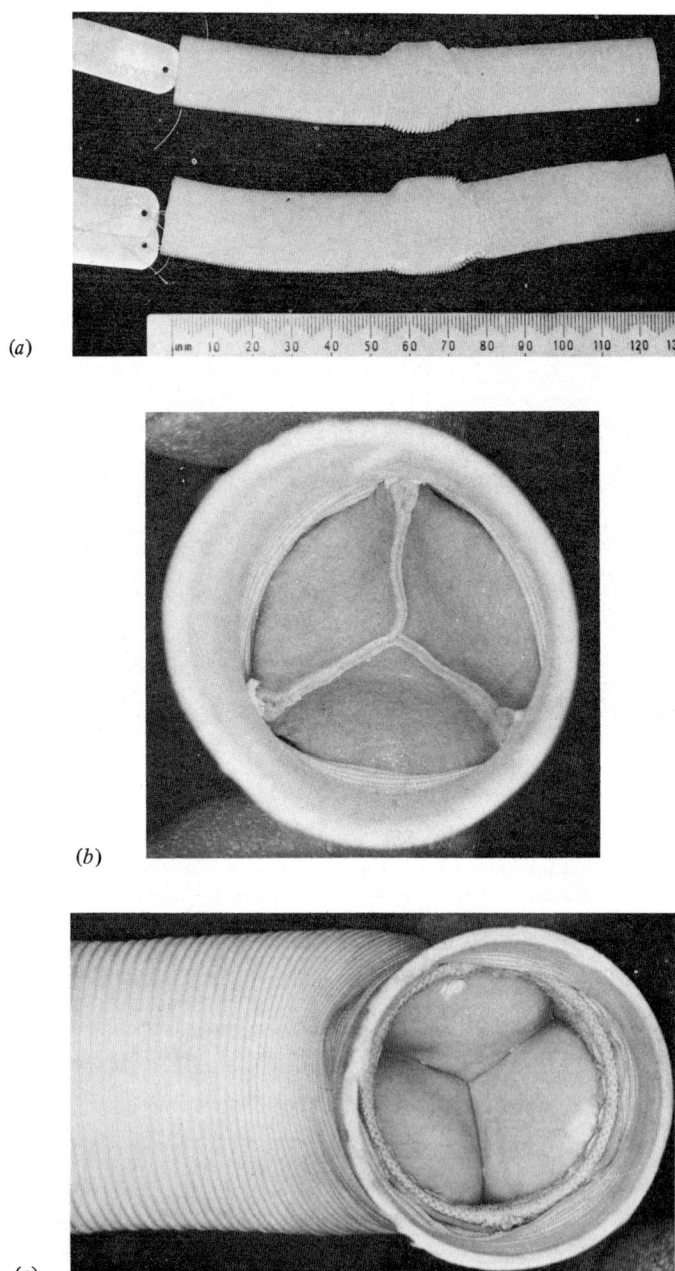

Figure 9.2 Pericardial pulmonary valve conduits. The low porosity woven Dacron tube prosthesis incorporates sinuses of Valsalva (*a*) and contains a three-cusp pericardial xenograft (outflow (*b*) and inflow (*c*) aspects of the valve). The valve is made of calf pericardium stabilized with purified glutaraldehyde and the entire conduit is stored in buffered formaldehyde. (Reproduced by courtesy of Shiley Laboratories Inc., Irvine, California)

length of the incision in the right ventricle and pulmonary artery and tailored in a diamond shape. During the preparation and insertion of the patch an attempt was made to ensure that the position of the monocusp was such that it coapted with the remnants of the patients' own pulmonary valve cusps. The patch was then sutured distally to the pulmonary artery and proximally to the right ventricle (*Figure 9.3*).

The pericardial pulmonary valve conduit was inserted as described in Chapter 8 for composite grafts.

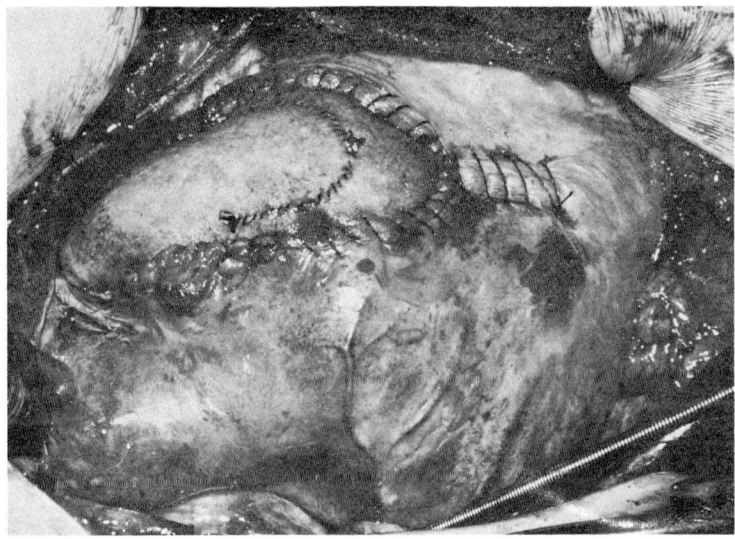

Figure 9.3 Operative view of a pericardial monocusp patch bypassing the sub-pulmonary obstruction and the conduction system of a patient who underwent septation of a primitive ventricle. To the right the inferior end of the ventriculotomy has been repaired and the proximal end of the pericardial patch sutured to the margins of the incision. To the left, the distal anastomosis with the pulmonary artery is obscured by the transposed aorta. The suture line by which the monocusp is attached to the pericardial patch is clearly seen

Post-operative investigations

British patients were followed up by regular physical examination, chest radiographs and electrocardiogram. Patients residing abroad were either followed in the same manner, or else by correspondence with the referring physician. Post-operative cardiac catheterization and angiocardiography were carried out in all patients where this was geographically feasible, and there was informed consent from the patient, parents, or both. Six patients consented to a second post-operative cardiac catheterization. In no case was the need for cardiac catheterization determined by the immediate physical condition of the patient.

Standard right (and left, if indicated) heart catheterization was carried out with the patient fasting, supine and premedicated with 1 ml/20 lb body weight of a mixture containing 25 mg pethidine, 6.25 mg of chlorpromazine and 6.25 mg of promethazine HCl/ml (maximal adult dose 2.5 ml). Resting cardiac output was determined by the direct Fick method, with oxygen consumption being measured using either the standard one-way valve technique, or the flow-through method[7]. Despite problems previously found in quantifying pulmonary regurgitation after fascia lata graft insertion[11], an attempt was made to achieve this by pulmonary angiography or double sampling dye dilution techniques.

RESULTS

Immediate surgical results

There were two hospital deaths (10.5 per cent mortality). One patient with double outlet right ventricle developed complete heart block three weeks postoperatively, which persisted and required pacemaker implantation.

Late complications

The period of observation ranged from 10–70 months (mean 53.6 ± 4.6 months) and the total follow-up is 912 patient months. There were no late deaths. The patient with primitive ventricle required resuturing of leaks around the septation patch 11 months after the first operation[5], and then developed complete heart block requiring pacing six months later. At the time of re-operation the pericardial monocusp patch appeared as fresh as on the day it had been inserted.

Status when last seen

All patients are presently asymptomatic, though the patient with primitive ventricle requires anti-failure medication. Twelve patients have complete right bundle branch block, but all except the two detailed above are in sinus rhythm. On chest radiographs, the mean pre-operative cardiothoracic ratio (CTR) was 0.59 ± 0.02. At six months following operation this had become 0.58 ± 0.02, and at 52 ± 2.5 months post-operatively, in 12 patients, the mean CTR was 0.56 ± 0.02 (*Figure 9.4*). None of these figures are significantly different statistically.

Post-operative findings at cardiac catheterization

Pre-operative and post-operative findings from the ten patients who had at least one post-operative cardiac catheterization are compared in *Table 9.4*. There was a highly significant ($p < 0.001$) reduction in the right ventricular (RV) systolic pressure, and in its relationship with the systemic arterial (SA) pressure. The mean post-operative pressure gradient between the right ventricle and the pulmonary artery was 9.3 ± 1.7 mmHg, thus demonstrating almost complete relief of the pulmonary obstruction. Resting flow through the graft was within normal limits (3.2 ± 0.4 ℓ/min/m²). The mean right ventricular end-diastolic pressure (RVEDP) was 5.0 ± 1.1 mmHg. The mean pulmonary artery diastolic pressure was 6.0 ± 0.9 mmHg. However, in individuals, the two pressures were

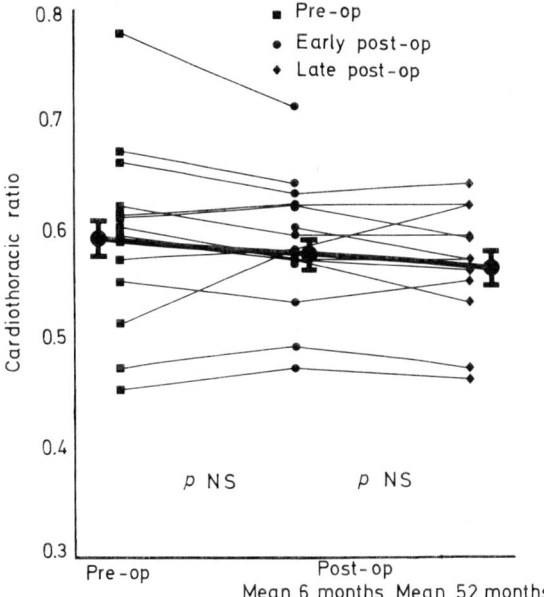

Figure 9.4 Cardiothoracic ratio of patients with right ventricular outflow tract reconstruction. The pre-operative values are displayed together with those obtained at six and 52 months post-operatively. The mean values for the group ± standard error of the mean are in solid lines

within 2 mmHg of one another in only two patients. One of them had a small residual ventricular septal defect.

Analyzing the sub-group of six patients who had two sequential post-operative cardiac catheterizations (*Table 9.5* and *Figure 9.5*), the findings are as for all ten patients except that in this sub-group there was a significant ($p < 0.05$) reduction in right ventricular end-diastolic pressure at the first post-operative catheterization (2.5 ± 1.0 mmHg) as compared with the pre-operative value (4.2 ± 2.0 mmHg). However, this trend was reversed at the second post-operative catheterization (RVEDP = 3.5 ± 1.0 mmHg). The fall in RV/SA systolic pressure in between the first and second post-operative catheterizations is entirely due to repair of leaks around the ventricular septation patch in one patient. Of more importance is the lack of change (strictly, a non-significant fall) in the right ventricular–pulmonary artery pressure gradient, despite a rise in cardiac output from 2.5 to 3.0 ℓ/min/m^2 between the two post-operative investigations performed at 16.7 ± 1.9 and 51.8 ± 2.0 months.

Angiocardiography demonstrated freely mobile, thin valve cusps in both the monocusp patches and the three-cusp valved conduit; indeed in some patients the leaflet appeared as fine as that of a normal pulmonary valve cusp (*Figure 9.6a* and *b*). In no patient was calcification observed.

Assessment of pulmonary regurgitation was attempted by pulmonary angiography, but comparison of right ventricular and pulmonary angiograms showed clearly that the catheter, however fine, pushed the anteriorly situated monocusp away from the patients' own pulmonary valve, thus holding it open during

TABLE 9.4
Pre- and post-operative findings in ten patients with one post-operative cardiac catheterization*

	Systemic index† (ℓ/min/m²)	O_2 uptake (ml/min/m²)	Right ventricle (mmHg)		Pulmonary artery (mmHg)			RV-PA gradient (mmHg)	RV/SA S ratio	TPR (m²)
			S	EDP	S	D	M			
Pre-operative	3.1 ±0.5	151 ±13.9	99.4 ±7.4	6.0 ±1.3	24.0 ±3.9	7.0 ±1.5	15.0 ±2.9	81.5 ±6.9	0.86 ±0.09	4.2 ±0.2
Post-operative (39.9 ± 6.6 months)	3.2 ±0.4	150 ±13.3	39.4 ±3.8	5.0 ±1.1	30.0 ±3.3	6.0 ±0.9	15.0 ±1.3	9.3 ±1.7	0.31 ±0.04	4.6 ±0.6
P value	NS	NS	<0.001	NS	NS	NS	NS	<0.001	<0.01	NS

* Results are expressed as mean ± standard error of the mean
† Post-operative pulmonary index given in the presence of left to right shunt

D = diastolic pressure, EDP = end-diastolic pressure, M = mean pressure, NS = not significant, P = statistical probability, PA = pulmonary artery, RV = right ventricle, S = systolic pressure, SA = systemic artery, TPR = total pulmonary resistance

TABLE 9.5

Pre- and post-operative findings in six patients with two post-operative cardiac catheterizations*

| | Systemic index† (ℓ/min/m²) | O_2 uptake (ml/min/m²) | Right ventricle | | Pulmonary artery | | | RV-PA gradient (mmHg) | RV/SA S ratio | TPR (m²) |
			S (mmHg)	EDP	S	D (mmHg)	M			
a. Pre-operative	2.6 ±0.2	149.0 ±12.1	100.5 ±11.0	4.2 ±2.0	21.2 ±2.4	7.2 ±1.5	12.0 ±1.2	89.6 ±3.7	0.91 ±0.14	4.1 ±0.2
b. 1st post-operative (16.7 ± 1.9 months)	2.5 ±0.3	174.0 ±14.0	38.0 ±4.1	2.5 ±1.0	25.0 ±2.9	3.0 ±0.5	13.0 ±1.3	12.5 ±2.7	0.34 ±0.04	5.1 ±0.7
c. 2nd post-operative (51.8 ± 2.0 months)	3.0 ±0.4	138.0 ±10.6	35.7 ±2.6	3.5 ±1.0	26.7 ±2.4	5.0 ±0.8	14.0 ±0.8	9.0 ±1.2	0.27 ±0.02	4.8 ±0.5
Statistical significance										
a and b	NS	NS	< 0.01	< 0.05	NS	NS	NS	< 0.001	< 0.01	NS
b and c	NS	NS	NS	< 0.05	NS	NS	NS	NS	< 0.05	NS

*Results are expressed as mean ± standard error of the mean

†Post-operative pulmonary index given in the presence of left to right shunt

D = diastolic pressure, EDP = end-diastolic pressure, M = mean pressure, NS = not significant, PA = pulmonary artery, RV = right ventricle, S = systolic pressure, SA = systemic artery, TPR = total pulmonary resistance

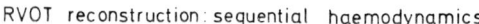

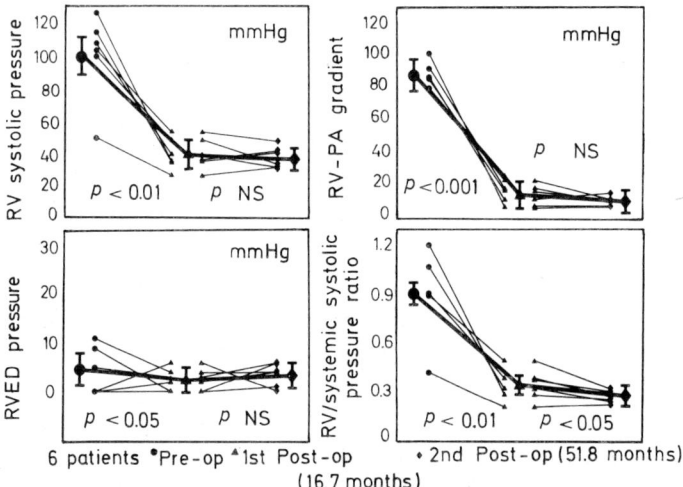

Figure 9.5 Graphic presentation of haemodynamic data from six patients who underwent three sequential investigations, one prior to operation and two following right ventricular outflow tract reconstruction (at mean post-operative intervals of 16.7 ± 1.9 and 51.2 ± 2.0 months respectively). The mean values for the group ± standard error of the mean are in solid lines. There were no statistically significant changes in these parameters between the first and the second post-operative investigations (RVOT = right ventricular outflow tract; RV = right ventricle; PA = pulmonary artery; RVED = right ventricular end-diastolic pressure; P = statistical significance; NS = not significant)

diastole. For this reason, double sampling dye dilution techniques for assessing pulmonary regurgitation were abandoned. On right ventricular angiography coaptation of the monocusp with the posterior wall of the pulmonary artery or with remnants of the patients' own pulmonary valve, was visualized, though in some patients cusp overlapping occurred.

Post-operatively, 11 patients (64 per cent) had a delayed decrescendo murmur of varying intensity, but always of short length, immediately following the snapping sound presumably related to 'closure' of the monocusp valve.

DISCUSSION

As has been made clear in Chapter 8, the history of conduits and right ventricular outflow tract reconstruction is one of a mixture of triumphs and unpleasant surprises. Fortunately, the triumphs have outnumbered the unpleasant surprises, but the rather high incidence of obstruction of grafts and conduits[8,17,20,23] particularly those made of autologous fascia lata[11] and the irradiated-frozen allografts[14,16], emphasizes the need for routine late cardiac catheterization in patients who have had any new type of operative intervention on the heart. There is no other way of obtaining adequate, objective, early warning of unexpected complications of the operation. Once the likely complications have been documented, other less invasive ways of assessing the problem may be appropriate, but the major question in the first instance is to know what to look for.

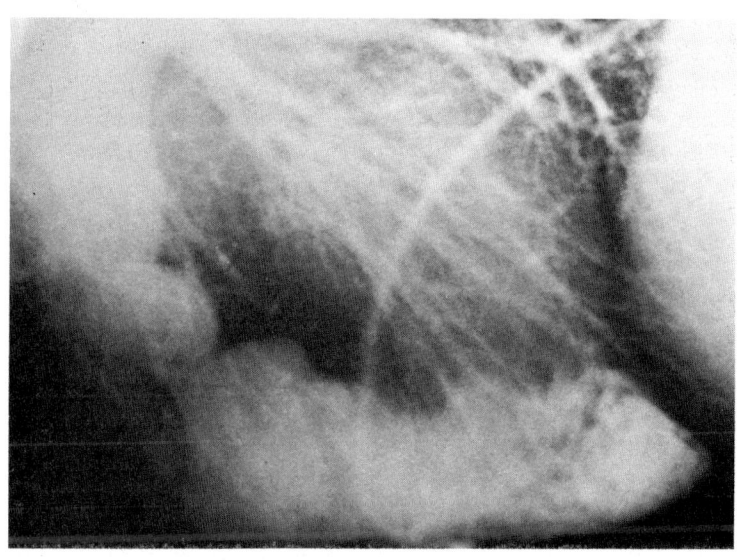

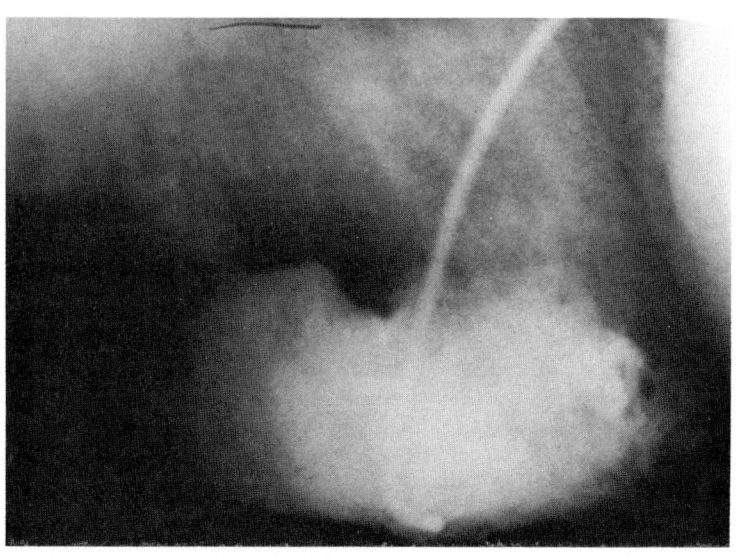

Figure 9.6 Angiocardiographic appearance of a monocusp patch in the right ventricular outflow tract. (*a*) Lateral view of the right ventricle in diastole early during the injection of contrast material. (*b*) Same view later on with both right ventricle and reconstructed pulmonary artery filled with contrast material. The anteriorly located monocusp is clearly visible as it moves towards the remnants of the pulmonary valve at the end of systole

The results of these post-operative studies have shown that the pericardial xenograft has relieved right ventricular outflow tract obstruction better than has been reported for standard repair of tetralogy of Fallot, with or without an outflow patch[6,18,19,21], aortic allografts (whether they be freeze-dried[23], irradiated[16], beta-propiolactone treated[8], or antibiotic sterilized[22]) or porcine xenografts[17,20]. However, this may not simply be a matter of material of the tissue valve; geometry of the graft may also be important, as indicated by the presence of gradients at either end of tubular conduits[13,17,20] and by the much higher rate of obstruction in otherwise identical aortic allografts when used to repair transposition of the great arteries as opposed to truncus arteriosus[16].

The primary aim of right ventricular outflow tract reconstruction must be maximal relief of right ventricular outflow tract obstruction, or else creation of right ventricular–pulmonary artery continuity without introducing obstruction. The evidence for this assertion comes from consideration of the results of classic repair of tetralogy of Fallot, where a high post-operative ratio of right-to-left ventricular systolic pressure has been shown to increase not only the immediate surgical mortality[10] but also late morbidity and mortality[18]. It is hard to believe that these data cannot be extrapolated to most complex forms of congenital heart disease.

No form of right ventricular outlet reconstruction has yet been achieved without pulmonary regurgitation in at least some patients[6,8,11,17,20,23]. Because of the technical problems of detecting and quantitating pulmonary regurgitation, which arise from the fact that most methods demand passage of a catheter through the pulmonary valve, clinical observation is probably the most reliable method of detection. Certainly the delayed, usually low-pitched, decrescendo diastolic murmur is unmistakable to the trained cardiologist. However, as with all physical signs, inter-observer differences are not negligible. Consequently comparison between the incidence of clinical pulmonary incompetence from different centres has marked limitations. These limitations become even more serious when quantitative clinical estimations are compared. All that can be said is that, given the fact that right ventricular outflow tract obstruction was almost completely relieved, and that only one patient had a small residual ventricular septal defect, the fact that the mean cardiothoracic ratio was 0.56 ± 0.02 at 52 ± 2.5 months after operation, indicates that on average, pulmonary incompetence was moderate. However, the fact that there was no significant increase in cardiothoracic ratio between six and 52 months strongly suggests that pulmonary regurgitation was not progressive. Isolated pulmonary regurgitation is usually, but not invariably, tolerated for long periods of time[1,4,15,24], albeit at the cost of a higher right ventricular mass[1], end-diastolic pressure[1,6], end-diastolic volume, and ejection fraction[2]. On the other hand, when it is associated with other defects, such as recurrent ventricular septal defects or pulmonary hypertension, the clinical picture is not so benign[4,25]. Obviously, if a valved conduit or graft is to be inserted, it is desirable that it should be competent, but not at the risk of introducing obstruction. The pulmonary incompetence in the patients reported herein was not due to valve shrinkage, as occurred with fascia lata grafts[11]. Angiocardiographic studies in this series and the findings at re-operation in one patient with recurrent ventricular septal defect, demonstrated the lack of shrinkage or dilatation of the pericardial preparations. Angiocardiography suggested that in most cases incompetence was due to poor coaptation of the monocusp valve with the remnants of the patients' own pulmonary valve. With greater attention to detail during surgery (*Figure 9.7*), this might have been

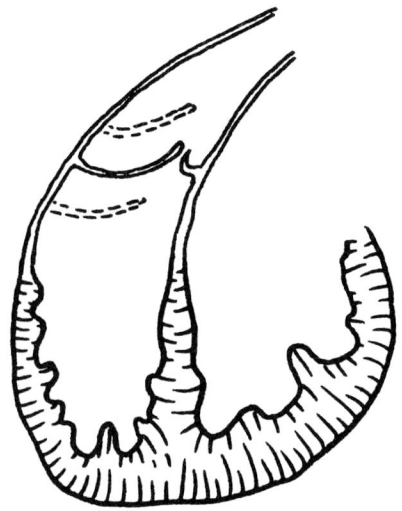

Figure 9.7 Schematic drawing showing the correct and incorrect positions of the mono-cusp valve. Unless perfect coaptation of the monocusp with the remnants of the patients own pulmonary 'cusps' is achieved, overlapping is likely to result in some degree of pulmonary regurgitation

reduced or even eliminated. In the small series of patients followed-up to 70 months (mean 53.6) there were no late deaths and only one patient (5.8 per cent) required re-operation for residual ventricular septal defect. These results compare favourably with other reported series. In a recent analysis of 85 operative survivors with external valve conduits the actuarial survival rate at five years' follow-up was 76.7 per cent and the actuarial re-operation rate at 5 years was 30.4 per cent[9].

Studies with glutaraldehyde stabilized pericardial xenograft valves in the mitral and aortic position have documented their almost complete freedom from thromboembolic and haemolytic complications, as detailed in Chapter 6. This study of the right ventricular outflow tract reconstruction has confirmed the durability of the glutaraldehyde stabilized pericardial xenograft valves also noted on the left side of the heart and this gives grounds for optimism about the future of the pericardial pulmonary valve conduit consisting of a three-cusped xenograft inserted within a low-porosity Dacron tube. This will almost certainly be competent, and therefore more suitable for use where post-operative pulmonary hypertension is anticipated. Hopefully it will relieve obstruction as well as the pericardial monocusp patch.

SUMMARY

Between May 1972 and May 1977 right ventricular outflow tract reconstruction was carried out in 19 patients with congenital heart disease. In 18 patients a pericardial monocusp patch was employed, constructed entirely of calf pericardium, stabilized in purified glutaraldehyde and sterilized with formaldehyde.

In one patient a pulmonary conduit consisting of a three-cusped pericardial valve within a Dacron tube was used.

There were two hospital deaths (10.5 per cent). Follow-up ranged from 10–70 months (mean 53.6 ± 4.6 months, total 912 patient-months). There were no late deaths. Recatheterization was carried out in ten patients an average of 40 months post-operatively and the right ventricular–pulmonary artery systolic gradient was 9.3 ± 1.7 mmHg. This was not significantly different in six patients who had a second post-operative catheterization at 51.8 ± 2.0 months post-operatively. Angiocardiography showed freely mobile, thin valve cusps. Clinical pulmonary insufficiency was detected in 64 per cent of patients. The cardiothoracic ratio decreased from the mean pre-operative value of 0.59 to 0.56 at 52 months following operation. In no patient was calcification of the pericardial xenograft observed.

These results compare well with those reported with other types of conduits, particularly with reference to relief of obstruction.

REFERENCES

[1] Burnell, R. H., Woodson, R. D., Lees, M. H. and Starr, A. 'Right ventricular performance in dogs following pulmonary valvectomy', *Surgery*, **65**, 952 (1969)

[2] Graham, T. P., Jr., Cordell, D., Atwood, G. F., Boucek, R. J., Jr., Boerth, R. C., Bender, H. W., Nelson, J. H. and Vaughn, W. C. 'Right ventricular volume characteristics before and after palliative and reparative operation in tetralogy of Fallot', *Circulation*, **54**, 417 (1976)

[3] Ionescu, M. I. and Deac, R. C. 'Fascia lata composite graft for right ventricular outflow tract and pulmonary artery reconstruction', *Thorax*, **25**, 427 (1970)

[4] Ionescu, M. I., Macartney, F. J. and Wooler, G. H. 'Reconstruction of the right ventricular outlet with fascia lata composite graft', *Journal of thoracic and cardiovascular Surgery*, **63**, 60 (1972)

[5] Ionescu, M. I., Macartney, F. J. and Wooler, G. H. 'Intracardiac repair of single ventricle with pulmonary stenosis', *Journal of thoracic and cardiovascular Surgery*, **65**, 602 (1973)

[6] Kaplan, S., Helmsworth, J. A., McKinivan, C. E., Benzing, G., Schwartz, D. C. and Schreiber, J. T. 'The fate of reconstruction of the right ventricular outflow tract', *Journal of thoracic and cardiovascular Surgery*, **66**, 361 (1973)

[7] Kappagoda, C. T., Greenwood, P., Macartney, F. J. and Linden, R. J. 'Oxygen consumption of children with congenital disease of the heart', *Clinical Science and molecular Medicine*, **45**, 107 (1973)

[8] Kawashima, Y., Naito, Y., Kitamura, S., Nakano, S., Miyamoto, T., Fujitino, M., Kazuka, T. and Manabe, H. 'Use of large homograft artery with semilunar valve for correction of tetralogy of Fallot', *Journal of thoracic and cardiovascular Surgery*, **67**, 685 (1947)

[9] Kirklin, J. W. and Bailey, W. W. 'Valved external conduits to pulmonary arteries', *Annals of thoracic Surgery*, **24**, 202 (1977)

[10] Kirklin, J. W. and Karp, R. B. *Tetralogy of Fallot from a Surgical Viewpoint*. Philadelphia; W. B. Saunders Company (1970)

[11] Macartney, F. J., Scott, O. and Ionescu, M. I. 'Late haemodynamic results of fascia lata reconstruction of the right ventricular outlet', *American heart Journal*, **89**, 195 (1975)

[12] Macartney, F. J., Tandon, A. P., Deverall, P. B. and Ionescu, M. I. 'Composite pericardial xenograft for right ventricular outlet reconstruction', (Abstract), *British heart Journal*, **39**, 925 (1977)

[13] Marcelletti, C., Mair, D. D., McGoon, D. C., Wallace, R. B. and Danielson, G. K. 'The Rastelli operation for transposition of the great arteries. Early and late results', *Journal of thoracic and cardiovascular Surgery*, **72**, 427 (1976)

[14] Merin, G. and McGoon, D. C. 'Re-operation after insertion of aortic homograft as a right ventricular outflow tract', *Annals of thoracic Surgery*, **16**, 122 (1973)

[15] Michl, L. and Shumaker, H. B. Jr. 'Pulmonary valvular incompetence in growing animals', *Surgery*, **73**, 412 (1973)

[16] Moodie, D. S., Mair, D. D., Fulton, R. E., Wallace, R. B., Danielson, G. K. and McGoon, D. C. 'Aortic homograft obstruction', *Journal of thoracic and cardiovascular Surgery,* 72, 553 (1976)

[17] Norwood, W. I., Freed, M. D., Rocchini, A. P., Bernhard, W. F. and Castaneda, A. R. 'Experience with valved conduits for repair of congenital cardiac lesions', *Annals of thoracic Surgery*, 24, 223 (1977)

[18] Poirier, R. A., McGoon, D. C., Danielson, G. K., Wallace, R. B., Ritter, D. G., Moodie, D. S. and Wiltse, C. G. 'Late results after repair of tetralogy of Fallot', *Journal of thoracic and cardiovascular Surgery*, 73, 900 (1977)

[19] Rocchini, A. P., Rosenthal, A., Freed, M., Castaneda, A. R. and Nadas, A. S. 'Chronic congestive heart failure after repair of tetralogy of Fallot', *Circulation*, 56, 305 (1977)

[20] Rocchini, A. P., Rosenthal, A., Keane, J. F., Castaneda, A. R. and Nadas, A. S. 'Haemodynamics after surgical repair with right ventricle to pulmonary artery conduit', *Circulation*, 54, 951 (1976)

[21] Ruzyllo, W., Nihill, M. R., Mullins, C. E. and McNamara, D. G. 'Haemodynamic evalution of 221 patients after intracardiac repair of tetralogy of Fallot', *American Journal of Cardiology*, 34, 565 (1974)

[22] Somerville, J. 'Homograft reconstruction of the right ventricular outflow tract in pulmonary atresia and extreme tetralogy of Fallot—Late results'. In *Second Henry Ford Hospital International Symposium on Cardiac Surgery*. Ed. by J. C. Davila, p. 349. New York; Appleton-Century-Crofts (1977)

[23] Somerville, J. and Ross, D. N. 'Long-term results of complete correction with homograft reconstruction in pulmonary outflow tract atresia', *British heart Journal*, 34, 29 (1972)

[24] Stafford, E. G., Mair, D. D., McGoon, D. C. and Danielson, G. K. 'Tetralogy of Fallot with absent pulmonary valve. Surgical considerations and results', *Circulation,* 57, *(Suppl. III)* 24 (1973)

[25] Weldon, C. S., Rowe, R. D. and Gott, V. L. 'Clinical experience with the use of aortic valve homografts for reconstruction of the pulmonary artery, pulmonary valve, and outflow portion of the right ventricle', *Circulation*, 37, *(Suppl. II)* 51 (1968)

10

The Chemistry and Biology of Aldehyde Treated Tissue Heart Valve Xenografts

E. Aubrey Woodroof

Si j'avais les main pleines de vérités, je me garderai de les ouvrir.
Bernard le Bovier de Fontenelle (1657–1757)

INTRODUCTION

Glutaraldehyde has been used effectively to stabilize connective tissue for clinical heart valve substitutes over the past eight years[1,10,22,34]. Its success as a biomaterial stabilizing agent has been widely recognized, although poorly understood. The purpose of this chapter is to review the rationale for the use of glutaraldehyde to stabilize tissue heart valves; the use of glutaraldehyde and formaldehyde as sterilizing agents; glutaraldehyde and formaldehyde toxicity; the effect of glutaraldehyde on the antigenicity of connective tissue; the chemistry of glutaraldehyde solutions and the reactions of glutaraldehyde with connective tissue proteins.

THE RATIONALE FOR THE USE OF GLUTARALDEHYDE TO STABILIZE TISSUE HEART VALVES

The parameters important in tissue stabilization (tanning) are glutaraldehyde concentration, time of exposure to glutaraldehyde, temperature, pH and the composition of the glutaraldehyde solution (the amount of monomer and various polymer components).

The kinetics of tissue stabilization as a function of glutaraldehyde concentration, when monitored by tissue thermal stability, are illustrated in *Figure 10.1*. Tissue tanning occurs very rapidly when exposed to glutaraldehyde at concentrations of 0.1 - 5 per cent, pH 7.4 and at room temperature. Within 1 h the reaction is 84 per cent complete with 5 per cent glutaraldehyde and 74 per cent complete with 0.1 per cent glutaraldehyde. Hardy reports that the absorbance at 265 nm of proteins being tanned (cross-linked) with glutaraldehyde continues to increase for up to seven days[20]. This observation in-

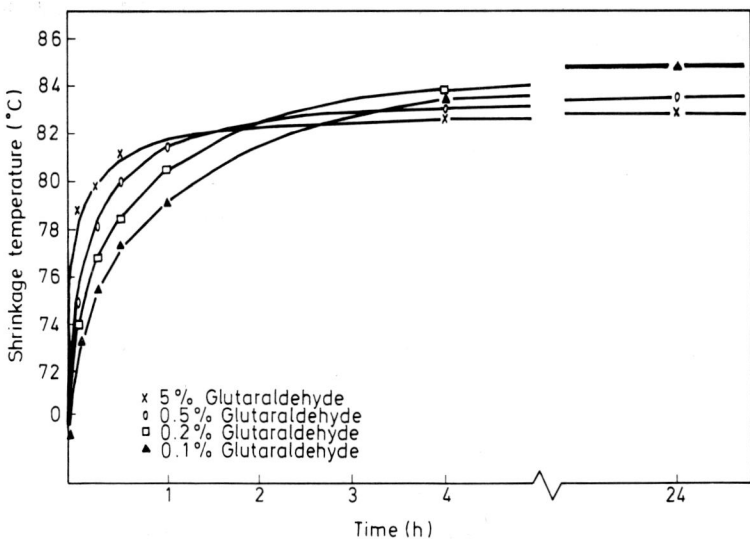

Figure 10.1 Thermal stability kinetics of porcine aortic valve cusp. The graph illustrates the shrinkage temperature versus the length of exposure of tissue to different concentrations of glutaraldehyde[36]

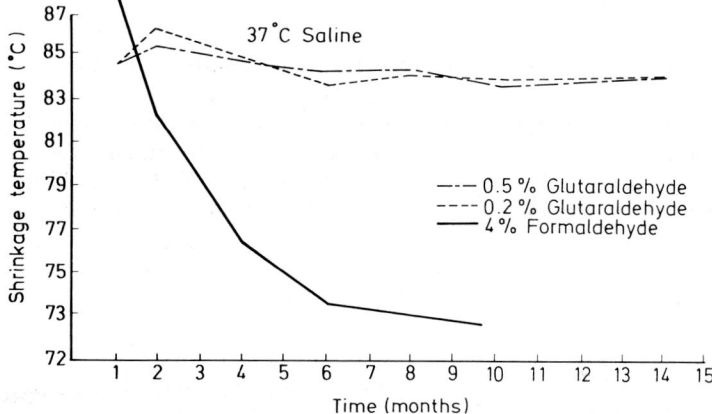

Figure 10.2 Thermal stability kinetics of porcine aortic valve cusp. The graph illustrates the shrinkage temperature of tissue treated with 0.5 and 0.2 per cent glutaraldehyde or with 4.0 per cent formaldehyde and then incubated in sterile normal physiological saline at 37 °C for various periods of time up to 14 months[36]

dicates that changes in the nature of the cross-links continue to occur even though the cross-link density, as measured by tissue thermal stability, reaches equilibrium after a few hours.

The thermal stability of connective tissue is commonly assessed by the change in length of tissue samples as the temperature of the surrounding aqueous solution is slowly increased. A dramatic shortening of tissue length is observed at the critical 'temperature of shrinkage'. This change in length is due to the transition of long asymmetric collagen molecules to random coils.

Figures 10.2 and *10.3* illustrate the kinetics of porcine aortic valve cusp tissue shrinkage temperature after one month's fixation in aldehyde solutions and subsequent incubation in sterile normal saline at 37 and 50°C[36]. We have

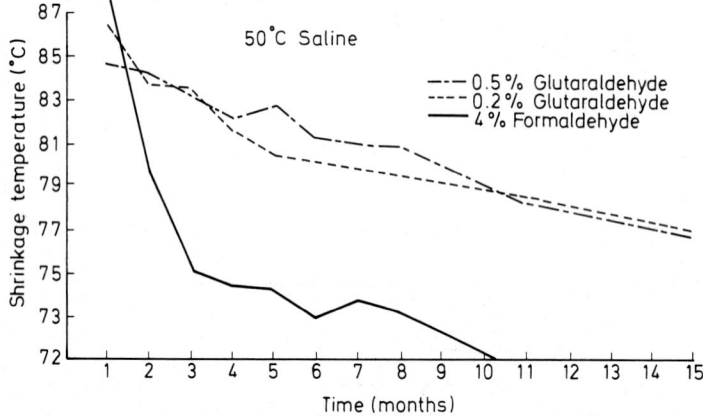

Figure 10.3 Thermal stability kinetics of porcine aortic valve cusp. The graph illustrates the shrinkage temperature of tissue treated with 0.5 and 0.2 per cent glutaraldehyde or with 4.0 per cent formaldehyde and then incubated in sterile normal physiological saline at 50°C for various periods of time up to 15 months[36]

found porcine cusp tissue treated with glutaraldehyde concentrations of 0.2 per cent to have slightly higher initial shrinkage temperatures (1 - 2 °C) than tissue treated with 0.5 per cent glutaraldehyde. When the tissue specimens are incubated in sterile saline at 37 or 50°C, the curves of the shrinkage temperature values for tissue fixed in 0.2 per cent and 0.5 per cent glutaraldehyde merge and are no longer significantly different. Tissue fixed in 4 per cent formaldehyde tends to have a high initial shrinkage temperature which rapidly decreases after incubation in sterile saline. Due to the apparent instability of formaldehyde–collagen cross-links, as evidenced by the shrinkage temperature decay, formaldehyde, as initial fixation solution, is no longer used for the preparation and manufacture of heart valve substitutes[2,9,21].

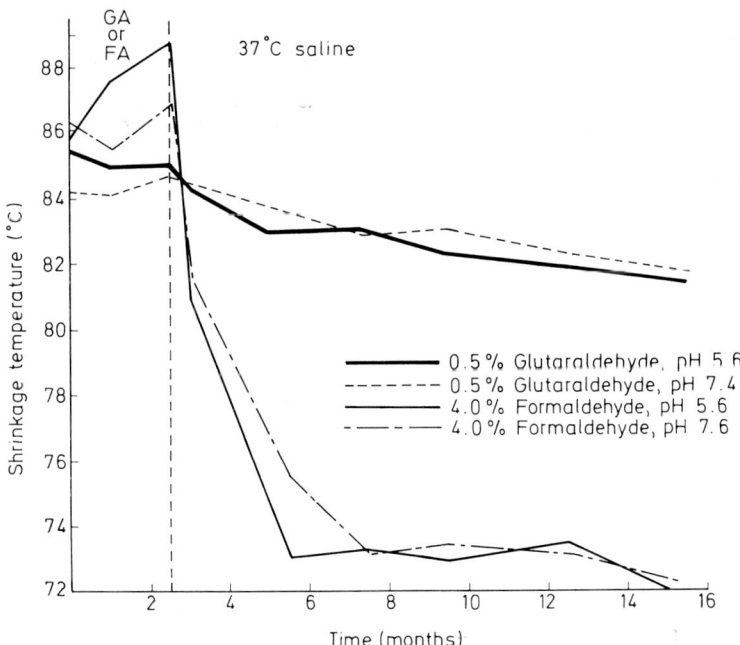

Figure 10.4 Thermal stability kinetics of bovine pericardial tissue. The graph illustrates the shrinkage temperature of pericardial tissue treated with 0.5 per cent glutaraldehyde or 4.0 per cent formaldehyde (at two different pHs) and then incubated in sterile normal physiological saline at 37°C for various periods of time up to 16 months[36]. (GA = glutaraldehyde, FA = formaldehyde)

Although the cross-linking of collagen by formaldehyde is not as stable as glutaraldehyde cross-linking, formaldehyde is a highly effective sterilization and storage medium for tissue which has been previously stabilized with glutaraldehyde. *Figure 10.4* presents the results of shrinkage temperature stability for bovine pericardial tissue stabilized in either glutaraldehyde or formaldehyde and then incubated in sterile normal saline at 37 °C. Clearly, the glutaraldehyde cross-link stability, as measured by shrinkage temperature is greater than that of the formaldehyde cross-links. The results are much different,

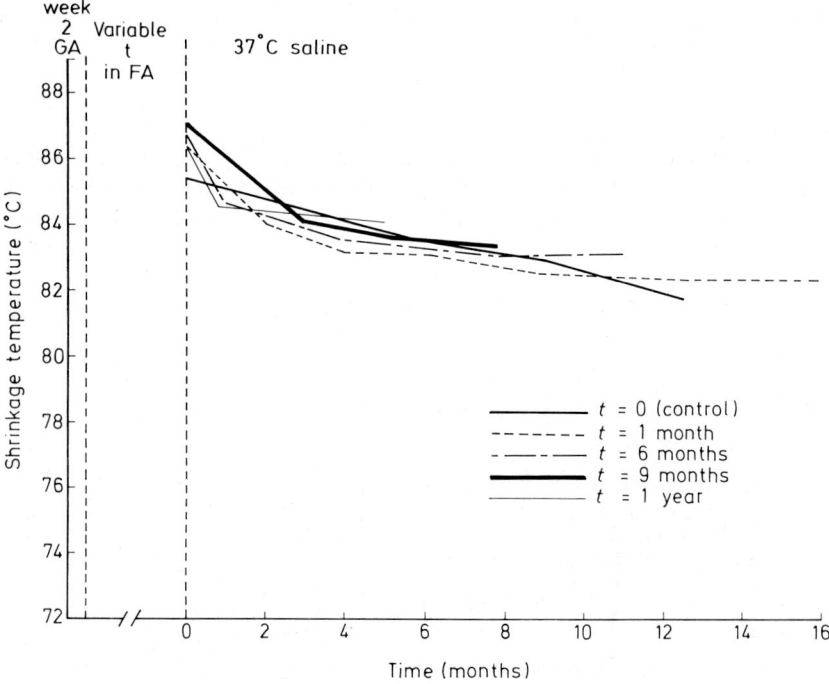

Figure 10.5 Thermal stability kinetics of bovine pericardial tissue. The graph shows the shrinkage temperature of pericardial tissue stabilized with 0.5 per cent 'Purified Glutaraldehyde' for two weeks and stored in 4.0 per cent formaldehyde for various time intervals (one month to one year). Following this treatment the pericardium was incubated in sterile normal physiological saline at 37 °C for periods of time up to 16 months[36] (GA = glutaraldehyde, FA = formaldehyde, *t* = time)

however, when pericardial tissue is stored in formaldehyde after initial fixation in glutaraldehyde. *Figure 10.5* shows the shrinkage temperature stability of pericardial tissue processed in this manner. Tissue stored in 4 per cent formaldehyde following glutaraldehyde fixation possesses the same long-term shrinkage temperature stability as tissue fixed in glutaraldehyde and not exposed to formaldehyde. Thus, the formaldehyde storage does not appear to cause a reversal of the stable glutaraldehyde bonds formed during the glutaraldehyde treatment. Although some collagen–formaldehyde cross-linking probably takes place, it does not seem to affect the stability of the initial glutaraldehyde-collagen cross-linking.

A final consideration is the configuration of the porcine aortic roots during the initial tanning process. We feel that it is important to preserve the shape of each porcine aortic root as close to the original *in vivo* configuration as possible. To accomplish this, the initial tanning step is performed under pressure with the aortic root in its natural shape and this is further maintained in the finished valve by an anatomically shaped stent that closely matches the configuration of each porcine aortic root.

THE EFFICACY OF GLUTARALDEHYDE AND FORMALDEHYDE AS STERILIZING AGENTS

Alkaline glutaraldehyde has been successfully used as a disinfectant and sterilizing agent for surgical equipment and instruments for more than 15 years. The best known glutaraldehyde solution used for this purpose is 'Cidex' manufactured by Arbrook, Inc.*. Numerous reports have been published documenting the efficacy of glutaraldehyde as a sterilizing agent for bacterial, fungal and viral micro-organisms[4,5,12,13,26,30,31,40]. In general, the efficacy of glutaraldehyde solutions to kill microbes is a function of the glutaraldehyde concentration, pH, temperature and time of exposure. As each of these parameters is increased, the ability of glutaraldehyde to sterilize is augmented[24].

Studies of the efficacy of glutaraldehyde (0.2 and 0.5 per cent) at pH 7.4 and of formaldehyde (4 per cent) at pH 5.6 to kill *Mycobacterium chelonei, Bacillus subtilis, Clostridium sporogenes, Aspergillus niger, Candida albicans, Escherichia coli, Pseudomonas aeruginosa* and *Staphylococcus aureus* have been performed. Each solution was maintained at $20\,^\circ$C. Approximately 10^6 organisms were exposed to one of the glutaraldehyde or formaldehyde solutions for various time intervals and the number of surviving organisms after treatment were quantitated using appropriate microbial assay techniques. Log plots of survivors against time of exposure were made for each organism and solution tested. 'D' values were calculated. The 'D' value is the time in hours required to kill 90 per cent of the

TABLE 10.1

Average 'D' value (h/log) for various micro-organisms treated with aldehyde solutions†

| Micro-organism | Glutaraldehyde | | Formaldehyde |
	0.5 per cent	0.2 per cent	4 per cent
Mycobacterium chelonei	1.06×10^{-1}	1.75×10^{-1}	1.05×10^{-1}
Bacillus subtilis	9.30	25.4	2.48
Clostridium sporogenes	1.95	2.90	2.48
Aspergillus niger	8.61×10^{-2}	4.63×10^{-1}	3.09×10^{-2}
Candida albicans	3.46×10^{-2}	22.2×10^{-1}	6.01×10^{-3}
Escherichia coli	1.29×10^{-3}	2.00×10^{-2}	2.98×10^{-3}
Pseudomonas aeruginosa	1.32×10^{-3}	2.29×10^{-3}	1.32×10^{-3}
Staphylococcus aureus	1.37×10^{-3}	4.04×10^{-3}	2.38×10^{-3}

†'D' value = time in hours to kill 90 per cent of micro-organisms

initial number of micro-organisms treated. *Table 10.1* outlines the results obtained. Our results[36] are generally consistent with the observations reported by others[4,5,12,13,26,30,31,40], demonstrating the efficacy of both glutaraldehyde and formaldehyde to kill a wide range of micro-organisms. However, we found that the death kinetic curves for *Mycobacterium chelonei* are non-linear at low glutaraldehyde concentrations (0.2 per cent) and these results indicate that the sterility confidence level (using death kinetic and product microbial bioload data) is insufficient when low concentrations of glutaraldehyde are exclusively used for the sterilization of porcine xenograft valves. In order to minimize microbial contamination of such tissue valve products it is recommended that the tissue

*Arbrook, Inc. is a division of Johnson and Johnson

should be exposed to a glutaraldehyde solution of at least 0.5 per cent for 72 h at room temperature. We have observed that vegetative microbial forms are 10-1000 times easier to kill than spores (*B. subtilis* and *C. sporogenes*). Dr. John McDowell of Arbrook, Inc., has made similar observations[24].

GLUTARALDEHYDE AND FORMALDEHYDE TOXICITY

The toxic effects of glutaraldehyde or formaldehyde on cells of any type are apparent at very low concentrations (greater than 25 parts/million[36]). When using a tissue heart valve stored in 0.5 per cent 'Purified Glutaraldehyde' or 4 per cent formaldehyde, it is imperative to use an adequate rinse protocol to remove residual glutaraldehyde or formaldehyde from the heart valve substitute prior to its clinical use. We recommend a protocol of three separate rinses in 500 ml of sterile normal saline for 2 min each with gentle agitation. Using this protocol, we have determined several facts of great practical significance. The glutaraldehyde concentration of the final (third) rinse solution was less than 1 part/million and the final rinse was neither pyrogenic nor toxic. The first rinse solution had a glutaraldehyde concentration of about 40 parts/million and was shown to be both pyrogenic and toxic. The properly rinsed tissue valves elicited no detectable toxic response when tested subcutaneously in rabbits[36]. Incompletely rinsed valves may cause a sterile, necrotic destruction of the host tissue annulus which may result in perivalvular leaks.

EFFECTS OF GLUTARALDEHYDE ON THE ANTIGENICITY OF CONNECTIVE TISSUE

Both porcine aortic valves and bovine pericardial xenografts treated with glutaraldehyde have been clinically used as heart valve substitutes for over seven and a half years with no detectable rejection phenomena[1,10,22,34,35].

The reduction in cellular or tissue antigenicity by treatment with glutaraldehyde has been reported by Tavis *et al.*[37,38,39] on modified bovine skin collagen; by McMaster *et al.*[25] on chicken and rabbit tendon; by Deng and Beutner[14] on antigens reactive with pemphigus antibodies and by Bubbers and Heeney[8] with mastocytoma cells treated with 0.3 per cent glutaraldehyde.

Extensive exposure of tissue to dilute glutaraldehyde solution results in a stable, insoluble biomaterial with enhanced resistance to proteolytic digestion[35,38,42]. Soluble proteins mildly treated with glutaraldehyde (bovine serum albumin, ovalbumin and human gamma globulin) have been shown to cross-react with antibodies formed against the native (untreated) proteins[17,41]. There are reports of complete, as well as incomplete, antigenic suppression when tissue or soluble proteins are treated with glutaraldehyde or formaldehyde.

Collaborative studies with Dr. P. K. Bajpai on characterization of the antigenicity of porcine aortic roots, fresh and treated with 0.5 per cent glutaraldehyde; and with bovine pericardium, fresh and treated with glutaraldehyde or treated with glutaraldehyde and formaldehyde, have been performed. Several methods were employed for detecting serum antibodies including passive haemagglutination, capillary tube precipitation and anaphylactic shock techniques.

Results obtained with passive haemagglutination and anaphylactic shock techniques will be subject to a subsequent publication[33]. The results of the studies performed with capillary tube precipitation indicated that the antigenicity of both porcine aortic valve tissue and bovine pericardial tissue is reduced but not abolished by treatment with aldehyde cross-linking agents. However, bovine pericardial tissue stabilized with glutaraldehyde and subsequently treated with formaldehyde results in lower tissue antigenicity than tissue treated with glutaraldehyde alone[33]. This may prove to be a significant clinical advantage for heart valves treated with glutaraldehyde and subsequently stored in formaldehyde. The level of antigenicity of aldehyde treated or untreated tissue is low compared with the antigenicity of bovine serum albumin when tested in rabbits.

In the clinical situation, serum antibodies may be produced against the aldehyde treated tissue but apparently not at levels sufficient to cause rejection. The mechanism of aldehyde reduction of tissue antigenicity is not known but may be related to the resistance of aldehyde treated tissue to proteolytic digestion[35,38,42].

THE CHEMISTRY OF GLUTARALDEHYDE SOLUTIONS

Aqueous solutions of glutaraldehyde are complex mixtures of free aldehyde, mono and dihydrated monomeric glutaraldehyde, monomeric and polymeric cyclic hemiacetals and various alpha, beta unsaturated polymers. Whipple and Ruta[41] and Halloway and Dean[18] have shown that the cyclic hemiacetal is the major component of commercial 25 per cent glutaraldehyde solution. The composition at 25 °C is approximately 4 per cent free aldehyde, 16 per cent monohydrate, 9 per cent dihydrate and 71 per cent cyclic hemiacetal (two isomers). The 235 nm absorbing alpha, beta unsaturates were present in small amounts[23]. Monomeric glutaraldehyde can be separated from the alpha, beta unsaturated polymer components by either distillation under vacuum or by multiple extractions with activated charcoal[16,27]. The ratio of absorbance of ultraviolet light (280/235) by a purified glutaraldehyde solution after either of the above treatments is typically between 1.5 and 2.5.

Hemiacetal-type polymerization reactions

Free monomeric glutaraldehyde reacts with water to form first a monohydrate and then a dihydrate linear monomer (*Figure 10.6*). The dihydrate can then cyclicize to form a hemiacetal (*Figure 10.7*)[3,16,18,19,20,23,27,28,41].

Free aldehyde functional groups absorb light weakly at 280 nm[23], whereas hydrated aldehydes absorb ultraviolet light very weakly at 280 nm (if at all). Reversal of the above reactions (reformation of the free aldehyde) is enhanced by heating[41].

In concentrated glutaraldehyde solutions, 25 per cent or 50 per cent, the hemiacetal monomer may polymerize by dehydration to form dimers, trimers or tetramers[19]. Upon dilution, these components rapidly revert back to an equilibrium mixture of monomeric glutaraldehyde[23].

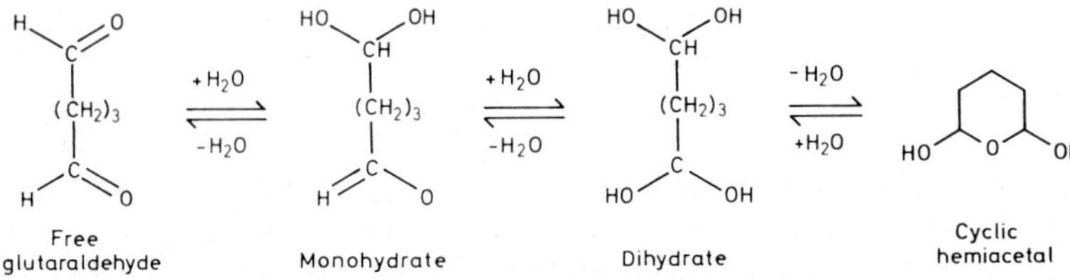

Figure 10.6   Monomeric forms of glutaraldehyde

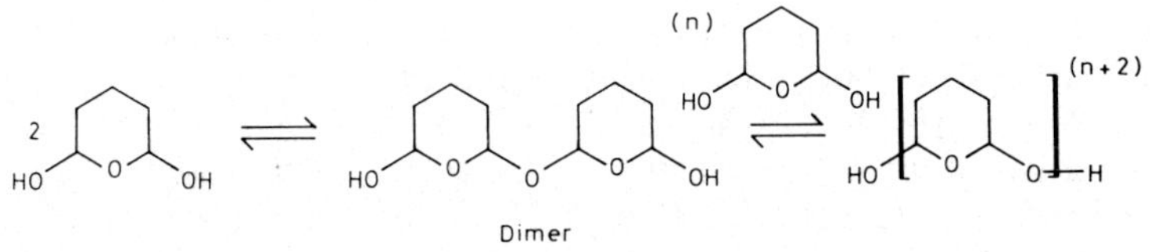

Figure 10.7   Hemiacetal polymer formation

Aldol condensation and polymerization reactions

Free glutaraldehyde can also polymerize into alpha, beta unsaturated dimers, trimers or larger polymers by aldol condensation reactions[27,28,29]. The rate of reaction increases exponentially as the pH, temperature or glutaraldehyde concentration are increased and may be monitored by measuring the absorbance of light at 235 nm. A small amount of alpha, beta unsaturated components cause appreciable absorption at 235 nm. Korn, Feairheller and Filachione[23] found that the worst commercial glutaraldehyde solutions contain no more than 1 per cent of alpha, beta unsaturated components. Examples of aldol condensation products are illustrated in *Figure 10.8*. In general, with increasing molecular weight, these polymers become increasingly insoluble in aqueous solutions.

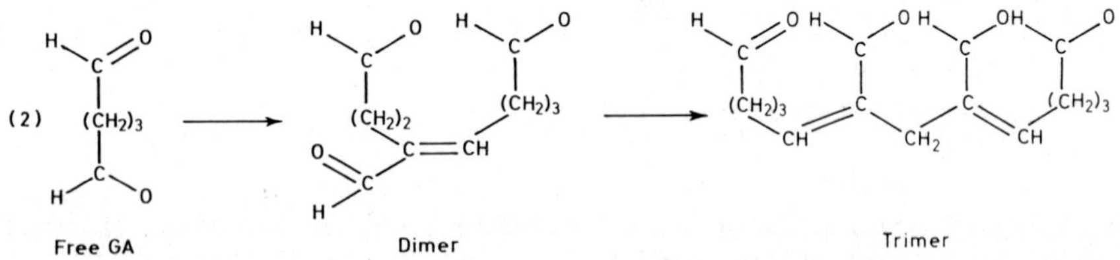

Figure 10.8   Alpha, beta unsaturated polymer formation (GA = glutaraldehyde)

Combinations

Reactions between hemiacetal and aldol polymers may occur to form heterogeneous polymers[3]. However, the contribution of these components to the total composition of aqueous glutaraldehyde solutions is insignificant.

REACTION OF GLUTARALDEHYDE WITH PROTEINS

There still exists considerable controversy concerning the mechanism[5] of glutaraldehyde reaction with proteins. The reactive species present in these solutions is apparently the free glutaraldehyde and not a condensation polymer as has been suggested by Richards and Knowles[20,28]. The reaction of the reagent with proteins appears to involve mainly lysinyl residues but is complicated in nature, yielding a mixture of at least three products[23].

Of the 34 mol of primary amines/10^5 g of collagen, approximately 26 mol appear to be available for the binding of glutaraldehyde, 20–22 of these, under favourable conditions, are involved in cross-linking, leaving 4–6 mol involved in unipoint bonds[7]. The molecular size of glutaraldehyde appears to be particularly suitable for bridging the gap between amino groups of the polypeptide chains of collagen.

Glutaraldehyde not only introduces more cross-links into collagen than other aldehydes (formaldehyde, acrolein, dialdehyde starch, succinaldehyde, etc.) but the glutaraldehyde cross-links are more stable. Boiling water and treatment in acid solution have little effect on the glutaraldehyde cross-links but cause appreciable reduction in those formed by other aldehydes[7].

Several types of glutaraldehyde cross-links have been proposed to explain the mechanism of glutaraldehyde-protein interactions and these are briefly outlined below.

Classic Schiff base reactions

Primary amines of either lysine, hydroxylysine or N-terminal amino acid residues present in proteins can react with free aldehydes to form a Schiff base. Schiff bases are relatively unstable at neutral pHs and may revert to the free amine and aldehyde upon increases in temperature or decreases in pH. A Schiff base may be reduced enzymatically or non-enzymatically[32] to form a secondary amine. In addition, Schiff bases may react with a free aldehyde (similar to the Mannich reaction) to form a secondary amine (*Figure 10.9*). Secondary amines are expected to be stable at physiological temperatures and pHs.

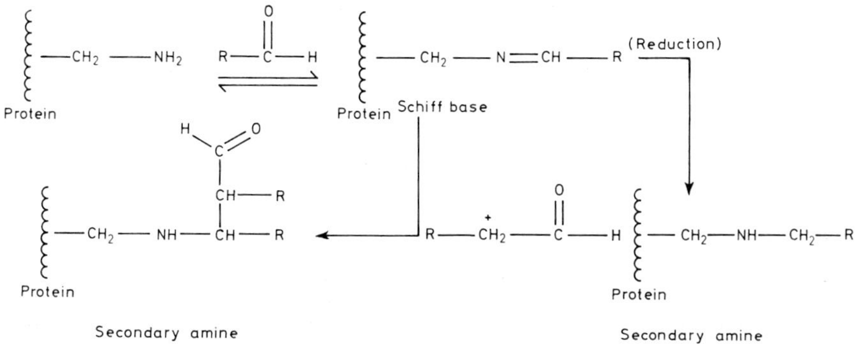

Figure 10.9 Formation of secondary amines via Schiff base intermediates

Alpha, beta unsaturated addition reactions

Cavins and Friedman[11] have demonstrated that primary amines react with methylacrylate or acrylonitrile to form stable secondary amine linkages (*Figure 10.10*).

$$R—CH_2—NH_2 + CH_2 = CH—C \equiv N \longrightarrow R—CH_2—NH—CH_2—CH_2—C \equiv N$$

Figure 10.10   Reaction of acrylonitrile with a primary amine

Richards and Knowles[28] proposed that proteins are cross-linked by a similar reaction between an alpha, omega polymer of glutaraldehyde and a primary amine of the protein (*Figure 10.11*). Their proposal has been recently refuted on the basis of misinterpretation of their C^{13} NMR data[20,23].

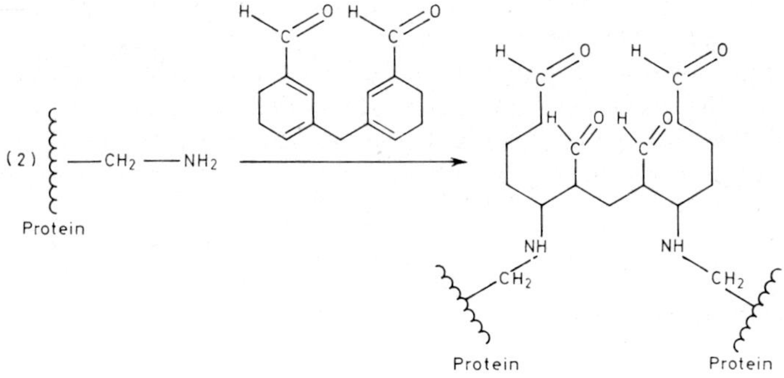

Figure 10.11   Reaction of a protein primary amine with an alpha, omega glutaraldehyde polymer

Pyridinium type cross-links

Recently Hardy, Nicholls and Rydon[19,20] have proposed a new mechanism to explain the nature of glutaraldehyde-protein cross-links. The reaction of free glutaraldehyde with a primary amine of the protein is followed by condensation of additional free glutaraldehyde and leads to the formation of a 1, 3, 4, 5 substituted pyridinium salt analogous to the amino acid desmosine. Hardy's proposed mechanism corroborates the observation of a new absorption peak at 265 nm as proteins are cross-linked with glutaraldehyde. The lability of the pyridinium type cross-link to reduction with sodium borohydride and alkaline hydrolysis is very similar to protein-glutaraldehyde cross-links, when treated in the same manner. An outline of the proposed pyridinium cross-link is illustrated in *Figure 10.12*. Hardy points out that the pyridinium linkage is not the only type of cross-link in glutaraldehyde treated proteins. It most likely represents a significant portion of the cross-links but other possibilities must exist.

Korn, Feairheller and Filachione[23] claim an average of four glutaraldehyde/ primary amine residue. To reconcile Korn's data and the data of Bowes and Carter[7], an average of 9–15 glutaraldehydes would have to be bound at single point protein attachments for the overall average to be four glutaraldehydes/

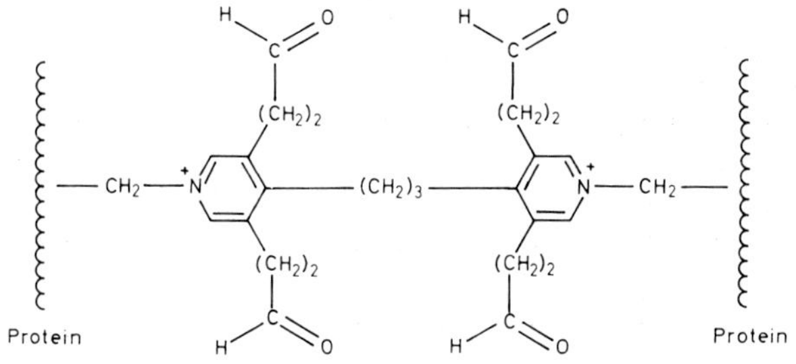

Figure 10.12 A protein pyridinium cross-link

primary amine. This seems unlikely and some glutaraldehyde must be non-covalently bound.

The overall picture of glutaraldehyde–protein cross-linking is not clear at this time. However, it would appear that Hardy has added a key piece to this intriguing puzzle. The combination of pyridinium type cross-links and secondary amine cross-links via an initial Schiff base intermediate most likely account for the structural stability of glutaraldehyde treated tissue.

REACTION OF FORMALDEHYDE WITH PROTEINS

Formaldehyde reacts with primary amines to form hydroxymethyl–secondary amines which can react with a free amide (asparagine or glutamine) to form an inter- or intramolecular cross-link (*Figure 10.13*). This reaction has been demonstrated with model compounds by Fraenkel-Conrat and Olcott[15] and by Bowes and Carter[7]. However, the reaction product is unstable to acid hydrolysis and has not been isolated from a protein cross-linked with formaldehyde.

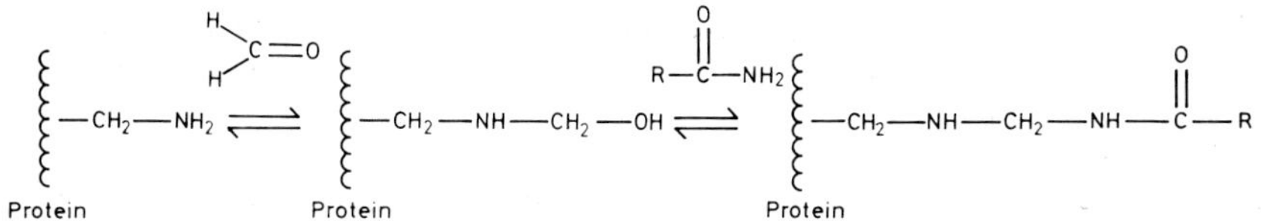

Figure 10.13 Formaldehyde protein interactions

In general, formaldehyde–protein bonds or cross-links have been demonstrated to be unstable by chemical kinetic studies as well as by practical clinical experience[2,6,9,21,36]. The use of formaldehyde for processing tissue heart valves is recommended for storage and for maintaining a higher degree of sterility, but formaldehyde should be used only after preliminary tissue stabilization with glutaraldehyde.

SUMMARY AND CONCLUSIONS

In choosing the optimal glutaraldehyde solution for stabilizing and sterilizing tissue heart valves, each of the following parameters should be considered: glutaraldehyde concentration and composition, pH and ionic strength, time and temperature of tissue exposure to glutaraldehyde, and the tissue configuration during the initial fixation. No single glutaraldehyde solution could either optimize the durability and flexibility of the tissue treated, or reduce its antigenicity and also provide the most effective degree of sterility. The importance and priority of each of these parameters for the clinical performance requirements of a tissue heart valve must be established and the most appropriate balance reached. At Shiley Scientific Inc. we utilize the highest quality of commercially available glutaraldehyde and subsequently purify this glutaraldehyde in our laboratories using a selective technique to control the glutaraldehyde monomer–polymer composition.

Both glutaraldehyde and formaldehyde have been shown to be effective wet sterilizing agents with more than adequate safety margins. Bacterial spores are 10–1000 times more difficult to kill than vegetative micro-organisms under identical conditions (pH, temperature, glutaraldehyde or formaldehyde concentrations, time of exposure).

Both glutaraldehyde and formaldehyde are toxic to cells at levels of 25 parts/ million. When using tissue heart valves stored in glutaraldehyde or formaldehyde, it is imperative to use an adequate rinse protocol to remove the residual glutaraldehyde or formaldehyde from each component of the valve, particularly the sewing flange. Incompletely rinsed valves may cause sterile necrotic destruction of the host annulus tissue and perivalvular leakage.

Glutaraldehyde has been shown to reduce the antigenicity of connective tissue. The mechanism of this antigenic reduction is not clear but is probably related to the enhanced resistance of the glutaraldehyde cross-linked tissue to proteolytic digestion. Pericardial tissue treated with glutaraldehyde and subsequently exposed to formaldehyde results in lower tissue antigenicity than tissue treated with glutaraldehyde alone.

Aqueous solutions of glutaraldehyde are complex mixtures of free glutaraldehyde, mono- and dihydrate glutaraldehyde, cyclic monomer and polymer glutaraldehyde and alpha, beta unsaturated glutaraldehyde polymers. The composition of these solutions can be controlled by purification (either vacuum distillation or extraction with activated charcoal) and by controlling the pH and temperature of the purified solutions.

Interaction of glutaraldehyde with tissue results in the formation of unusually stable cross-links. The nature of these cross-links has received considerable attention from many scientific disciplines over the past ten years. The 'glutaraldehyde cross-link' is probably not a single type but consists of at least three different chemical species. Hardy's recent proposal of a 'pyridinium type cross-link' seems to be consistent with the plethora of published data on this subject. Another type of cross-link is a secondary amine linkage which can be formed by reduction of a Schiff base. Both of the above cross-links would be stable at physiological pHs and temperatures and could explain the excellent *in vivo* durability of glutaraldehyde treated porcine and bovine xenograft heart valves. Richards and Knowles proposed the theory of a stable secondary amine cross-link which could be formed by an additional reaction between a primary amine and an alpha, beta unsaturated polymer of glutaraldehyde. The contribution of this type of cross-link to the observed *in vivo* stability of glutaraldehyde treated tissue valves is believed to be insignificant.

The use of formaldehyde to process tissue heart valves is recommended for maintaining sterility during storage but only after preliminary tissue stabilization with glutaraldehyde.

Ongoing research at Shiley Scientific Inc. and other places is directed towards elucidating the glutaraldehyde cross-linking mechanism. An understanding of this mechanism will be important in optimizing stable cross-link formation and thereby improving the durability of glutaraldehyde treated tissue heart valves.

Acknowledgements

I thank Bruce Fettel, George Johnson, John Darnall, Rebecca Zadro and Lucinda Jacobs for their comments and suggestions.

REFERENCES

[1] Angell, W. W., Angell, J. D. and Sywak, A. 'Selection of tissue or prosthetic valve. A five-year prospective, randomized comparison', *Journal of thoracic and cardiovascular Surgery*, 73, 43 (1977)

[2] Angell, W. W., deLanerolle, P. and Shumway, N. E. 'Valve replacement: present status of homograft valves', *Progress in cardiovascular Diseases*, 15, 589 (1973)

[3] Aso, C. and Aito, Y. 'Studies on the polymerization of bifunctional monomers', *Makromolecular Chemistry*, 28, 195 (1962)

[4] Borick, P. M., Dondershine, F. H. and Chandler, V. L. 'Alkinized glutaraldehyde, a new antimicrobial agent', *Journal of pharmaceutical Sciences*, 52, 1273 (1964)

[5] Borick, P. M. 'Chemical sterilizers (Chemosterilizers)', *Advances in applied Microbiology*, 10, 291 (1968)

[6] Bowes, J. H. and Elliott, R. G. H. 'Tanning with formaldehyde in the presence of organic compounds', *JALCA*, 57, 374 (1962)

[7] Bowes, J. H. and Carter, C. W. 'The reaction of glutaraldehyde with protein and other biological material', *Journal of the Royal Microscopical Society*, 85, 193 (1966)

[8] Bubbers, J. E. and Henney, C. S. 'Studies on the synthetic capacity and antigenic expression of glutaraldehyde-fixed target cells', *Journal of Immunology*, 114, 1126 (1975)

[9] Buch, W. S., Kosek, J. C., Angell, W. W. and Shumway, N. E. 'The role of rejection and mechanical trauma on valve graft viability', *Journal of thoracic and cardiovascular Surgery*, 62, 696 (1971)

[10] Carpentier, A., Deloche, A., Relland, J., Fabiani, J. N., Forman, J., Camilleri, J. P., Soyer, R. and Dubost, Ch. 'Six-year follow-up of glutaraldehyde-preserved heterografts', *Journal of thoracic and cardiovascular Surgery*, 68, 771 (1974)

[11] Cavins, J. F. and Friedman, M. 'New amino acids derived from reactions of epsilon-amino groups in proteins with alpha-beta unsaturated compounds', *Biochemistry*, 6, 3766 (1967)

[12] Collins, F. M. and Mackaness, G. B. 'The relationship of delayed hypersensitivity to acquired antituberculous immunity', *Cellular Immunology*, 1, 253 (1970)

[13] Collins, F. M. and Montalbine, V. 'Mycobacterial activity of glutaraldehyde solutions', *Journal of clinical Microbiology*, 4, 408 (1976)

[14] Deng, J. S. and Beutner, E. H. 'Effect of formaldehyde, glutaraldehyde and sucrose on the tissue antigenicity', *Applied Immunology*, 47, 562 (1974)

[15] Fraenkel-Conrat, H. and Olcott, H. S. 'The reaction of formaldehyde with protein. Part V cross-linking between amino and primary amide or guanidyl groups', *Journal of the American Chemical Society*, 70, 673 (1968)

[16] Gillett, R. and Gull, K. 'Glutaraldehyde–Its purity and stability', *Histochemie*, 30, 162 (1972)

[17] Habeeb, A. J. and Hiramoto, R. 'Reaction of proteins with glutaraldehyde', *Archives of Biochemistry and Biophysics*, 126, 16 (1968)

[18] Halloway, C. E. and Dean, F. H. 'C-NMR study of aqueous glutaraldehyde equilibria', *Journal of pharmaceutical Sciences*, 64, 1078 (1975)

[19] Hardy, P. M., Nicholls, A. C. and Rydon, H. N. 'The hydration and polymerization of succinaldehyde, glutaraldehyde and adiopaldehyde', *Journal of the Chemical Society*, (*Perkin II*), 2270 (1972)

[20] Hardy, P. M., Nicholls, A. C. and Rydon, H. N. 'The nature of the cross-linking of protein by glutaraldehyde. Part I', *Journal of the Chemical Society*, (*Perkin I*), 958 (1976)

[21] Ionescu, M. I., Pakrashi, B. C., Mary, D. A. S., Bartek, I. T. and Wooler, G. H. 'Long-term evaluation of tissue valves', *Journal of thoracic and cardiovascular Surgery*, 68, 361 (1974)

[22] Ionescu, M. I., Tandon, A. P., Mary, D. A. S. and Abid, A. 'Heart valve replacement with the Ionescu–Shiley pericardial xenograft', *Journal of thoracic and cardiovascular Surgery*, 73, 31 (1977)

[23] Korn, A. H., Feairheller, S. H. and Filachione, E. M. 'Glutaraldehyde: nature of the reagent', *Journal of molecular Biology*, 65, 525 (1972)

[24] McDowell, J. Arbrook Inc., personal communication (1977)

[25] McMaster, W. C., Kouzelos, J., Liddle, S. and Waugh, T. R. 'Tendon grafting with glutaraldehyde fixed material', *Journal of biomedical Material Research*, 10, 259 (1976)

[26] Navarro, J. M. and Monson, P. 'Etude du mecanism d'interraction du glutaraldehyde avec les micro-organismes', *Annals of Microbiology (Paris)*, 127B, 295 (1976)

[27] Rasmussen, K. E. and Albrechtsen, J. 'Glutaraldehyde. The influence of pH, temperature and buffering on the polymerization rate', *Histochemistry*, 38, 19 (1974)

[28] Richards, F. M. and Knowles, J. R. 'Glutaraldehyde as a protein cross-linking reagent', *Journal of molecular Biology*, 37, 231 (1968)

[29] Robertson, E. A. and Schultz, R. L. 'The impurities in commercial glutaraldehyde and their effect on the fixation of the brain', *Journal of Ultrastructure Research*, 30, 275 (1970)

[30] Rubbo, S. D. and Gardner, J. F. *A Review of Sterilization and Disinfection*. London; Lloyd-Zuki (1975)

[31] Saitanu, K. and Lund, E. 'Inactivation of enterovirus by glutaraldehyde', *Applied Microbiology*, 29, 571 (1975)

[32] Siegal, R. 'Collagen cross-linking. Synthesis of collagen cross-links *in vitro* with highly purified lysyl oxidase', *Journal of biological Chemistry*, 251, 5786 (1976)

[33] Slanczka, D. J., Bajpai, P. K. University of Dayton, Department of Biology and Wright State University, Department of Physiology, School of Medicine, Dayton, Ohio. *Clinical Research*, 26, 124A (1978)

[34] Stinson, E. B., Griepp, R. B., Oyer, P. E. and Shumway, N. E. 'Long-term experience with porcine aortic valve xenografts', *Journal of thoracic and cardiovascular Surgery*, 73, 54 (1977)

[35] Strawich, E., Hancock, W. D. and Nimni, M. E. 'Chemical composition and biophysical properties of porcine cardiovascular tissues', *Biomaterials in medical Development of artificial Organs*, 3, 309 (1975)

[36] Studies conducted by Shiley Laboratories (1975–1978)

[37] Tavis, M. J., Harvey, J. H., Thornton, J. H., Woodroof, E. A. and Bartlett, R. H. 'Adherence to de-epithelialized surfaces: a comparative study', *Surgical Forum*, 25, 39 (1974)

[38] Tavis, M. J., Harvey, J. H., Thornton, J. H., Woodroof, E. A. and Bartlett, R. H. 'Modified collagen membrane as a skin substitute: preliminary studies', *Biomedical material Research*, 9, 285 (1975)

[39] Tavis, M. J., Harvey, J. H., Thornton, J. H., Woodroof, E. A. and Bartlett, R. H. 'Graft adherence to de-epithelialized surfaces: a comparative study', *Annals of Surgery*, 184, 594 (1976)

[40] Thomas, S. and Russel, A. D. 'Temperature-induced changes in the sporicidal activity and chemical properties of glutaraldehyde', *Applied Microbiology*, 28, 331 (1974)

[41] Whipple, E. B. and Ruta, M. 'Studies of aqueous glutaraldehyde', *Journal of organic Chemistry*, 39, 1666 (1974)

[42] Wood, J. G. 'The effects of glutaraldehyde and osmium on the protein and lipids of myelin and mitochrondria', *Biochemica et Biophysica Acta*, 329, 118 (1973)

Index